Rehabilitation of the Severely Disabled

2—Management

Rehabilitation of the Severely Disabled

2—MANAGEMENT

P. J. R. NICHOLS
M.A., D.M.(Oxon.), M.R.C.P., D.Phys.Med.(Lond.)
Consultant in Physical Medicine,
Nuffield Orthopaedic Centre,
Headington, Oxford; Director of
Mary Marlborough Lodge
Disabled Living Research Unit,
Nuffield Orthopaedic Centre,
Headington, Oxford

with the assistance of

E. A. HAMILTON, M.A., B.M., B.Ch.

and

E. M. HOLLINGS, M.A.O.T.

NEW YORK
APPLETON-CENTURY-CROFTS
Division of Meredith Corporation

LONDON
BUTTERWORTHS

Suggested U.D.C. Number: 616-089.1

Suggested Additional Numbers: 362.65
615.851.3

ISBN 0 407 38512 6

Printed in Great Britain
at the Pitman Press, Bath

So many worlds, so much to do
So little done. . . . . . .

In Memoriam Alfred, Lord Tennyson

Contents

List of Appendices

Preface

The long-term rehabilitation of disabled patients should ideally be the concern of all doctors, medical ancillary workers, social workers and members of the welfare service. Such rehabilitation demands a sustained interest in the social and the industrial re-integration of these patients. It also entails a close liaison between hospital doctor, general practitioner, industrial medical officer, medical officer of health and all the workers in this field, but neither the sustained interest nor the close liaison is at present universal.

The production of both interest and liaison is hampered by the difficulty which many patients have in communicating with their doctors, and by the scant time which most doctors can devote to the exploration of all the implications of total rehabilitation. An increased integration of the work of the para-medical professions is necessary to overcome this problem.

In this book, which is based upon experience in a Disabled Living Research Unit, an attempt has been made to analyse some of these problems. Such analysis has called for a multi-disciplinary approach and yet one which is very individual. Since generalizations are frequently inappropriate, much of this book is based upon actual case histories describing the assessment and treatment of individual patients, whether successful or unsuccessful in outcome. It is hoped that they may lead to a wider appreciation of the problems of the severely disabled, a more practical and active approach to their rehabilitation, and a closer understanding between the many and various workers in this field.

This book is written in an attempt to share some of the experiences and knowledge gained by such a Unit with others working in the same field.

Clinical practice is necessarily always changing as further knowledge becomes available, and the feed-back of information from the follow-up study has had many repercussions on the practical handling of patients in the Unit, and caused several changes of policy. Thus, although it is recognized that there can be no substitute for comprehensive clinical care, it has become apparent that frequently the tragedies of the physically handicapped are attributable to social and welfare difficulties coupled with administrative complications, and that increased and unremitting effort to integrate the work of a unit with the work of the welfare services is essential if these tragedies are to be averted.

So much more could be done in an all-perfect society. So much more can be done in our present far from perfect society if the problems are recognized and the will to solve them exists.

P. J. R. NICHOLS

OXFORD

Acknowledgements

A book of this nature inevitably draws upon the experience and skills of many people. The management of the severely disabled is a particular example of the team approach and this book is the outcome of considerable team effort from all who have worked in Mary Marlborough Lodge since its opening. Some have now left the department, others visit only occasionally, but many have contributed to the sum of experience and knowledge which has lead to the writing of this book. In particular, Miss G. McCay, M.C.S.P., Miss F. Cowie, M.A.O.T., and Miss R. Wilshere, M.C.S.P., Compiler of Equipment for the Disabled.

The staff of the Nuffield Orthopaedic Centre has always taken a great interest in the Unit, particularly Professor J. Trueta, who supervised the building, opening and early years until his retirement, and his lecturer Dr. M. Agerholm. More recently, Professor R. B. Duthie, Mr. J. C. Scott, Mr. R. G. Taylor, Mr. E. W. Somerville, Mr. J. D. Morgan, and Mr. J. W. Goodfellow have contributed considerably by their help and advice with patients and by referring their patients for rehabilitation, while Dr. F. H. Kemp and Dr. J. L. Boldero have given freely of their time to help with the often difficult radiology of the patients.

Colleagues at the United Oxford Hospitals have also referred many patients and helped with advice and collaborated with the complex problems of management; in particular, we would like to thank Professor W. Ritchie Russell, Professor A. Crampton-Smith, Dr. J. M. K. Spalding, and Mr. J. C. Smith.

Patients are referred from many departments and most severely physically disabled patients attend more than one hospital department. It is often uncertain who is most directly clinically responsible and this makes it difficult to acknowledge all those who might be concerned with patients whose histories we have quoted. We are, however, indebted to all our colleagues who have referred patients and would particularly acknowledge permission to quote from histories of patients referred by: Dr. P. Boyle, Dr. D. A. Brewerton, Professor R. B. Duthie, Mr. J. W. Goodfellow, Dr. W. Goody, Mr. M. M. Harrison, Dr. T. Keeble, Mr. P. Lenton, Mr. R. S. M. Ling, Dr. J. Morgan, Dr. D. R. L. Newton, Mr. G. Parkes, Dr. J. G. Parish, Mr. E. W. Someville, Mr. L. H. F. Walton, Dr. J. J. Walsh, Dr. W. G. Wenley, and Dr. C. Westropp.

Many of the appliances and adaptations to appliances discussed in this book were designed and made in the Research Workshops at Mary Marlborough Lodge. The technicians make a considerable contribution in the assessment of patients and the general rehabilitation of both in-patients and out-patients. I would like to make particular acknowledgement to Mr. T. S. Strange, Chief Technician, Mr. G. Codling, and Mr. F. Molden.

Many organizations have been most co-operative in giving permission to publish details of patients in their care and in providing up-to-date information. In particular we should like to mention Greenhill House, the Oxfordshire Cheshire Home; the Grove Cheshire Home, Norwich; and the Welfare Department of the City and County of Norwich.

We are grateful to the National Fund for Research into Crippling Diseases for permission to publish photographs of Patient M.M.L. No. 445. The London Borough of Bexley was most helpful in enabling us to publish sketch plans of alterations carried out to one of their flats. We gratefully acknowledge the drawings of this flat provided by Mr. C. Wycliffe Noble, F.R.I.B.A., who provided the photograph (*Figure 8.2*) on page 292. Most of the other photography was carried out by the Department of Medical Photography, Nuffield Orthopaedic Centre.

Several of the staff of Mary Marlborough Lodge owe much to the Rancho Los Amigos Hospital, Downey, California, for inspiration and help, and it is a pleasure to thank the Occupational Therapy Department in particular for permission to publish their 'Check List for Hand Splints' (*see* Appendix V).

We are particularly indebted to Dr. D. A. Brewerton and Miss G. McCaul for making available to us material which they had collected and had at one time considered publishing.

The Medical Social Workers of the Nuffield Orthopaedic Centre, Miss M. Kennedy (now retired), Mrs. B. Taylor, and Mrs. P. Cattell have been indefatigable in their efforts on behalf of our patients and of great help and inspiration in the development of techniques of managing the severely disabled.

The nursing staff have to bear much of the burden while patients are in the Unit, and Sister C. Lake and her staff have not only nursed the patients but made a very considerable contribution to the assessment and rehabilitation of the patients and the training of their relatives.

Mrs. L. C. Allen, the Librarian of the Nuffield Orthopaedic Centre helped considerably with literature and references.

The main bulk of the secretarial work for this book was undertaken by Mrs. J. Bolongaro, to whom we are considerably indebted.

Finally, we wish to thank our patients, their families and friends who have taught us so much about themselves. We would particularly like to acknowledge those to whom we have made direct reference and who have allowed us to reproduce their photographs.

1—Introduction

SOURCE OF MATERIAL

Introduction

British social legislation has opened the doors of medical institutions to comprehensive care of all patients so that rehabilitation services of all kinds have become overwhelmed by the vast load of degenerative disorders which constitute a high proportion of the severely disabled and the elderly.

Too often the naïve opinion expressed is that the physically disabled represent a great reservoir of unlimited potential waiting to be released from the shackles of disability. It seems more than likely that the physically disabled do include a proportion of the highly endowed, similar to the general population, but there are also similar proportions of the lazy, inept and unsocial. Furthermore, physical disability reacts upon personality, and many conditions, for example multiple sclerosis, cerebrovascular accidents and old age, carry a concomitant organic brain damage.

Many disabled, their families and their advisers are often unrealistic in their view of their ultimate capabilities. They often believe that with gadgets, aids, appliances, more help at home or special housing, the patient can live a normal life, but such faith in physical aids is misplaced because aids and appliances cannot usually solve social and welfare problems. Furthermore, rehabilitation cannot add to what was present before the onset of disability, it can only attempt to approach the pre-morbid situation. One cannot blame the patient or the family for grasping at any mechanical or prosthetic device; however, it is inexcusable to provide equipment without adequate assessment of the patient and his environment, adequate rehabilitation and training in the use of necessary gadgets and prosthetics and adequate follow-up.

A patient with a physical disability may or may not be handicapped, but there will be certain things he cannot do and certain places he cannot reach without help. Often the patient is best served by helping him to accept his handicap. This training is part of the processes of rehabilitation and emphasizes the need for comprehensive assessment of the patient from clinical, functional and social aspects and in the context of his home environment, education, family and available training. It is also necessary to assess the patient's intellect, personality and motivation.

Many severely disabled patients are relegated to chronic wards, day hospitals, or institutions for the chronic sick. Those who are referred to hospital departments usually finish up attending the Occupational Therapy and Physiotherapy departments. Few organizations are able to spend time and devote staff to the detailed reappraisal of the problems of the chronic disabled. Some hospitals have been able to set up Functional Assessment Units, usually within the Occupational Therapy department, and through these units to contribute considerably to the management of the common disabilities.

Mary Marlborough Lodge

The material for this book has been largely derived from experience at Mary Marlborough Lodge, a Disabled Living Research Unit which was opened in 1960 at the Nuffield Orthopaedic Centre, Oxford.

It was built by the National Fund for Research into Crippling Diseases and financed by the National Fund during its early years. Additions were provided by the Disabled Living Activities Group of the Central Council for the Disabled and also by the Lady Hoare Thalidomide Appeal Fund. By 1964 it was absorbed into the National Health Service and became part of the Nuffield Orthopaedic Centre and administered by the Oxford Regional Hospital Board.

Mary Marlborough Lodge was originally built to take 12 residents in 2 single rooms, 4 double-rooms, and a 2-bedded self-contained flat; the flat being available for assessing independence, or for the training of a relative or companion with the patient. Apart from the day-room and dining-room, there is a kitchen with adjustable fitments providing facilities for assessing and training in domestic activities, and a work-room where the therapist can train and assess patients' functional capabilities.

More recently, the facilities have been extended to give a total of 18 beds, and Mary Marlborough Lodge is attached to the Oxford Regional Artificial Limb and Appliance Centre, sharing the gymnasium facilities, and providing the rehabilitation programme for amputees.

There is a large range of both simple and complex equipment available for assessment and training purposes, including a range of simple aids to daily living and electrically operated beds and hoists;

for it is only through practical trial of such appliances that a true assessment of their value can be achieved.

Associated with Mary Marlborough Lodge is a research bungalow, given by the Disabled Living Activities Group of the Central Council for the Disabled. This provides a research workshop in the form of parts of a house with moveable walls and flexible fitments so that various architectural requirements can be studied in relation to disabled patients. It has facilities for gardening for the disabled with a special garden area which has raised beds and greenhouses adapted for wheelchair and ambulant disabled. This unit also houses a complex Information Centre originally compiled from the detailed records and data used in the publication *Equipment for the Disabled*, and now providing a valuable ongoing service for patients and staff.

Where special equipment and personalized appliances are used, comprehensive workshops are an essential part of the establishment. The workshops of Mary Marlborough Lodge are concerned with the making of special splints and appliances, adapting standard equipment for special needs and carrying out design and research projects associated with equipment and aids for the disabled. Experience with one group of problems frequently leads to solutions for others and the close integration of therapists and technicians enables both groups to help each other in solving physical problems for patients.

Thus, Mary Marlborough Lodge is a functional assessment unit, a therapeutic department, a training centre, and a research department where physiotherapist, occupational therapist, technician, nursing sister and medical social worker can collaborate in the assessment and rehabilitation of the severely disabled.

Rehabilitation team

The rehabilitation team comprises clinicians, physiotherapists, occupational therapists, nursing officers, medical social workers and technicians. In the closely integrated atmosphere of a Disabled Living Unit the activities of the members of the team may seem to overlap, but their main spheres of influence can be clearly outlined.

The physiotherapist is primarily concerned with the following:

(1) the physical assessment;

(2) the physical problems of transferring (bed to chair, chair to toilet, and so on) and logically progresses to mobility, whether this includes walking re-education or the use of lifts, hoists and other apparatus.

The occupational therapist is concerned primarily with the following:

(1) functional assessment;

(2) dressing, feeding, washing, and toilet management;
(3) housing (design and alterations);
(4) training for work or limited activity and hobbies.

The nursing sister is primarily responsible for the nursing care of the patients, but she and her staff contribute considerably in the rehabilitation and training of patients and relatives. In particular, the nursing staff are concerned with the prevention of bed sores in patients who are paralysed or have sensory loss, the management of urinary incontinence, the care of the bowels in patients unable to defaecate and the general care and management of the more severely disabled. Much of their work involves teaching and training the patient and their relatives or other attendants, when satisfactory nursing and care routines have been established.

The technicians concentrate on design, development and manufacture of apparatus and appliances, ranging from simple aids to complex powered appliances. The technicians have a considerable role to play in contributing towards the general assessment of the patient and their capabilities as well as designing, developing, making and fitting the necessary aids, appliances and splints.

The medical social worker must add the social and domestic assessment to the sum of information collated about the patient. Secondly, she assists in the management of the patient by discussion with them, helping them to sort out current problems at home, practical and financial, demonstrating to the patient that there are ways and means of surmounting most problems. Finally, she co-operates with the rest of the team in planning the final resettlement. Without the social worker, the translation of the problem into a practical domestic solution would frequently be impossible.

Between September 1964 and December 1968, the admissions to the Disabled Living Research Unit, Mary Marlborough Lodge, Nuffield Orthopaedic Centre, Oxford, were at a rate of approximately 200–250 a year, with out-patient attendances at approximately double that rate (this is, 400–500 per year). Many patients are admitted on more than one occasion, and most out-patients attend more than once. Approximately 500 individual patients have been admitted, and 700 attended as out-patients in the period between September 1964 and December 1968, and it is upon our experience with these 1,200 patients that the opinions described in this book are based.

The majority of the patients admitted or seen as out-patients at Mary Marlborough Lodge during the years 1964–1968 inclusive are listed in Table 1.1.

These patients represent the most commonly occurring severe

TABLE 1.1

Major Groups of Disabilities Referred to Mary Marlborough Lodge 1964–1968

Diagnosis	*Number as in-patients*	*Number as out-patients*	*Total*
Rheumatoid arthritis (including Still's disease)	62	110	172
Poliomyelitis	63	63	126
Hemiplegia	46	72	118
Muscular dystrophy	68	45	113
Amputees (including children with multiple congenital limb deformities)	56	53	109
Osteoarthritis	15	91	106
Degenerative neurological disorders	29	52	81
Multiple sclerosis	25	41	66
Cerebral palsy	19	44	63
Tetraplegia	39	16	55
Paraplegia (including spina bifida)	24	19	43
Total	446	606	1,052

physical disabilities and have formed the large proportion of our practice.

The remaining 200 or so patients seen during this period cover some 30 separate clinical diagnoses within the general classification of disorders of the locomotor system.

The patients may be admitted from other wards of the Nuffield Orthopaedic Centre for a period of functional assessment or for rehabilitation prior to discharge, or they may be referred from other hospitals in the region or beyond, for assessment or for solving particular physical problems.

Out-patient assessment clinics and wheelchair clinics for both in-patients and out-patients are a feature of the work, thus extending the clinical and practical experience.

THE DISABLED POPULATION

The incidence of the physically disabled in the general population is not accurately known, but there are various surveys which enable an indirect calculation to be made.

In Britain, about 1½ million people (3 per cent of the population) are found in official administratively defined categories of the disabled.

Nearly 700,000 people were on the Department of Employment and Productivity's Disabled Persons' Register in 1968. Of these over 400,000 were disabled pensioners from the two World Wars still alive, and about 200,000 industrial injury disablement pensioners. An analysis of the Department of Employment and Productivity statistics shows amputations and limb injuries account for 30 per cent disabilities, spinal injuries for 5 per cent and rheumatics for a further 4½ per cent. Industrial accidents in 1966 totalled 296,000 and road accidents in 1966 were over 390,000 with nearly 100,000 classified as seriously injured.

In 1966 the local authorities' registers included over 200,000 physically disabled in addition to the blind and partially sighted (approximately 140,000). There are about 205,000 patients residing in hospitals for the chronic sick and mentally disabled, the majority of these being subnormal or psychologically disturbed. For the country as a whole, an enquiry showed that in April 1967, there were 4,223 chronic sick patients in the age range 15–59 years in non-psychiatric hospitals within the National Health Service. About 56 per cent of these were aged 50 years or over and some were occupying beds for terminal rather than long-stay cases. Half the total, including 74 in the age group 15–34 years were, however, accommodated in the wards of geriatric departments or in chronic sick wards; 1,300 were in general wards, and of the remainder about 500 were in younger Chronic Sick Units and 300 patients were accommodated by means of contractual arrangements. There are 76,000 handicapped children including 32,000 at special schools or in special units.

But all these figure are incomplete and frequently overlap and give little insight into the quality of the disability. From all available evidence it seems likely that between 3 and 6 per cent (between 1½ and 3 million people) of the population suffers from some degree of physical disability which is, or is likely to become, a physical handicap.

The quality of the disability is more relevant and some assessment of this can be gained from studying the diagnostic labels accorded the patients in the various administrative groups and patient surveys. For example, analyses of wheelchair users indicate that the arthritides and the neurological disorders are the most potent source of invalidism. Cardiovascular and respiratory disease are the next most common sources of disability.

If all the available surveys are analysed, it is possible to list the commonest disorders which are associated with prolonged physical disability in their approximate order of incidence. (*See* Tables 1.2 and 1.3.)

TABLE 1.2

Common Disorders Causing Physical Disability, Listed in Approximate Order of Incidence

Osteoarthritis
Rheumatoid arthritis
Multiple sclerosis
Hemiplegia
Respiratory infections
Cerebral palsy
Paraplegia; traumatic; congenital (spina bifida)
Tetraplegia
Other neurological disorders, particularly Parkinson's disease
Other muscular disorders, particularly muscular dystrophy
Amputation
Results of trauma, particularly fractures of femur

TABLE 1.3

Common Disorders Causing Physical Disability, Listed According to Age of Onset

Children	Paraplegia (spina bifida) Cerebral palsy Muscular dystrophy Rheumatoid arthritis (Still's disease)
Young adults	Paraplegia (traumatic) Tetraplegia Fractured femur
Middle age	Rheumatoid arthritis Multiple sclerosis Hemiplegia
Elderly	Osteoarthritis Lower limb amputation Bronchitis

There is evidence that rheumatoid arthritis, osteoarthritis and multiple sclerosis are the most common locomotor disorders leading to hospital admission in middle age (40–60 years). In the older age-group, these same disabilities persist, in addition to hemiplegia, Parkinsonism, peripheral vascular and respiratory disorders. In young adults the most frequent cause of long-term disability is fracture of the femur, but in this age of high-speed travel, traumatic paraplegia, tetraplegia and head injuries are on the increase. Probably about 5 million people in Great Britain suffer from some clinical degree of osteoarthritis, and another 1½ million have, or have had, active rheumatoid arthritis. Informed estimates indicate that in Great Britain there are 40–50,000 patients with multiple sclerosis and over 20,000 with muscular dystrophy.

The largest group of disabled persons is among the elderly; in 1968 about 25 per cent of all those over 65 years of age had some form of disability or infirmity. At present, the elderly population (that is, those over 65 years of age) in the United Kingdom is nearly 7,000,000.

Other features of the disabilities leading to handicap are related to the conditions, natural history and to the associated manifestations. The majority of the disabilities leading to handicap are progressive, sometimes remittant, but usually the trend is inexorably downwards, for example, in rheumatoid arthritis, multiple sclerosis, osteoarthritis, muscular dystrophy and Parkinson's disease. The majority of the lower limb amputations are associated with progressive peripheral vascular disease, and most strokes are manifestation of progressive vascular disorders. The major static disabilities, paraplegia and quadriplegia, are beset with intercurrent infection of the urinary tract, and for the tetraplegias, chest infections are an added hazard. Among the common disabilities, apart from the results of trauma, only cerebral palsy presents a non-progressive condition.

Poliomyelitis used to feature high in the disability classification, but since the introduction of vaccine, its incidence has dropped dramatically. However, there are still many patients with severe paralyses who will continue to present with functional problems over the next decade or so.

For the most part, the physically disabled make up a significant proportion of the population, and most are suffering from disorders the incidence of which is little affected by living standards or occupation, and although the majority can be helped by treatment, they cannot at present be cured.

DISABILITY AND HANDICAPPED

Impairment of function is the inevitable accompaniment of many diseases and syndromes and of old age. The impairment derives from the physical disability which accompanies the disorders of age, and the individual's reaction to the disability in his or her particular mode of living. The loss of function may be due to reduced power, reduced range of joint motion or reduced endurance, to deformity or to a combination of one or all of these defects. The loss may be anatomical, physiological or psychological. The disability producing this functional loss is likely to be a chronic or remittent clinical condition which defers or interrupts normal physiological and psychological processes, and thus imposes a functional limitation or an ordinary activity. This limitation may be simply a loss of physical capability, such as the inability to negotiate stairs or an inability to achieve self-care.

However, the disability may impose patterns of behaviour which are unacceptable outside the individual's immediate domestic environment; ataxia, inco-ordinated movements and speech defects are particular examples. Even minor disabilities can impose an altered financial and social status. The middle-aged man with osteoarthritic hips may no longer be able to compete on the factory floor or cope with commuting to work, and this could force him to accept a lower status.

Thus physical disability is a medical identifiable condition causing impairment of function whether through reduced power, loss of co-ordination, reduced endurance, or deformity. If the impairment encroaches upon the individual's inability to live a normal life, then it constitutes a handicap.

Disability is specific, handicap is non-specific and represents the inability to overcome the obstacles imposed by the disability or the cumulative effect of several disabilities.

Certain specific problems face patients with specific disabilities, for example the blind, or those liable to fall or have fits. Some respiratory cripples have special requirements for ventilation, and many disabled are limited only by heavy lifting, or negotiation of flights of steps. Other patients have special requirements, particularly for managing their toilet activities (for example, those with urinary incontinence, or patients with colostomy or ileostomy). A proportion of the disabled have dietary requirements which need special provision such as access to refrigeration.

There are two main areas of difficulty for all disabled persons:

(1) Difficulties in handling domestic equipment or in performing certain actions, such as lifting and bending, due to loss of strength or skill or due to deformity or pain. Patients particularly prone to these difficulties are those with arthritis of the upper limb, and most neurological disorders.

(2) Difficulties of access and progression, mainly associated with

steps, stairs and long distances. These face all wheelchair users, patients with lower-limb arthritis or amputation; respiratory or cardiac cripples and the elderly.

The majority of the disabled population are affected by one or other or both of these two groups of difficulties.

Disability frequently reduces a person's choice of alternatives, whether these be places to live, careers or friends; but such limitations are the basis of social handicaps and also denote some degree of social deterioration. This loss of function, the translation of disability into handicap is, however, more often due to non-medical factors than to intrinsic disease processes.

Although certain disorders carry with them socially unacceptable features, or are accompanied by intellectual deterioration, the majority of handicaps are imposed by architectural, administrative and financial barriers, transport problems and many other extrinsic superimposed restrictions.

Although the disability is often specific, the resulting handicap is non-specific, and represents that individual's inability to overcome the disability in a particular set of circumstances. Thus, when assessing the quality of a disability or a handicap, it is necessary to establish the inter-relationship between the two. Disability evaluation must include a full appraisal of the clinical, functional, and social features of the patient. By studying these in the context of the particular patient's environment, a functional assessment can be made. The detailed assessment of the clinical disability and the functional handicap must run hand in hand when managing the severely disabled.

PRINCIPLES OF PHYSICAL REHABILITATION

The general principles of rehabilitation consist of maintaining and improving the mobility of joints, preserving and improving muscle power and actively restoring and developing muscle function. The maintenance and preservation of function is a major contribution during periods of enforced inactivity or immobilization, and this phase must be followed by active re-establishment of function and the utilization of residual capability. When there is irrevocable loss of function, the rehabilitation must employ substitutes to achieve optimum function, and must include training the patient to use these substitutes. These principles were established in relation to limb fractures and the other results of trauma, but they can equally well be applied in the management of any dysfunction of the locomotor system.

For generations physiotherapy has been widely used in the treatment of the chronic neurologically disabled, but there is little evidence that it affects the natural history. Clearly, twice-weekly attendances at a physiotherapy department for the application of heat, massage and a few passive exercises has no physical value, although psychologically it may help the patient by continuing to give him hope, and by forcing him to get out of his home.

The prevention of flexion deformities, contractures and bed sores is a primary responsibility of those nursing the patient, and the relatives can be taught the necessary manoeuvres easily and quickly. Passive stretching, turning and general movement must be given at least once daily if they are be effective. Unfortunately, it is often difficult to persuade parents or relatives to carry out the manoeuvres with sufficient vigour and frequency as they are often reluctant to disturb the patient, or to produce the discomfort which naturally accompanies the defeat of muscle spasm.

Specific muscle re-education and academic attention to range of movements and muscle power lose significance after the initial acute illness is over, and functional activities and maintenance of morale assume the greater importance. Independence of activity is the aim; whether this is obtainable by voluntary effort, by altered methods of practice, or by the use of aids or gadgets, is immaterial. In this field, the activities of the physiotherapist and occupational therapist are both supplementary and complementary.

Most simple fractures and minor disabilities regain full function without much formal rehabilitation providing the patient is adequately instructed in home management and has no inhibiting fears or pains which he does not understand. In different language, a good patient with good motivation usually recovers from minor disabilities without the aid of intensive rehabilitation. Patients with relatively minor disabilities, but who require a high degree of physical fitness for their work, and patients with multiple or complex injuries or disabilities will benefit from a more intensive full-time rehabilitation regimen; but this may not be possible without the provision of special facilities.

Rehabilitation of common disabilities can be conducted on an in-patient or out-patient basis, at a day hospital or a residential centre, depending on the facilities available and the local circumstances.

The main needs for rehabilitation are space and adequate well-trained staff. A large open gymnasium and treatment pool should be the basis of a comprehensive physiotherapy department. Small individual treatment areas, expensive electrical treatment machines and complex passive therapy apparatus are largely irrelevant.

Purposeful activity and functional movement are the mainstay of treatment.

Before World War II only a few centres had applied the rehabilitation principles laid down by Robert Jones in his 'curative workshops', but the Royal Air Force established the modern approach of full-time intensive orthopaedic rehabilitation by converting 'convalescence' into 'rehabilitation'. This pattern was developed by grouping patients with similar disabilities, narrowing the remedial aims of the group, and increasing the number of groups or classes to produce graduated progression through the classes as each patient improved. Each class had an activity programme based on a few remedial exercises, for example, quadriceps setting, or hip abduction or shoulder mobilizing. Management was augmented by specific physiotherapy, occupational therapy and hydrotherapy, where it was necessary.

Because of urbanization and the concentration of population in Great Britain, most rehabilitation is carried out on an out-patient basis. Full-time rehabilitation in special centres is reserved for the severe and complex disabilities. In rural communities and underdeveloped countries the difficulties of day treatment are probably greater than the difficulties of providing hostel accommodation suitable for full-time rehabilitation.

Of those patients who require rehabilitation following accident or illness or reconstructive surgery to achieve a good functional result some are expected to regain their former functional capability, and some who may have suffered from complex multiple injuries will be left with a permanent residual disability.

Finally, there are patients who need an extension of the rehabilitation service. These are patients whose disability is progressive or who have severe permanent disability, such patients require a special approach and management if they are to achieve maximum functional capability.

REHABILITATION OF THE SEVERELY DISABLED

The long-term rehabilitation of the severely disabled must be based on a detailed assessment of the patient's physical disability and a pragmatic appraisal of their possible capability. This assessment must be made in the context of the natural history of the disability (for example, stable or unstable), the severity of their handicap, their psychological make-up and their intellectual capabilities in the context of their possible ultimate environment, social and financial.

Without a full assessment in context, much of the effort of staff and patient may be misdirected. Physiotherapy is the basis of much rehabilitation for the period of time when definitive improvement can be obtained and it may sometimes be justifiable for long periods of time. However it is easy to unwittingly continue such treatment for longer than necessary. For example, there are patients who attend departments for excellent physiotherapy but return home exhausted and have to be provided with assistance to achieve domestic independence. Such misdirection can be avoided by pragmatic assessment.

The total reappraisal of severely disabled patients is a complex and time-consuming activity requiring the concentrated efforts of an experienced team. Successful rehabilitation depends on maximal patient co-operation, and this is only forthcoming when the patient understands enough to become a member of the rehabilitation team. The atmosphere of group therapy of a rehabilitation unit can often instil the will to improve and also the preparedness to accept the degree of disability. Unfortunately, such units are in short supply and many hospital departments are under such pressure that time cannot be given to adequate assessment and rehabilitation.

Having made the assessment, a realistic approach to resettlement can be planned drawing on available physical aids, such as wheelchairs, hoists and other specialized fitments and appliances. The designing of special splints and gadgets may need to be undertaken and the patient then trained in their use. Finally, social readjustment, retraining, rehousing or permanent institutionalization must be arranged. Even in a sophisticated and mature society, which has financially accepted the responsibility for supporting its disabled, this can be a complex and often frustrating exercise, and trained social workers are essential members of the rehabilitation team.

This book sets out to describe the 'rehabilitation approach' to the management of the severely disabled. Assessment of the patient, the disability, the patient's functional capabilities and the possible environment, form a large part of the text, for adequate management can only be based on adequate assessment. Further sections deal with specific clinical problems and functional problems which tend to recur time and again in the management of the severely disabled. The general principles of management and resettlement are outlined. Case histories are quoted to illustrate the problems.

Each patient is an individual, and each severely disabled patient needs individual care. Although techniques of management may tend to become standardized, this is because the patterns of disease and disability often recur. However, for optimal results, the patients must be gently led and guided along appropriate lines by unhurried exploration of possibilities. Many severely disabled patients have lived with their handicap for many years, many suffer pain and all suffer frustration. They are not always amenable to new ideas, and conversely they may well set their sights beyond what is possible or practical. Practical trials, whether successes or failures, are part of the assessment, providing factual evidence for therapists, patients and relatives. It is often difficult to deny an appliance or line of management, but a practical demonstration of its lack of value is much more acceptable than either an ex-cathedra refusal, or a compliance which leads to a wrong decision. It is this slow, practical appraisal that is so time-consuming and needs specialized Units and staff.

AIDS, APPLIANCES AND EQUIPMENT FOR THE DISABLED

In general, the majority of disabled patients manage to continue to live an active life without any aids, apparatus, appliances or special equipment, indeed many of the consultants who have most to do with such patients spend more time advising them how to do without such aids, than they do in prescribing them. This approach is the correct one, for disability does not necessarily mean handicap. The functional handicap is a reflection of many other factors, architectural, mechanical, domestic, social, financial and welfare. It is not possible to solve the social and welfare problems with aids and appliances. Mechanical aids should only be prescribed when they are really needed.

Although it is difficult to obtain accurate statistics, the figures available make it clear that a high proportion of all devices supplied, whether they are artificial limbs, wheelchairs, walking aids, orthopaedic appliances, or simple personal aids, are not used by the patient at home. Patients are reluctant to admit this when they are reviewed in hospital, but a domiciliary follow-up will reveal the true use obtained from mechanical aids which have been supplied. This lack of appreciation of the utilization of appliances is in part due to the inadequacy of the appliances provided, and in part due to inadequacy of evaluation of the patient's real needs.

It is reasonable to provide certain small simple aids in the possibility that a patient might find them of value, but the more complex and expensive the appliance, the more necessary it is to be able to assess the patient adequately, and also to provide adequate training in the use and application of the apparatus.

The more sophisticated and specialized the aid, the more personal its design and fitting needs to be. The more complicated the appliance, the more difficult the patient may find it to learn to operate successfully. Unless the appliance gives the patient a practical advantage either in the immediate or foreseeable future, he is unlikely to persist in the use of the appliance or to co-operate fully in entering into a prolonged training programme. This attitude is seen very clearly in amputees or patients with brachial plexus injuries. The loss of an arm, or the paralysis of an arm can be overcome relatively quickly by learning to become one-handed. Once the patient has done this, it is very difficult to get him to learn to use an artificial arm; it takes longer and requires more effort to use the appliance than to do without it. Acceptance of such an appliance may depend on vanity for the patient who wants a cosmetic effect to overcome an obvious physical disability, or it may be that they really can see a need for the appliance, as for a specific job. The latter reason is less common than the former.

Acceptance of any appliance or aid depends on early decisions, an efficient appliance, understanding and co-operation from the patient and the motivation of the patient towards that appliance.

Classification

It is convenient to classify mechanical aids into appliances, personal aids and equipment. Appliances are devices which are made to fit the patient for the purpose of correcting a deformity or increasing a function. They include corsets, calipers, surgical footwear and splints. Personal aids are usually small items prescribed to assist functional ability and include pick-up sticks, bath aids, toilet aids, eating aids, adapted household gadgets and adapted clothing. Equipment refers to larger mechanical aids such as mechanical beds, hoists, adapted kitchen equipment, special chairs and remote-control apparatus.

Some aids may well be difficult to classify, particularly walking aids, and this makes the supply complicated. The difficulties arise because generally speaking appliances and aids which are needed for continued active treatment of patients are the responsibility of the hospital service, and these services are mandatory. But articles required for home nursing or for more social or welfare activities are the responsibility of the local authorities and their powers are permissive.

For hospital and specialist services the responsibility is placed firmly on the consultant's shoulders. He may prescribe whatever he considers necessary for the patient's condition; furthermore, if there is disagreement as to liability for supply, or doubt as to whether the appliance is needed for continued treatment or home nursing, then it is the hospital's responsibility to accept liability to supply. The situation becomes more difficult when the patient's needs are more attuned to social and welfare activities, and aids are needed to help him return to work, or to increase his independence. Under these circumstances, it may be difficult to argue that they are needed for continued treatment or indeed for home nursing, and yet it may be obvious that it is to the patient's advantage to increase his activities and independence.

The discretionary powers of the local authorities are very wide, ranging from the provision of simple personal aids to architectural reconstruction of the patient's house, building ramps, widening doors, installing hoists and so on. But the financial arrangements very considerably from authority to authority, and the controlling influence may or may not be directed by informed professional advice.

Thus, although legislation is comprehensive, and it is theoretically possible to provide any patient with any apparatus or appliance he needs, it is often very difficult to negotiate the administrative labyrinths leading to such provisions, and indeed it is often very difficult to persuade some authorities to undertake the complex arrangements to support severely disabled patients. It is frequently much easier for all concerned if the patient is admitted to an institution caring for the permanently physically disabled. Such a solution to the problem salves the public conscience, is seen to make necessary provision, but commits the patient to a life of dependence and often frustration. For these reasons, if no other, a Unit capable of undertaking comprehensive clinical and functional assessments is the most useful means of determining the patterns of resettlement of disabled patients. Such Units can bridge the gap between hospital management and local authority responsibility, and working in collaboration with the local authority and general practitioners can lead to reasonable patterns of management of the severely disabled patient in the context of the individual circumstances, both clinical and social.

Units staffed with personnel experienced in rehabilitation and management of the severely disabled, with a large range of aids and appliances available for trial, and with technicians available to carry out necessary alterations or to devise and make individual appliances, can make an outstanding direct contribution. Through comprehensive follow-up services such Units can provide a realistic approach to the long-term solutions.

The provision of mechanical aids is a complex exercise in prescribing, and must be preceded by a detailed assessment of the patient's needs in the context of their physical disability, their motivation and general social background. Furthermore, there is an urgent need for the dissemination of information concerning the design of aids and their provision between hospital and specialist service, the general practitioner and the local authority and welfare services.

MOTIVATION OF THE PHYSICALLY DISABLED

The onset of illness needing medical care and admission to hospital, combined with the possibility that reduced capacity or even severe disability may result, produces anxieties in all people. Many people cope with them through their own resources and those of their families. Some people however, though normally quite capable of managing their own affairs, will need help with problems which are, for some reason, especially hard for them as individuals. The nature and extent of the difficulties which patients and their relatives feel in meeting illness and its consequences depend on such factors as personal make-up, the family, and the economic situation.

The disabled population has its natural scatter of personality types; the intellectual, the eager, the indolent and the workshy. There is no specific evidence that personality types are associated with particular disabilities, but reaction to disability is largely determined by the underlying personality and intellect.

Correlations between mental status and physical trauma, physical deterioration or chronic disability are urgently needed to help in the assessment of physically handicapped patients. There is an increasing awareness of the part which clinical psychologists can play in the management of the physically disabled.

Evaluation of the pre-morbid personality presents the clinician with much more of a detective problem, and it is in this area that the general practitioner, close relatives, friends and neighbours can offer help. For children, school reports, and teacher's personal comments can help considerably. The interpretation of all this information is complex and requires considerable experience. Even if the general education of all doctors in psychological recording was considerably improved, this field would need considerable expertise. But the therapists experienced in working with the physically disabled develop an instinctive interpretation of their relationship with these patients. When there is opportunity for open discussion between therapist, social worker, nursing staff, welfare worker, education authority as well as clinician, then it is often possible to achieve a realistic appraisal of the limits to which rehabilitation should be pursued. One person can frequently be misled but the team approach allows a wider scope and is helpful in delineating the framework in which each member of the team can contribute.

Perhaps the most important outcome of this type of practical approach is that each specialist tends to limit the activities of his colleagues. Thus objectives become more clear-cut and pragmatic, and therefore more easily attainable. The best rehabilitation approach is one which sets limited objectives, attains that objective, re-assesses the situation and then moves forward to the next objective. Patients who are set unattainable targets lose faith and hope.

It is more difficult to establish the presence of altered or altering intellectual competence; nowhere is this more clearly demonstrated than in multiple sclerosis. The euphoric, laissez-faire, attitude of these patients is well recognized, but the lack of insight is often misinterpreted as courage and determination to overcome disability. However, after early depression, many patients with multiple sclerosis develop an increasing intellectual deficit, and the euphoria is pathological and associated with the intellectual deterioration. Clinical psychologists can help to define such changes and should be integrated into the rehabilitation team both as regards establishing a diagnostic assessment and also with the view to planning long-term rehabilitation and resettlement.

REFERENCE

Agerholm, M. (1966). *Equipment for the Disabled*, 2nd edn. London; National Fund for Research into Crippling Diseases

2—*Assessment of the Severely Disabled*

GENERAL ASSESSMENT

One of the most difficult problems in the management of the severely disabled is to establish an assessment of the long-term prognosis. Many of the disorders leading to severe disability have their own unpredictable variations (for example, rheumatoid arthritis). Others, which are known to be progressive, such as muscular dystrophy and motor neurone disease, proceed at varying rates. So-called static disabilities (for example traumatic paraplegia) are subject to intermittent intercurrent problems, particularly urinary infections, which have a dominant influence on the patient's capabilities, while others, such as multiple sclerosis, are associated with many other disabilities deriving from the same underlying pathology. Furthermore, there is increasing evidence that many disorders are polymorphic and the disability is an interaction of environmental and inherent factors which will interact differently, according to the circumstances. The complexity of these factors makes a comprehensive appraisal not only very important but also very difficult. With physical limitation of rehabilitation services and shortage of staff, it is necessary to indicate quantitatively which patients will benefit from rehabilitation and which patients are likely to remain uninfluenced.

Walking can be said to be dependent upon strength and endurance, rather than co-ordination, whereas upper-limb function is more dependent on co-ordinated muscle activity. Difficulties in walking may arise from many possible causes; for example, hemiparetic patients may have interference with balance, or muscle weakness, or spasticity. Balance may be disturbed by lesions of the cerebellar systems or the visual system. Muscle weakness of trunk, abdomen, hip, knee or foot muscle groups may all seriously affect walking. Similarly, spasticity in lower-limb muscle groups, flexors or extensors, will seriously impair locomotor function. Walking ability is also related to mental alertness, but incontinence, cardiovascular disease, joint degeneration and sensory deficit may individually or collectively have a significant effect. Thus the assessment of patient's mobility potential must include an appraisal of all these motor and sensory aspects of the patient's condition.

The functions assessed under the activities of daily living are relatively standardized; feeding, dressing, personal hygiene, writing, typing and simple manual tasks. Charts of activities can be graded to indicate levels of activity, and if correlated with the initial level of function, successive assessments will give a record of changes and indicate the degree of recovery or the effectiveness of rehabilitation measures.

Most occupational therapy departments have their own charts of activities of daily living and many departments have added to these records a system of scoring. Quantitative assessments expressed numerically offer the attraction of ready comparison; patient with patient, or capability with capability. But the assumption that the physical assessment of competence in activities of daily living provides a simultaneous assessment of a patient's functional capacilities is merely naïve. The practical domestic situation is much more complex.

As yet, there is no detailed analysis of the inter-relationship of clinical records, muscle charts, joint range and competence in activities of daily living. There is no analysis of the inter-relationship between competence in, say, putting on a vest, eating bread and butter, and controlling a wheelchair. Furthermore, competence in any particular activity achieves different levels of significance in different sets of circumstances. For example, the ability to walk from wheelchair to toilet may have more significance for domestic independence than the ability to walk from house to shops.

In order to obtain a comprehensive functional assessment, detailed records of function are necessary; but these can become so complex that processing the data presents almost insuperable problems, outweighing the value of the possible results. But functional assessment can provide a comprehensive index of a patient's capability, giving a realistic appraisal of the patient, more relevant than simple records of joint range and estimation of muscle power.

The primary object of assessment is not necessarily description or classification, but an exploration of the functional variables which may serve to help predict responses to treatment. By reviewing daily living activities in near real-life situations, it is possible to achieve a considerable exposure of the important but intangible and immeasurable variables which are often the most important; the patient's willingness to co-operate, his tolerance of failure, levels of aspiration, ability to understand new situations, awareness of limitations and capabilities, his level of intelligence and education, in short, his motivation.

Such practical tests as the occupational therapist can carry out in assessing activities of daily living can be developed into graded orders: ability to adapt to decisions made, accuracy and endurance. They can give a very clear understanding of the patient, although they do not provide an I.Q. or a 'mental status' quotient. In all functional assessments the patient's capabilities are more important than their disabilities and the changing patterns of competence present a pragmatic measure of recovery.

Successful response to treatment depends very largely on the patient's ability to understand, adjust and accept the treatment. For this reason emotional and intellectual status influence the final result. There are likely to be definite patterns in the pre-morbid state, and an understanding of the patient's normal mode of living and capabilities obtained by direct questioning of relatives and neighbours when compared with his current ability will lead an experienced therapist to a shrewd quantitative assessment of the standard of attainment which can be achieved.

Sometimes clues can be derived from social or welfare workers, sometimes from direct personal knowledge such as school reports, and all possible sources should be explored to enable a firm appraisal of the pre-morbid personality.

Patients' potentials for recovery and for rehabilitation are as diverse as the patients themselves and their disorders, ranging from the achievement of a single function, such as the ability to 'transfer', to the return to full-time employment. There are no objective criteria available by which the clinician is enabled to predict the potential of rehabilitation or to determine which patients will achieve much and which patients will achieve little. The most a detailed clinical reappraisal will yield is general guidance regarding the progress of the disability.

PHYSICAL ASSESSMENT

After the general clinical assessment, attention can be directed towards the patient's independence and functional capability. The physical features of the patient's clinical condition determine the intensity of rehabilitation activities and delineate the aims of management. Because of the complexity of problems inherent in the management of the severely disabled, a full clinical examination and record is essential. For many patients, a muscle chart (usually graded 0–5 in accordance with the Medical Research Council scale) is a useful base line. But also it is important with many severely disabled patients to record muscle contractures as these may determine handicap and may be amenable to improvement by physiotherapy or surgical measures (a useful chart is given in Appendix D).

Flexion deformity of the wrists, whether from changes consequent upon rheumatoid arthritis or a congenital deformity such as radial club hand, may put the hand in a functional position as regards feeding. Very careful assessment of function is necessary because correction of the deformity may render the patient unable to feed, although producing a meaningful improvement in power of grip. To compensate for the correction of wrist flexion, an increase in elbow or shoulder range may render the patient once again independent for feeding. The flexed wrist compensates for loss of elbow flexion and conversely in the presence of limited elbow movement, correction of the wrist deformity demands a functional improvement in elbow movement to retain function.

Furthermore, it is only by detailed clinical reappraisal that the effectiveness of various alternative methods of management can be compared. Much time can be spent in devising complex wheelchairs or gadgetry, or in altering the domestic situation, whereas it may be possible to achieve some significant improvement in function by a surgical procedure. Sometimes an appropriate splint can be devised to simulate the end-result which surgery hopes to achieve and a functional assessment of the efficacy of this splint indicates the improvement which surgery is likely to produce.

For this purpose, simple splintage materials, such as mallable plastic (Prenyl or Plastazote), or metal (Duralumin), or plaster-of-paris, can be employed by physiotherapist or workshop technicians. For therapist, clinician and patient alike, practical tests are always of more value than theoretical discussions based on charts of muscle activity or daily living activities. Surgeons especially find these charts difficult to accept, and appreciate the direct impact of a demonstration, photograph or film.

FUNCTIONAL ASSESSMENT

Clinical assessment is based on a stylized system of 'history taking', clinical examination, muscle-power charting and so on, without which significant details may be missed. Functional assessment can be systemized and formalized, based on Activities for Daily Living charts and graded activities. Although much information can be acquired by questioning, observation of activities is more helpful. A patient may state that he is completely independent for dressing and undressing and yet under direct observation, it may soon be clear that either he has taken a certain amount of help for granted, or he cheats by failing to complete some aspects of the task, or he is unrealistic (euphoric) and lacking in insight about his handicap. This distinction is only available after direct functional assessment and may give the clinician quite a different appraisal of the situation from that which he gained in the out-patient department or on examining the patient in a hospital ward. Sometimes it is sufficient to know that the patient is able to carry out a particular activity, but on other occasions it is essential to record the details of how the task is performed as trick movements may be a risk if new techniques are introduced or the functional anatomy altered by surgical procedures. It is in this field, that film records can be invaluable, allowing for careful study of movements without overtiring the patient, and allowing for repetitive analysis.

Preliminary functional assessment can be directed towards the main areas of activity as follows:

Personal care	Nursing Feeding Toilet Dressing
Mobility	Walking Wheelchairs Transfers
Household	Cooking Housework
Hobbies/recreation	
Outdoor activities	
Work	

Enquiry will enlarge upon some of these activities, particularly home conditions, general mobility and upper-limb function.

Home conditions

Type of house, flat, bungalow, Residential Home
Main problems, access-steps, stairs, bathroom upstairs and so on
Family living at home, relatives or friends near

Mobility

General pattern
Lie, sit, stand, walk
Walking unaided, aids, appliances
Implications at home, ramps, steps, kerbs, distances
Lie, sit, wheelchair, method of transfer, suitable chair
Method of propulsion
Outdoor transport, private, public

Upper-limb function

Reaching, lifting, carrying, handling

Having obtained an over-all impression of the patient's problems, direct detailed observation will enable the therapist to build up a picture of the patient's handicap under the following headings:

Personal care

Washing, including hair, nails, shaving or make-up
Toilet
Bath
Dressing
Eating and drinking

Communication

Speech, telephoning, writing, typing
Public transport, shopping, social functions

Domestic activities

Basic meal preparation and housework where applicable for men and women.

Work/education/training

Including job of running a home
Problems related to patient's particular job and place of work or education.

Leisure activities

Personality and mental attitude:
Positive or negative attitude
- Quick or slow reaction
- Anxious or relaxed
- Co-operative or resentful
- Dependent or independent

These headings form the basis for the therapists' preliminary assessment (*see* Appendix A).

When the main problems lie in personal independence a more

detailed analysis of activities of daily living is called for (*see* Appendix E).

As far as home conditions are concerned, it is always preferable for a therapist to carry out a domiciliary visit, but where this is not practical, it is probably simpler to ask the domiciliary occupational therapist employed by the local authority or the appropriate welfare officer, or social worker to complete a prepared questionnaire so that relevant details are not missed. Appendix C sets out a sample proforma for domiciliary assessment.

Shortened assessment questionnaires can be prepared for patients with limited disabilities, or for use in units concerned with particular disabilities. For example, osteoarthritis of the hip is a common disability frequently referred for surgery, in which the patients' functions are of significance in deciding the type of surgical treatment and the post-operative rehabilitation. A functional assessment record of lower-limb disability is included in Appendix F.

Similarly with the current interest in reconstructive surgery for rheumatoid hands, hand function tests are particularly relevant. Assessment of hand function is one of the most difficult parts of the physical appraisal of a patient, and to present the findings in a meaningful and reproduceable fashion is even more difficult. A simple form of functional assessment using standard objects with space for comments has been found of value. These activities can be readily interpreted by other therapists, or by surgeons considering reconstructive operations (*see* Appendix J).

Amputees present an interesting and relatively simple assessment problem. Upper-limb function tests can readily be used, either for children or for adults (Appendix H), and these demonstrate particularly how tests can become training regimens, or training regimens can be utilized as tests for record purposes. When the performance of upper-limb amputees in exercises carried out primarily for training purposes is timed (for example, typing, writing, assembling construction outfits), it will give an objective record of competence. Any improvement in time and accuracy gives a measure of the patterns of improvement and functional capability.

With more-sophisticated appliances, such as powered artificial limbs supplied to children with severe limb deformities, these tests lead to the establishment of 'learning curves'. If appropriate improvement does not occur, and this is readily evident on the learning curve, then attention is immediately drawn to the need to study reasons for lack of improvement (for example, whether the appliance is inadequate for the task, or the control of the appliance too complex for the child to master). Without objective records, the need to reassess the appliance and the training programme may not become readily obvious.

Assessment of lower-limb amputees is simple; distance, and the time taken to traverse a distance are easily recorded and are much more reliable than clinical impression or the patient's casual comments (Appendix I).

For more detailed functional assessment, graded tests can be devised, but it is particularly important that these activities should be planned in the context of the patient's disability, home conditions, social background and likely resettlement. The process of getting up in the morning; sitting up in bed, getting out, going to the toilet, washing, dressing and grooming, may appear to repeat many of the functions observed in the preliminary assessment; but as a related sequence of events to be performed in reasonable time, this requires considerable perseverance and may uncover factors such as fatigue, pain or spasm not apparent when these activities are performed separately. As well as observing the physical function involved, step by step, points such as the following should be noted:

(1) How much of this sequence could the patient manage safely without help?

(2) Could any accident risk be reduced by the provision of aids such as grab rails?

(3) Would adjustment in heights of his bed, chair, or toilet help him?

(4) Would simple adaptations to his clothes help him?

(5) Was any pain, fatigue, or spasm noticeable and if so, was this due to any particular task in the sequence, or was it due to the sustained effort?

(6) Could the routine be simplified to make it less tiring or to reduce the time required?

(7) What was the patient's attitude, did he give up easily or did he persevere?

(8) Was he distressed by failure, was he angered by it or did he accept his limitations?

Household tasks such as planning and cooking a family meal, or washing, hanging out clothes and ironing can be used in a similar way.

ASSESSMENT FOR WORK

It is seldom possible to simulate the patient's job in an occupational therapy department, except perhaps for home-making, but it is possible to examine his work potential. Firstly, it is necessary to carefully go through the patient's daily routine by question and by definitive practical tests where necessary and when possible

Patient's occupation
When last at work
Getting up in the morning; can this be done in reasonable time
With or without help
Main difficulties
Mobility; walking, with or without aids
Wheelchair; independent or needs help negotiating kerbs, crossing street
Leaving the house; steps, slopes, rough grounds
Public transport; distance to bus stop or train
Mounting bus or train
Any problem sitting in bus or train
Distance from transport stop to place of work
Private transport; car, invalid tricycle
Getting in and out; with or without help
Getting wheelchair into vehicle
Difficulties with driving
Adaptations needed
Parking; distance from parking place to work
Sufficient space to off-load and transfer into wheelchair
Access to place of work and circulation; steps, slopes
Heavy swing-doors, narrow doors
Narrow passages, awkward corners
Circulation within working area
Atmosphere; heat, cold, damp, exposure to weather, any problems
Toilet; distance to toilet
Access to toilet; walking/wheelchair
Independent or needing help for toilet
Clothing; any difficulty with protective or special clothing
Food; distance and access to canteen
Any difficulties in eating
Confidence to eat in public
Facilities for eating packed meal

The general patterns of work activity need to be considered both as related sequences and as a series of tasks in separate contexts.

Architectural hazards are numerous and situations similar to those at work can usually be found without much difficulty. Specific work situations, prolonged standing, carrying, lifting, manual dexterity and so on may be tested by mock-up in an experienced rehabilitation centre. A therapist who has assessed the patient and seen him at work in the physiotherapy department and occupational therapy department can often tell directly what are the likely problems. A visit to the place of work and discussion with the employer, or employees in similar work may be of considerable help. Although these situations are more relevant to the less severely disabled, the principles apply to all disabled patients, at the stage when resettlement in work is being planned.

To avoid mistakes, frustrating to patients, therapists and employers alike, detailed assessment and planning is essential. For example, office work does not only involve typing or writing; filing letters handling small cards, telephoning and taking down messages while sitting at a desk, lifting down and handling books, interviewing other people are all involved. Most patients have never had to consider and analyse work in this detail and often may find it difficult to describe or demonstrate it without the help of systematic enquiry. Successful resettlement can be a complex activity for patient, therapist and rehabilitation or resettlement officer.

SOCIAL ASSESSMENT

Social and welfare problems often predominate among the problems of the severely disabled. Once adequate clinical care has been instituted, the social and welfare aspects become increasingly important, particularly in the home situation. The majority of the severely physically disabled are cared for at home, and the family bears the brunt of the load of nursing and general care. The amount of support which the family receives depends on the family, and on the local organization. This varies considerably from area to area.

The majority of the problems are either concerning the handling of the disabled patient, particularly during the day when the able members of the family have to be at work or at school, and the housing. Patient-handling can be eased by the provision of various aids and appliances, hoists, commodes, special beds and by assistance from district nurses, domiciliary therapists and services such as Meals on Wheels. Most of the housing problems derive from difficulties of access and lack of manoeuvring space. The patients are often amenable to alterations, either minor or major structural changes, or to rehousing.

Rehousing may often appear to be an attractive solution from the physical handicap aspect of the problem; but such recommendations should be made only after careful assessment of the family relationships, and the likely support for the patients from the family and neighbours. Conversely the lack of family and local support is equally of importance in the over-all appraisal, because rehousing may not be helpful if it means leaving the neighbourhood where the patient has friends, neighbours and family connections. For the physically handicapped, much can be done with grip rails, ramps, re-hanging doors and the installation of suitable washing, toilet and bathing aids. The majority of housing adaptations are carried out within a year of recommendation, but rehousing takes considerably longer in most instances.

Adequate social assessment of a family, and it usually must be a whole family assessment, is a complex and difficult activity. It is frequently unsatisfactory when tackled only from the hospital angle, and a broader approach is needed. Local knowledge can be invaluable. The general practitioner should be able to provide much background information, and when he has district nurses, domiciliary occupational therapists and social workers collaborating with him, then much of the assessment of disabled patients can be done at a domiciliary level. Many of the referrals to hospitals units are required because of the current regulations relating to the prescription and provision of certain items of equipment which can only be prescribed by hospital consultants; or because the influence of a hospital consultant is thought more likely to produce results from the various departments of the local authority.

The hospital assessment unit may have to rely heavily upon the local workers for much of the social and welfare aspects of the assessment. Many hospital departments prefer to send their own workers out into the community to achieve an adequate assessment. This is good for the hospital department and helps them to achieve a realistic appraisal, but it often duplicates the work and becomes time-consuming and expensive if the unit is admitting patients from widely scattered areas. Undoubtedly, however, a personal observation is often of greater value than a second-hand report. In this sphere, the practice of multi-disciplinary domiciliary consultations has much to offer, with the physician, therapist, and social worker carrying out a domiciliary visit together with the general practitioner and the local workers. In this way, undoubtedly, many admissions to hospital units could be avoided, and problems delineated more clearly and more quickly than in the clinical atmosphere of an outpatient department or the somewhat isolated surroundings of a rehabilitation unit.

No matter how the social assessment is achieved, it is a *sine qua non* in the total assessment of a severely physically disabled patient.

PERSONALITY AND INTELLECT ASSESSMENT

Some authorities consider that many of the patient's personal characteristics are the result of external factors and that if the social environment and family background are supportive, the outcome of rehabilitation is likely to be successful. But lack of achievement may be associated with a lack of personal drive and endeavour as well as lack of opportunities or support from family, friends or community. The patient's reaction to the combination of all the relevant factors is often referred to under the general term 'motivation'. There is no evidence that there are particular personalities associated with specific disabilities, but some physical conditions have a direct organic effect upon the brain and central nervous system and thus may be associated with changes in intellect and personality.

It becomes important to record these faculties, never an easy task but doubly difficult in the case of disabled patients for whom many of the available 'test-batteries' are unsuitable. It is inappropriate to ask a wheelchair-bound patient dependent upon others to move him from place to place, about his aspirations for action and community activities.

Patients with painful joint conditions such as rheumatoid arthritis, voluntarily restrict their activities to avoid pain, and thus enquiries related to achievement and activities may produce inapposite answers. Standard questions such as 'Would you be unhappy if you were prevented from making numerous social contacts?' are clearly inappropriate.

Physical disability, whether painful or not, will undoubtedly induce a reactive depression in many instances; furthermore, severe disability in childhood will interfere with education and thus influence the assessment.

There is evidence that some of the most severely physically disabled patients have stable personalities, because they no longer have to struggle, they are cared for. But progressive lack of social activities accompanying disability is often associated with an increasingly introverted personality.

The correlation between educational levels and achievement is definite. Patients who have had a higher education are predominant among those who achieve maximal activity in spite of severe disability. This feature is closely linked with the social status and the consequent opportunity or support for education. Certain disabilities, particularly strokes and multiple sclerosis, are associated with organic damage, intellectual deterioration and personality change, impairment of memory, lack of insight into the disability, and an inability to adapt or to accept training, all of which mitigate against rehabilitation techniques; and it is an essential part of the total assessment of the patient to delineate these features. A full psychological assessment can often give a clear indication regarding the possible outcome of rehabilitation or indicate the particular lines of management likely to give best results.

There is a need to establish standard personality, educational and intellectual status tests applicable to the physically disabled and there is a wide field of activity for collaboration with clinical psychologists in the field of physical rehabilitation.

RECORDS, REPORTS AND COMMUNICATION

Assessment forms, check lists, practical trials, learning curves, domestic assessment and reports are of little value unless they are accurately and concisely recorded and presented in an acceptable fashion to those to whom they have significance. Many complex and comprehensive assessments are locked up in clinical notes, and filed away in hospital departments or doctors' surgeries.

Details of assessments must be summarized and the relevant positive and negative findings (capabilities and disabilities) listed and cross-referred to the clinical findings. Such documentation can form the most valuable means of communication between all those concerned with the management of the patient: hospital medical staff, general practitioners, local authority medical officers, social workers, welfare workers, appliance medical officers, voluntary organizations are all likely to be involved.

A copy of the clinical summary and the relevant details or summarized functional assessment sent to all concerned can be invaluable. They will delineate the reasons for the various recommendations and prevent garbled information being transmitted by the patient, relatives, friends and so forth. Furthermore, integrating clinical with functional assessment and domestic assessment may well obviate the need for repeating assessment, examination, trials by other auxiliaries or doctors, and thus increase the efficiency of the rehabilitation and resettlement service.

A clearly set out assessment of functional activity and the other relevant factors can be a more useful record of handicap and achievement than lengthy muscle charts and clinical examinations. The example given here illustrates how such a report gives a complete picture of the patient against which all therapy and management can be appraised.

OCCUPATIONAL THERAPIST'S REPORT

Preliminary Assessment: date...

Name: Mr. B... Age: 50 Ward G Diagnosis: Rheumatoid arthritis

Home conditions

Lives in an old cottage with his wife, who works as a secretary, and son aged 16 years who is studying for 'O' levels. Three steps at front door; patient can no longer manage these. Outside toilet, approach slippery and uneven. Mr. B sleeps downstairs. Neighbours bring him his midday meal.

Mobility

Patient is virtually chairbound and only stands and shuffles three or four steps to transfer from bed to wheelchair and wheelchair to toilet. Has 8G wheelchair and Invacar.

Upper-limb function

Generalized loss of power and loss of precision function of both hands. Loss of joint range in shoulder and elbows limits his reach to mid-range.

Personal care

Can wash face and hands only, shaves himself, wife washes him. Bathroom upstairs. Cannot get off toilet. Has difficulty cleaning himself.

Dressing

Dependent on his wife, who dresses him before she goes to work every morning.

Communications

Has to be helped into Invacar, but does go out to friends. No other problems.

Work

Was an electrician, and was still working part-time until 15 months ago.

Mental attitude

Mr. B. resents being dependent on others, and is worried because his wife is the wage earner. He is friendly, easy in manner and appears eager to get some work.

Suggestions

Occupational therapist to meet domiciliary occupational therapist and welfare officer at cottage *re* roughened concrete path to toilet and (?) sloped concrete path from gate to back door. To try out toilet heights and grab-rails. To look into dressing and clothing problems. Possibility of some part-time work discussed with medical social worker. Occupational therapist to test his aptitude for figures (his writing is clear though slow) and (?) adding-machine and typing.

The need for repeated reassessment

Assessment is not an isolated single episode, but a continuing sequence of examinations, studies, consultations, appraisals, and reviews of the patient's capabilities, disabilities and handicaps, based upon complete evaluation of the physical, functional, educational, psychological and social attainments. The personnel involved in obtaining this comprehensive review is large, and only relatively few patients require the full range of studies. Therefore, it is probably appropriate that such assessments should be carried out in special centres which are closely associated with a regional clinical centre. Because of their special experience, such centres should also be able to provide postgraduate training for therapists and other ancillary staff. The first task lies in identifying the problems. The initial selection of the patients is important, referral being necessarily selective, and this is followed by the comprehensive assessment, then the planning of rehabilitation in all its aspects, therapy, appliances, training and resettlement. From the centres, there would emerge continuing studies of the disabilities, and a continuing programme of teaching and research. But for the work to remain clinically and practically orientated, the most important step is the follow-up. This only becomes realistic if it is taken right into the patient's home, or other place of domestic resettlement. For it is at home, about a year after the last admission, that the real test of success or failure lies.

The need for continued detailed reassessment is illustrated by the two case histories, No. 582 and No. 54.

M.M.L. No. 582 born 1946 male

Diagnosis: Osteogenesis imperfecta

This young man was a classical example of osteogenesis imperfecta. He was small, intelligent with a relatively large head and characteristically high-pitched 'metallic' voice.

His limbs were small and deformed from numerous fractures and his trunk foreshortened with a marked kyphoscoliosis and 'keeling' of the chest wall. He had a remarkably objective view of his disability and of life in general.

Throughout his life, he had been cared for by his mother, and had achieved an educational level suitable for university entrance. The problem now was whether he could achieve enough independence to take up his university place. Clearly, the two main problems were mobility and personal care.

After many discussions, a university was found which could both offer him a course suitable to his academic capabilities and interest, and also was prepared to collaborate in organizing suitable accommodation.

At this time, he was using a child-size front-wheel-drive self-propelling wheelchair and a Barret light-weight outdoor motorized tricycle. He was unable to get his wheelchair into the tricycle and his parents were lifting him for all transfers. He needed help with washing and toilet, and having led a very sheltered life, was somewhat unrealistic both about the problems he might face and possible solutions.

The first problem was that of the wheelchair and his transfer techniques. Eventually, after much practice, a special chair was ordered with the following specifications:

Wheels.—20 in (50 cm) diameter front propelling wheels with solid tyres; 8 in (20 cm) castor wheels at the rear

Seat.—13 in (32 cm) × 13 in (32 cm) and 18 in (46 cm) height from the ground

Cushion.—2 in (5 cm) hard based

Back.—'Zip' back with the zip set 4 in (10 cm) from the right-hand side of the back canvas. The zip to be operated from the front and to open from the top downwards, and to have 2 in (5 cm) overlength to ease replacement after opening.

He was able to lift objects of up to 3 lb (1·36 kgm) in weight, so from a household point of view, he could manage to cook light meals. Long-handled pick-up appliances made him independent for many other activities. A pair of specially made portable ramps were also provided and enabled him to achieve universal access to home and university. This chair was based on a lightweight folding frame and proved to be highly successful. With this chair he was able to transfer independently, using a sliding board, into bed and in and out of his outdoor tricycle.

The toilet was a problem, but he could transfer on and off through the back of the chair providing the seat was between 20 and 22 in high (50–57 cm). On the toilet he used a 'child's' seat. If the toilet was lower than 20 in (50 cm) he used a specially made 'overseat', which was 20 in (50 cm) high at the front and 22 in (57 cm) at the back (the University toilet seats were 17½ in (44 cm) high).

Washing was achieved with a long-handled sponge. He was independent using a wash-basin 26 in (66 cm) high with 21 in (52 cm) clearance underneath for the wheelchair. Bathing was accomplished by a double bath seat made to fit the bath available at home and at college. An occupational therapist from the Unit went with the patient and a local social worker to the University and discussed all the likely problems with the medical and welfare authorities.

The University was able to allocate special accommodation and make some minor structural alterations once they were convinced that the assessments made were realistic. For example, the wardrobe doors were altered so that he could reach the handle, the mirrors were lowered, and gantry tables were provided at the correct height. His special toilet seats were provided in two suitable toilets and in one the door was removed and a curtain provided.

Comment

A detailed assessment and comprehensive plans of function followed by willing collaboration from University authorities and local authority social and welfare authorities, enabled him to achieve university education.

At follow-up a year later, he had moved out of the special accommodation into some standard quarters which he found himself and could manage. This brought him into the general life of the University rather than segregating him in special accommodation and isolating him from University community life. This illustrates how the well-motivated patient will progress with his independence once given the facilities and help to take the first steps.

M.M.L. No. 54 born 1947 female

Diagnosis: Poliomyelitis; Keratoconus; Eczema; Ehlers-Danlos syndrome

At 2 years of age, this girl had an attack of acute anterior poliomyelitis which left her with severe weakness of both legs. She eventually was able to walk with crutches and calipers, and various orthopaedic procedures were undertaken to maintain her mobility. At the age of 10 years she had rotation osteotomy of the right femur and at 15 years of age she had transplantation of tibialis anterior to the os calsis.

Her childhood was spent mostly at a school for physically handicapped children, She rarely went home as her mother had remarried, achieved a new family, and found it increasingly difficult to manage her. Her schooling had frequently been interrupted by treatment and she was pleasant but a rather frustrated, agressive and difficult child.

While in hospital, she began to have recurrent dislocation of the right hip, and later the same year this was arthrodesed. She had great difficulty during her post-operative rehabilitation period. Her sight was deteriorating because of keratoconus, eventually requiring a corneal graft in 1965. She was by now having repeated dislocation of the left hip and a pseudarthrosis was performed.

From 1965 onwards, she was admitted to the Disabled Living Unit at intervals, usually during each school holiday. On the first admission, she was supplied with a semi-reclining self-propelled wheelchair with elevating footrests and 25 in (63 cm) diameter rear wheels. It had to be reclining with elevating legrests, because of the arthrodesis of the right hip and cushioning was complicated. At this time, she was able to transfer from bed to chair by means of a sliding board, and direct from chair to toilet if the seat was at 21 in (52 cm), and had an old-fashioned wooden surround.

She was accepted as a pupil at a special school for physically handicapped older girls; she settled in very well and achieved G.C.E. 'O' levels in English language, English literature and history. However, her increased activity precipitated painful symptoms in her right shoulder. The apparent weakness was at first thought to be due to muscular dystrophy, but estimation of the serum creatokinase and electromygraphy were normal, and clinically it was considered that she was a mild case of Ehlers-Danlos syndrome.

By December 1966, she was having so much trouble with her shoulder that self-propelling was an increasingly slow and painful procedure. It was therefore considered justifiable to issue her with an electrically-powered indoor chair, with a similar frame and cushioning to the self-propelled one.

She was now doing well at school, the electric chair gave her considerable independence and opened up many possibilities for her. On total review, it was decided that her future lay only in a wheelchair existence and thus it was reasonable to convert the previously arthrodesed right hip to a pseudarthrosis and to fix the painful snapping scapula, and these operations were carried out during the school holidays.

These two operations and the subsequent rehabilitation produced further over-all improvement. She returned to school and achieved a total of 6 G.C.E. 'O' levels. After she left school in the summer of 1968, she was accepted for further education at a technical college to work for G.C.E. 'A' levels. Much of the education was planned to be done on a correspondence basis and with visiting tutors, and with transfers organized by hospital friends she attended the college weekly for practical sessions.

In January 1969, she entered a residential home to make a new life, continuing her further education, contributing to the life of the Home and ultimately making a career for herself.

Although severely physically disabled and with very poor sight (officially registered as a blind person), she is an excellent cook with active hobbies of reading, needlework, cookery, music (including playing the clarinet).

This outcome was the combination of repeated re-assessments, orthopaedic surgery and rehabilitation, adapting her appliances and independence techniques to her current capabilities and finally undertaking surgery to allow her to adapt to increasing disability.

3—Clinical Problems

INTRODUCTION

Each major disability group is associated with patterns of handicap determined by the pathological changes and the natural history of the disease. But when the degree of disability becomes severe, these patterns become less easily distinguishable and whatever the underlying cause the impairment of function which results is similar in each case. Although this tends to make differentiation less distinct as far as total practical physical management is concerned, there are many specific clinical problems which are particularly characteristic of each disease group and which affect the functional handicap. It is some of these problems which are discussed in this chapter.

POLIOMYELITIS

Poliomyelitis was first made notifiable in the United Kingdom in 1912 and from then until 1947 the annual notifications varied from 250 to 1,600 patients each year. The epidemic of 1947 brought the annual notification for that year to 8,000 and it is estimated that in the succeeding 5 years, 20,000 patients died or were disabled by the disease. Since the general introduction of vaccination in 1960, the disease has become virtually non-existent in the United Kingdom, although new acute cases may occur sporadically or be brought here from overseas. Because the majority of patients with residual paralysis following poliomyelitis were young when they contracted the disease, they still constitute a significant section of the disabled population and from time to time may present as problems of rehabilitation.

Two main groups of these patients may still require help. Firstly, patients with widespread residual disabilities who through increasing age or other infirmities, require reappraisal of their functional capability, and secondly, those who having been weaned completely or partially from respiratory aids, may exhibit symptoms of increasing pulmonary insufficiency.

Permanent disability

Until the general availability of vaccination, a high proportion of orthopaedic surgery was concerned with the resolution of residual orthopaedic problems resulting from poliomyelitis. Reconstructive surgery, tendon transplantation, arthrodesis, arthroplasty, osteotomy, the design, making and fitting of appliances and physical and social rehabilitation were all needed in their full range.

Patients with poliomyelitis often become masters of trick movements, developing skills which enable them to obtain a high degree of independence even when severely disabled. With the passage of time, acute poliomyelitis has ceased to be a common problem and experience in managing such patients is being lost. When they present for review or reappraisal because of intercurrent illness, accident or the onset of symptoms associated with degenerative changes in the joints, the opportunity of reassessing their detailed needs must not be missed. At this late stage, the introduction of classical splints, fixed, lively or powered is not easily tolerated. The patients are often so skilful with their trick movements, that any apparatus tends to impede function rather than increase it, and reconstructive surgery may, even at this late stage, offer a more appropriate solution.

Vascular disturbance

One feature of paralysis of the lower limbs which tends to cause increasing trouble as the patients grow older is the cold, blue and swollen leg. Chilblains are common and the skin may break down and ulcerate. Massage, contrast baths and various rubifacients are often advised, but for a patient who spends all day in a wheelchair either at home or at work, these techniques only add to the daily burden of the attendant, and at best, give only temporary relief from symptoms. Elastic bandages or tubular elasticated dressing, applied while the patient is still in bed, may control the oedema to some useful degree. If the paralysis is incomplete, patients should be encouraged to utilize any remaining muscular power in their legs, propelling their wheelchairs with their feet, or deliberately exercising any active muscles for several minutes every hour, thus promoting venous return and helping to reduce postural oedema. Sheepskin-lined boots may give considerable relief from chilblains, and occasionally, sympathectomy is necessary.

Case history No. 424 illustrates the complexities of rehabilitation and resettling a severe case of poliomyelitis.

M.M.L. No. 424 born 1939 male

Diagnosis: Anterior poliomyelitis

Whilst overseas working as a schoolmaster, this patient contracted acute anterior poliomyelitis. He had a severe generalized infection, and was nursed in a respirator for some weeks. He was brought back to the United Kingdom suffering from residual paralyses of all limbs and trunk. His legs, shoulders and elbows were completely flail, but he regained some active movements in both hands. His general recovery was complicated by urinary retention, and severe urinary infection, but eventually this was cleared and he regained control of micturition.

It was nearly 10 months after the onset of the disease before he had recovered sufficiently to be transferred to the Disabled Living Unit for the later stages of his rehabilitation.

The first problem was to achieve comfort in a wheelchair; this could only be attained by a chair with a reclining back and elevating footrests with a 4 in (10 cm) cushion and special cut-away area to prevent pressure over his coccyx. The trouble in seating was because of his size (6 ft, 1·8 m), his flail legs, his weak abdomen and lower spinal musculature. However, having achieved comfort in the chair, the next stage was to fit ball-bearing arm supports. Reclining brackets, special bowed proximal arms, standard distal arms and standard troughs enabled him to start using his hands in a functional position. T-bars were necessary for feeding and special extensions were added for typing.

Once he could begin to use his hands again, his ultimate potential began to emerge. The reclining chair was replaced by a reclining electrically-powered indoor chair with the same fittings; he could operate the standard Powerdrive control box.

At first it was difficult, as he was depressed and appeared to be quite prepared to let others do everything for him. Over a period of several months, he gradually came to realize that he was capable of working and might indeed become self-supporting. While he was still a patient in the Disabled Living Unit he was encouraged to take in proof-reading for a local publishing house, and also tutoring both for special students and for a correspondence course.

The next step was to find a possible place to live in the locality. Eventually, a house was found in which the garage could be converted into a suitable room in which he could work. The remainder of the ground floor was adapted for his bedroom. A housekeeper was engaged, and she came to the Unit to learn how to cope with his nursing and appliances. Eight months after admission to the Disabled Living Unit, and 18 months after the acute illness, he was discharged and installed in his house.

He slept on an electric Egerton bed and was transferred by means of a portable hoist with an all-in-one split-leg sling. He was completely dependent for washing, dressing and bathing. He could use a 'spork' (spoon with prongs) for solid and semi-solid food, but it had to be cut up for him. Liquids were drunk through a straw from a glass fixed in a special holder. He worked 6–8 hours a day and was soon earning a living wage.

Eighteen months later, after many disappointments, he was given a full-time appointment as a school-teacher in a small grammar school. This involved moving house and re-establishing himself and his housekeeper; but this was accomplished with the minimum of outside help and he has now settled down to his new job.

Comments

It would be difficult to be more disabled than this patient (apart from respiratory paralysis) and yet achieve full-time employment. His full resettlement was only achieved after considerable effort on behalf of the patient by professional and lay people of many disciplines. There were many times when the plan appeared to be unrealistic and there were many times when repeated failure was depressing and frustrating to all concerned. However, there was a conviction that he had enough intellectual competence and drive to achieve a working status and that the mechanical problems of handling him were all capable of solution. Difficult though these problems were to solve, it is significant that the main recurrent problem was in convincing first the patient and then likely employers and local authorities that it was worthwhile.

HEMIPLEGIA

Hemiplegia is one of the commonest physical disabilities; there are probably about half a million patients in the United Kingdom surviving after a stroke. Most patients survive their first stroke, and about 85 per cent survive for more than two years. The greater the residual damage, the less the life expectancy; similarly, the younger the patient the better the prognosis.

The commonest causes of hemiplegia are cerebral thrombosis associated with hypertension and arteriosclerosis, embolism and cerebral haemmorrhage. The onset may be insidious or sudden. Initially, the paralysis in flaccid with absent tendon jerks, within a few days it becomes hypertonic with exaggerated reflexes. Persistent flaccidity seems to carry a poor prognosis. Spontaneous recovery starts soon after the initial episode and continues for many months, but usually the greatest degree of improvement in function is seen in the first few months. Subsequent recovery is slower and less likely to effect ultimate functional capacity.

Physical treatment in the acute stage is directed towards preventing deformities occurring, particularly 'frozen shoulder', by passive movements and supporting splints. As recovery begins, so active rehabilitation is introduced. Standing, walking and arm mobilizing supplemented by passive movements of those joints which the patient cannot move himself, form the basis of early active treatment. After the first few weeks, rehabilitation can be directed more towards functional activity, and it is at this stage that the complications and associated disorders may play a dominant part in determining the rate of progress in the pattern of achievement.

As many of the patients are in the older age-groups, the commonly associated disabilities include arteriosclerosis, hypertension, diabetes mellitus, cardiac insufficiency, degenerative arthritis, visual defects, hearing defects and the general frailties of the elderly.

The characteristics of the stroke itself are diminution of power, diminution of sensation, spasticity, visual-field defects, speech impairment, impaired perception of body image, and impaired cerebration.

Sensory defects are common and interfere with function, but loss of position sense and impairment of the body image are even greater barriers to successful rehabilitation.

Ankle instability is present in about half the patients and a double-iron below-knee caliper with a drop-foot spring or drop-foot stop is often necessary. Springs accentuate the problems of spasticity and a heel-stop may give a better functional result. Occasionally, full-length calipers are necessary to control a flail knee or to help overcome persistent knee flexion, but are poorly tolerated by most elderly hemiplegics.

Recovery is invariably greater in the leg than in the arm and thus concentration on the walking re-education dominates the first phase of active rehabilitation. But some patients will not achieve independent walking and will require a wheelchair; unfortunately, the co-ordination required to propel a single-hand controlled wheelchair is considerable and few elderly hemiplegics are able to achieve this skill. Some of them can, however, manage to control a wheelchair in their own environment by combined activity of one hand and one foot; the arm provides forward propulsion, albeit towards the opposite side and the foot controlling the direction, by acting as a brake and a pivot. Many younger hemiplegics can become very skilful with single-hand control chairs, but few can achieve outdoor mobility involving any slopes or rough ground.

The spastic arm is more difficult to manage and its chance of recovery is small. The spastic adducted shoulder can be mobilized by a combination of passive and active movements, particularly while in the warm treatment pool, or after injections of local anaesthetic and hydrocortisone if pain is a predominant feature. Ice packs are often used in relieving spasm and may be followed by several hours of reduced spasticity, during which time active and passive movements can be achieved. There are many varieties of slings and wrist splints, but usually passive stabilizing splints are more helpful than lively ones.

Intensive rehabilitation can achieve improved function in the majority of patients surviving the first few months after the acute cerebrovascular episode. About two-thirds of the patients should achieve personal independence and one-third are likely to be fit for employment. The end results of rehabilitation depend upon the patient's age; the older groups, often with associated pathology having the lower rehabilitation potential. Other factors associated with poor results are involvement of the dominant hand and severe speech defects.

Distinction must be made between spastic deformity and structural contracture. The spastic deformity disappears in sleep, and can be relieved by positioning or a slow passive stretch. Spastic deformity can be controlled by braces and splints, but no brace, whether static or dynamic, will control progressive spasticity. Surgical procedures aimed at rebalancing muscle power are equally doomed to failure. Infiltration of muscle with local anaesthetics, will enable the deformity to be analysed, and temporary reduction of spasticity by infiltration with 40–45 per cent alcohol can allow active rehabilitation to proceed. Non-progressive spacticity or fixed contractures are amenable to corrective surgery. Tendon lengthening, direct injection of the motor points or selective neurectomy are the procedures of choice. Heelcord lengthening for the spastic drop-foot, associated with tenotomies of toe flexors, if necessary, is often helpful. Split anterior tibial transfer can compensate for lateral dorsiflexion. Hamstring release for knee flexion contractures is more successful than the Eggers procedure. No surgical procedures will improve weak hip abduction and no surgical procedures can restore normal gait, for hemiplegia is a disorder in which imperfect motor control is inherent. Thus reconstructive procedures should aim at reducing deformity and improving standing and walking stability.

There are few procedures which will improve the upper limb. Release of the entire flexor muscle mass of the forearm from its origin, or injection of this muscle mass with phenol or alcohol will often improve the appearance of the hand and facilitate the use of splints, since splintage of a flail hand is easier than splintage of a spastic one. Similarly, injection of the biceps and brachialis relieves the flexor spasm of the elbow and prevents the ugly reflex flexion of the elbow which so often occurs during walking.

Most recovery will occur early, and deformities which are present at 3 months will usually persist. Surgery can achieve permanent correction of such deformities but is usually reserved for the younger hemiplegics whose clinical condition is unlikely to deteriorate.

In hemiplegia, interference with muscle power, muscle control and muscle tone all contribute to the disability. Motor defect alone is seldom a real bar to functional recovery. A patient with hemiparesis from polio may have complete independence and a patient with an arm and a leg amputated on one side, although clearly handicapped, can achieve considerable functional skill. Hemiplegia, then, is not necessarily a severe disability unless loss of motor power is associated with sensory deficit, speech impairment or impairment of cerebration.

Early assessment of the long-term prognosis is very difficult but is all important if realistic decisions and plans are to be made. The rehabilitation potential is dependent upon the severity of the illness, the degree and location of cerebral damage, as well as the level of the pre-morbid training, education and skill. Disturbance of balance may occur through involvement of the vestibulocerebellar system or impairment of visual spatial perception. Disturbances of postural fixation are usually indicated by inclination to the affected side while sitting or standing, with the eyes closed, and are associated with difficulty in walking re-education. Disturbances of the body image are common and lead to a sensation of instability associated with a fear of falling and an impairment of total function. Disturbance of the body image will mitigate against simple activities such as dressing and walking, and persistent attempts to achieve these activities in the gymnasium may be doomed to failure until the patient is taught to recognize, understand, and compensate for his disturbed body image. A simple test is to ask the patient to draw himself. A characteristically distorted drawing is a clear indication that the patient is likely to have difficulty in activities requiring an awareness of the paralysed side.

Successful rehabilitation of a hemiplegic patient depends largely upon his ability to adjust, comprehend and accept treatment, and this requires his active co-operation and participation. Thus the intellectual and emotional changes caused by the cerebrovascular accident must be ascertained, and this implies a study of the pre-morbid state as well as the situation during rehabilitation.

Although experienced therapists can evaluate the patient's likelihood to achieve realistic results, much can be learnt from clinical and education psychologists, and by applying the testing techniques capable of statistical analysis mentioned earlier (*see* Chapter 1). By the employment of objective techniques, variables such as motivation, frustration, co-operation and adaptability can be evaluated and analysed.

Sensory defects in hemiplegia due to brain damage may present as loss of limb sensation or defects of co-ordination. These latter are the more significant as they may hinder learning ability, or the patient's awareness and understanding of himself, or his ability to perform integrated actions. Aphasia and memory loss occur in a wide range of severity and clearly affect the patient's ability to learn. Dysphasia presents considerable problems as it is accompanied by intellectual impairment, shown even in the non-verbal tests of intelligence. Anoscognosia (lack of awareness of disease) or denial of the ownership of the paralysed limb is confined to right-handed people with lesions in the right (non-dominant) hemisphere and makes functional training difficult.

Apraxia is the inability to perform previously-learnt skilled tasks, and can be demonstrated by the patient's inability to copy simple drawings of various designs. It should be distinguished from ataxia, which is muscular inco-ordination. Agnosia means loss of ability to recognize the impact of sensory stimuli, and results in an inability to understand the function of articles which can be clearly described. Perseverance is a response which is more appropriate to previous instructions than current ones, and can be applied to speech and thought as well as action.

The presence of any of these disturbances of co-ordination is an indication that physical therapy and rehabilitation are likely to be unavailing. At best, training will take considerably longer than in the absence of such signs. Indeed, speech therapy, re-education of balance and deliberate training to understand the sensory deficits are probably the most important parts of rehabilitation for these patients.

One further indication of cerebral damage which has a poor prognosis is the persistence of emotional liability. Rapidly changing emotions, temper outbursts, attacks of inappropriate crying or laughter are all indications of loss of brain tissue. Although the pre-morbid personality will determine the emotional reaction of a patient to a major illness, in strokes the physical and mental effects of the illness must be carefully assessed. It is the patient's ability to change which is important and much more clinical and psychological data is needed to establish clear guide lines for the clinician and therapist.

Case history No. 881 illustrates the problems of hemiplegia in a young woman.

M.M.L. No. 881 born 1946 female

Diagnosis: Right hemiplegia

At the age of 20 years, shortly after the birth of her baby, this patient developed a dense right hemiplegia and dysphasia associated with a block of the left middle cerebral artery. She collapsed and developed a severe chest infection requiring tracheostomy. During the ensuing weeks, her condition slowly improved and the tracheostomy was closed. Six months after the original illness, she still had a dense right hemiplegia and severe dysphasia. The question then arose as to whether she was likely to achieve enough independent function to return home to look after her husband and baby, and she was transferred from hospital to the Disabled Living Unit. Later she was admitted to a rehabilitation hospital.

Nine months after the illness, she was able to walk well with a below-knee caliper, including going up and down stairs and getting on and off public transport. Her right hand and arm were useless, but with her left hand she was quite independent for all personal care (washing, bathing, toilet and dressing).

She was unable to cut up her food but was otherwise independent for feeding. She could cook, shop and carry out all the necessary activities for running a house with certain aids designed for the one-handed. She would have had difficulty managing a baby with one hand, and conversation was difficult because of the severe expressive aphasia.

However, her disability was not in the physical activities. Even after intensive training she was incapable of initiating activities or remembering details. She could not maintain interest or concentration long enough to finish preparing or cooking a meal. She was nervous of going out on her own, of meeting people, of using the telephone or taking part in group activities even with people she knew well.

The only occupation she enjoyed was reading children's books, and watching children playing. She seemed to want to have her own child with her but had little initiative to attempt to do anything with the child. Further months were spent in a rehabilitation centre nearer home with regular contact with the family, but even 18 months after the illness, there was no sign of the patient achieving enough recovery of higher brain function to return to independent domestic life.

When retested by the psychologist at this time, the formal tests showed no improvement over the previous year. Her reading age was $13\frac{1}{2}$ years and her full I.Q. was at the 7th percentile (borderline range). The verbal tasks were more affected than performance tasks. Memory tests showed a very limited span and verbal learning tests showed a very low recall and retention. She still had a severe memory deficit and a persistent slight expressive phasia.

However, she was sent home from the long-stay unit. Her child (now nearly 2 years of age) was cared for by her parents-in-law who lived in the same road. The patient remained at home all day, with the housework being done by a home-help.

She was incapable of running the home because of her lack of initiative and lack of insight. She would cook a meal, but had no idea of time, so would dish the meal to the table an hour before her husband arrived home, quite unaware that it would be cold by the time he arrived. She repeatedly bought articles from door-to-door salesmen or mobile shops, running up bills which her husband could ill-afford to honour.

Her mother was dead; her father had remarried and was unable to offer practical help. Her mother-in-law was naturally more concerned about her son (the husband) and was pressing the idea of divorce. Although sorry for her daughter-in-law, she felt that her son and she had persevered long enough. Her son had 'no life' and she felt she could no longer accept the responsibility for her daughter-in-law, although she was prepared to look after the baby (her grandson) indefinitely.

The husband was caught between natural revulsion and a sense of responsibility. He felt lost and unable to cope. Although he had a feeling of responsibility, he did not see how he could continue and he had lost his affection for his wife.

The patient herself seemed to think she was a competent housewife and did not appreciate the difficulties nor show any anxiety about herself, her child or her husband.

(1) Should this patient remain at home and persist with the present family arrangement? This would entail considerable support from the local authority with daily visits to an occupational therapy centre in the hopes that she would slowly improve to a level at which she could acquire more housewifely competence.

(2) Should she be admitted to a residential home? This would be congenial as she is friendly and cheerful, but she was physically too competent for most local authority homes to accept her.

(3) Should she be admitted to a residential Sheltered Workshop? This would not be suitable as, although these units cater for the physically handicapped, this patient would not be capable of the necessary level of physical or mental skill required.

(4) Should she be admitted to a long-stay hospital or hostel for the young chronic sick? She is not intellectually defective enough to warrant admission to a mentally handicapped unit nor is she physically handicapped to a severity warranting admission to a chronic hospital.

If she was single, she could be admitted to a hostel or attend an occupational therapy centre, coping with simple routine work, and possibly graduate to sheltered employment if she improved over the years.

But what about the family? If the situation remained static, either the husband or mother-in-law would be likely to press for an issue or to succumb to depression or anxiety. If she was admitted to a residential home, they would probably press for divorce after the statutory period of three years.

Comments

When dysphasia or aphasia is present, assessment is always more difficult. It is the patient's capabilities in realistic situations which are more important than his disabilities and his abilities to overcome handicap, to understand problems and to initiate solutions which need to be exploited. When these higher capabilities are absent, the effects of rehabilitation are limited.

CEREBRAL PALSY

Among the physically disabled children in this country, the cerebral palsied, or spastics, form by far the largest group.

Cerebral palsy is the term used to describe a group of non-progressive disorders of motor function associated with brain disease or damage. Children suffering from cerebral palsy may have paresis, inco-ordination of voluntary movement or unwanted involuntary movements as their major handicap. The paresis may be spastic or flaccid and may be associated with mental impairment, epilepsy or disorders of sensation. The muscular imbalance frequently leads to skeletal deformities.

The clinical syndromes of cerebral palsy consist of one or more of the neurological syndromes of hemiplegia, diplegia, ataxia, dyskinesia or athetosis. These syndromes are seldom present as separate entities. More often, features of several co-exist in the same child, with some degree of co-ordination and unsteadiness is an almost constant finding.

There are two aspects of treatment of this condition: the general treatment needed by any chronically disabled child, and the specific treatment, demanded by cerebral palsy and its complications. The latter is aimed at training the child to overcome or circumvent its particular disability, and at preventing the development of secondary contractures. Intellectual assessment is of particular importance in the case of the cerebral palsy child, whose intellectual capability may be masked by physical inability to co-operate. Without such assessment, it is easily possible for the standard of education aimed at to be below the child's true potential. At present, it may be expected that between 33 and 50 per cent of those suffering from cerebral palsy will achieve employment in the competitive labour market, and another 10–20 per cent will achieve sheltered employment.

The type of employment and the level of training must depend not only on the intellectual capacity, but also on the type and severity of the physical disability. The bizarre manifestations of certain disabilities, such as ataxia and dyskinesia, are socially unacceptable rather than functionally restrictive, and children who suffer from them may be trained to follow activities demanding considerable manipulative skill. Both in training and employment, lack of mobility may be the inhibiting feature, and appropriate surgery, particularly for the lower limbs, may make a disabled child independent, and open up wider fields of education and employment for his adult life.

It has been suggested that as the deformities produced by cerebral palsy are due to muscle imbalance, surgical treatment should be directed towards strengthening the relatively weak antagonists of the spastic muscles. But the basic lesion of cerebral palsy lies in the damaged brain, not in the muscles themselves. Surgery is therefore more appropriately reserved for a salvage procedure if extensive and continuous physiotherapy is unsuccessful. Such physiotherapy should aim at preventing contractures by splinting, stretching, bracing and giving remedial exercises, and for the sake of continuity and frequency, is best carried out by the parents after initial instruction by a physiotherapist.

Thus, it is necessary to settle for simple results; for the attainment of stability rather than for complex alteration of functions. Comprehensive mental and physical assessment should be able to delineate the functional aims of the surgery. When the ankle cannot be dorsiflexed beyond 90 degrees while the knee is extended, gastrocnemius recession, or elongation of the Achilles tendon improve dorsiflexion and reduce the effective power of the calf muscle. Adductor tenotomy with or without obturator neurectomy, is usually successful in preventing dislocation of the hip, and iliopsoas transplantation may prevent the hip dislocating in those children with severe paralysis of the hip adductors.

Upper limb surgery is less often indicated; but wrist fusion for the severe flexion deformity, or tendon lengthening to achieve a tenolysis effect may have excellent results. In general, however, tendon surgery is unsuccessful in patients with athetosis. Where possible, a trial by splintage or infiltration of spastic muscles with local anaesthetic will help to establish the likely outcome of a particular surgical procedure.

The majority of spastic children are diagnosed early and become the subjects of considerable attention and skilful assessment and training organized by the combined efforts of parents, the Spastics Society and local authorities.

The aims of therapy are to improve hand function, to teach personal care and independence, to develop hobbies and interests, and to provide a system of training perception and social behaviour. Many cerebral-palsy children have speech defects, and speech therapists can help them to achieve the understandable diction, necessary for leading a normal life.

Probably the most important aspect of therapeutic training is the part played by the educational psychologist, as an accurate assessment of intelligence and ability for training will determine the remainder of the general management programme.

The major contribution to be made for cerebral palsy is by patient, persistent encouragement and training. Physical aids have little place, though children with severe motor disorders can sometimes achieve remarkable skills. For example, those who are totally unable to walk or use their hands, because of athetosis, may achieve considerable skill in propelling a wheelchair with their feet.

M.M.L. No. 193 born 1929 female

Diagnosis: Cerebral palsy

This woman has cerebral palsy with spastic quadriplegia. She had been cared for at home, in special schools, and eventually was admitted to a residential institution. She had never been able to use her hands but had become remarkably competent with her mouth. She occupied herself making jewellery using pincers, scissors, pencil and paintbrush each with mouth attachments.

Although physically severely handicapped, she had a remarkable verbal competence and was relatively easily intelligible. She was within the normal range of intelligence. However, her physical condition slowly deteriorated after reaching the age of 30 years.

She had obturator neurectomy and division of the motor supply of the left triceps in an attempt to relieve the pain and deformities

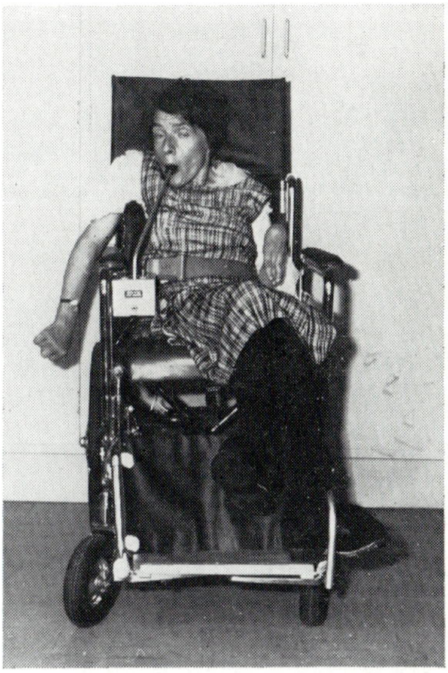

Figure 3.1. Patient No. 193 using an electrically-powered indoor chair operated by a mouth-stick. Spasms of the arms and legs are shown

associated with her spasticity. At the age of 35 years, she had a right chemopallidectomy. Over the years, she had increasing trouble with urinary infections and renal calculi; on several occasions, stones were removed and eventually she had to have a right nephrectomy.

The over-all pattern of upper-limb spasticity was one of extension. The left arm used to lock behind her body, but this was relieved by the chemopallidectomy. However, severe extension spasm remained and the shoulders were markedly retracted. She had severe spasms of both legs with contractures. The spasm had been slightly relieved by obdurator neurectomy and the chemopallidectomy, but it was still very difficult for her to sit comfortably in a chair because of the constant tendency to spasm.

Although in early life the patient had been able to stand and take a few steps with assistance, her independent function decreased as she grew older. The ability to make jewellery was a useful occupation, and she later was given an electric typewriter and began to learn to operate this with a mouth stick.

Eventually she was supplied with an electrically powered indoor chair with a simple 'joystick' control which, surprisingly she could operate very accurately with a mouth stick. This chair proved a great morale-booster for her and gave a degree of freedom which she had never previously experienced (*Figure 3.1*).

PARAPLEGIA

Rehabilitation of paraplegics has 4 aims.

(1) To prevent disuse atrophy, contractures and deformities in those muscle groups in which the innervation is still intact.

(2) To achieve the maximal degree of independence for each patient by training them in activities of daily living.

(3) To prepare each patient for an active life, with sufficient acceptance of the handicap of paraplegia to enable it to be used as a starting-base and not a stumbling-block.

(4) To introduce sufficient mental and physical conditioning so as to enable patients to be able to undertake retraining for employment, inside and outside the home.

The first major project to be initiated in the realization of these aims is the attainment of mobility, but the degree of mobility aimed at must be related to the total resources of the patient. Thus, while it may be a practical mechanical possibility for many paraplegics to walk, whether with crutches, calipers or aids, functionally it is usually such a fatiguing process that most patients give it up at an early stage. Most accept the philosophy that crutch and caliper walking is equivalent to a period of intense exercise, while a wheelchair is the more efficient mode of progression for normal activities and work.

Similarly, the ability to stand must be reviewed in context. Standing may be useful for transfers, but if it demands too much effort and time from the patient or his helpers, the transfers are better accomplished directly between bed and chair, chair and toilet.

Mobility is therefore to be aimed at not as an isolated entity, but as a means to an end, the accomplishment of useful or pleasurable activities and the realization of a patient's total potential.

The provision and acceptance of a wheelchair gives only a limited range of mobility, since the use of a wheelchair out of doors is curtailed by the fatigue of propelling on uneven surfaces, and the difficulty of manoeuvring repeatedly up and down steps and kerbs. A motor-car is therefore a *sine qua non* for a paraplegic with a life to lead.

The provision of outdoor transport is also an important factor in retraining for work and obtaining eventual employment, since suitable work is often difficult to find in the same location as a patient's home. Such retraining and employment are essential for the prevention of the economic wastage which paraplegia otherwise represents to both patient and to the community, and for the reconstruction of the self-esteem of the patient himself.

It is paradoxical that welfare and insurance provisions often make it unnecessary or unrewarding for the injured man to return to work. In these instances, early diversion into a stimulating and absorbing hobby is the only counterbalance to the stultifying and handicapping effects of social benefits for the disabled.

Conversely, those who are not entitled to such benefits need considerable help both practical and financial, in helping them to achieve independence against the odds of paralysis, spasticity and incontinence.

Pressure sores

The incidence of pressure sores in paraplegics is reported variously from 25 to 75 per cent of patients. Probably many of the sores start within the first few days of the spinal-cord injury during the period of spinal shock when nursing attention is largely directed towards the treatment of acute injuries and the preservation of life. At this time there may be local arterial collapse and vasoparalysis in addition to local pressure, moisture and superficial skin damage. Such conditions predispose to the development of the superficial bedsore, which has a relatively good prognosis, and also to the necrosis of deeper tissues, which is far more serious.

The only efficient method of preventing pressure sores is by varying the pressure distribution and protecting the danger areas. This can be done in the early phases after spinal injury by careful nursing with frequent turning, use of a turning bed or a plaster bed or Stryker frame. As the patient progresses, he must learn to vary the pressure himself as much as possible, assisted by tilting beds, alternating pressure cushions and sheepskins (*see* Chapter 4).

Limb spasticity

Immediately after a spinal injury, there is a state of complete or almost complete suppression of all reflex activity of the spinal cord below the level of the injury known as spinal shock. The more severe the injury and the higher the lesion, the longer is this period of shock. Improved nursing and early management of the paralysed bladder, reduce the duration of shock and its end is heralded by the appearance of reflexes whether physiological or pathological.

As spinal shock wears off, flexion activity supervenes and is never completely overcome by extension activity. Quite minor stimuli of certain areas of the extremities induce marked, sudden and painful flexor spasm. Over a period of months, extension spasms appear; these are slower in onset and can be induced mainly by positioning of the limb. Some paraplegics can utilize these extensor spasms to stand without support, However, most spasms are unpredictable and uncontrollable and are rarely a real advantage to the patient. About 1 in 5 paraplegics has spasms which are a definite hindrance to his rehabilitation or independence, constituting a significant hazard in the precipitation of skin damage.

In the treatment of such spasm, drugs of the chlorpromazine group are often employed. Diazepam is the drug usually chosen and is given in doses ranging from 5 to 40 mg daily. The optimal distribution of the dosage throughout the day must be determined by trial and error for each patient; but a large night dose (10–20 mg) possibly backed by a smaller dose (5 mg) at breakfast or lunchtime, is generally found most useful. Diazepam is an effective sedative, and in this dosage produces a good night's sleep, while its antispasmodic effect prevents disturbance by frequent painful spasms. Morning stiffness is decreased, and dressing, washing, hoisting and transferring are all facilitated. A larger daytime dose tends to cause unwanted sleepiness and inability to concentrate during the day (*see* Chapter 4).

Bladder involvement

The most serious complication of spinal-cord injury is the disturbance of bladder function. Less frequent is a disturbance of renal function, such as the diminution or cessation of urine production associated with spinal shock or renal hyperaemia secondary to splanchnic deficiency.

The bladder is innervated from both the sympathetic and parasympathetic nervous systems. Spinal injuries above the centre controlling micturition (that is, lesions above the 12th dorsal vertebra), give rise to an upper motor neurone type of reflex, neurogenic, autonomous bladder. In these cases, there is a reflex response to bladder distension and preservation of the bulbocavernosus reflex. During spinal shock, the bladder is atonic, the detrusor weakened and the sphincter contracted; thus there is a retention of urine. The bladder wall is unable to respond to stretch. As spinal shock wears off, the high lesion may allow an automatic bladder to develop, in which regular micturition occurs at relatively long intervals with a residue of 20 per cent or less. However, sooner or later, the contraction becomes more frequent and gains in intensity (the hyperplastic bladder). In lower lesions the autonomous bladder may develop in which evacuation may be precipitated and incomplete. Residual urine may be less than 10 per cent.

For long-term management, it is essential to achieve complete emptying if the risk of infection is to be avoided. Catheterization within 24–36 hours is rarely recommended or required, as it is these early catheterizations which are likely to cause havoc if infection is not prevented. All catheterizations of spinal-injury patients should be carried out with the strictest aseptic technique, as once an infection has been introduced into a neurogenic bladder, it is almost impossible to eradicate it. Unfortunately, intermittent catheterization is still the best method of managing these patients in the early stages and this imposes considerable responsibility and stress upon the Spinal Injury Unit concerned.

The eventual state of the tone of the bladder musculature may be atonic or hyperplastic. Either condition places the paraplegic patient at considerable permanent risk. The atonic bladder will distend until reflex evacuation or retention with overflow results, while the hyperplastic bladder responds to intrinsic and extrinsic stimuli by contracting at frequent intervals. When the tension within the bladder rises, during the intervals between evacuation, reflux into the ureters and infection of the renal pelves may occur.

Indwelling catheter

With the higher spinal-cord lesions, with complete cord lesions, and in female paraplegics, there is an increasing chance that eventually an indwelling catheter will be needed, with a serious risk of peri-urethral inflammation, abscesses and fistulae. Narrow-gauge soft catheters are less likely to cause trouble than the more rigid and the larger ones. The use of balloon catheters or Foley catheters may be necessary in females, but they successfully prevent complete drainage from the lowest part of the bladder.

The greatest danger of an indwelling catheter is that infection will be introduced into the bladder and this can only be avoided by observing the strictest sterile non-touch techniques on all occasions when the catheter is changed (usually every 7–14 days).

The collecting-bottles should contain adequate antiseptic and be adequately sterilized or frequently replaced. But probably the most important factor is the strict sterile technique of catheterization and adequate use of antiseptic during the procedure. Providing these principles are adhered to, the hazards of catheterization are less than those of imperfect bladder function and of operation for urinary diversion.

Role of surgery in managing the paraplegic bladder

Bladder training remains the mainstay of management of the neurogenic bladder whether the lesion is organic neurological disease or spinal injury. Drugs which stimulate or depress the detrusor muscle have their place in assisting training. The majority of patients will manage with reflex evacuation and manual expression, but some will fail to achieve satifactory bladder emptying and are liable to develop vesico-ureteric reflux.

A paraplegic patient can tolerate residual urine for many years in the absence of infection, but the combination of residual urine with an infection usually leads to pyelonephritis. Indications for surgery are largely governed by the persistence of infection in spite of conservative treatment.

In the longterm, these patients may develop hydronephrosis and suffer recurrent attacks of pyelonephritis, renal calculi and progressive renal damage. Unless free urine drainage is achieved, chronic renal failure is inevitable. However, it is easier to employ a urethral catheter, either intermittently or, when necessary, to leave it indwelling, than to embark on urinary diversion. It is only when obstructive signs do not improve after catheterization, or catheterization becomes difficult, or in the female with congenital paraplegia that surgery is indicated. Operation on the bladder neck, the external sphincter, the pudendal nerves and sacral plexus or a subarachnoid alcohol may help to reduce urethral resistance to evacuation of the bladder.

Urinary diversion is usually only necessary when the conventional and simpler methods have failed or when there is urethral complications leading to difficulty in catheterization. More recently, surgeons are regarding continuous incontinence in girls or women as an indication.

The ileal loop is the usual method of diversion now advocated for girls with paraplegia due to spina bifida or when there is obstruction to drainage causing reflux. The problem of the congenital paraplegic is different in that there has never been any bladder training established (*see* Myelomeningocoele). The operation must be planned to fit in with orthopaedic procedures, such as psoas transplant or femoral osteotomies. The ileal loop diversion is usually deferred until the other procedures are over and during which catheter management will be easier. When the child is old enough to manage the urinary ileostomy, and the child and parents accept the need for the operation, then this is the time to consider it. Usually this is between 6 and 7 years of age, but well may be earlier if circumstances dictate. There is little doubt that currently this appears to be the most effective method of controlling the female congenital paraplegic. The segregated colonic loop may be indicated when only the left kidney remains functional, but problems may arise where a daily reflex defaecation has been achieved and the operation risks interfering with this. Ureteric-colonic anastomosis is contra-indicated in paraplegics as bowel function is also defective.

Ureterostomy is an operation which can be carried out in advanced stages of renal failure and puts little additional stress on the patient. There is no need to open the peritoneal cavity and there is no bowel anastomosis. Disadvantages accrue from having to provide two appliances for collecting urine, and there are technical difficulties in providing an adequate spout, preventing stenosis of the orifice and tension on the ureter.

For women with multiple sclerosis who have paraplegia with incontinence, it is usual to provide continuous catheter drainage. Progressively larger catheters are usually needed to prevent leaking round the catheter. In such instances, the urethra can be cored out from the vaginal wall and brought out in the suprapubic abdominal wall (anteversion of the urethra); but for the fat woman with a short urethra, this is not suitable.

Occasionally, suprapubic cystotomy and vesicostomy may be considered when urethral lesions, such as stricture, recurrent periurethritis, periurethral abscesses, or fistulae lead to difficulties in catheterization. In young men and boys a small penis may give rise to difficulty in fixing condoms or catheters and a cystostomy may be the management of choice.

Results of rehabilitation

Many paraplegics return to work, and it was largely due to the remarkable results of the National Spinal Injuries Centre at Stoke Mandeville which drew attention to the general needs for rehabilitation of the severely disabled. Rehabilitation of the paraplegic to a full integrated life is now so common that it is only those with complicating clinical conditions or in whom routine measures have failed, or those with particular resettlement problems who come to specialized rehabilitation centres. An example of this type of problem is given in case history No. 112.

M.M.L. No. 112 born 1921 male

Diagnosis: Traumatic paraplegia

At the age of 36 years, this man was involved in an accident at his place of employment and sustained a complete paraplegia at the level of the 9th dorsal vertebra. He became a stable, well-adapted paraplegic, wearing a urinal and evacuating his bladder 4-hourly by abdominal contraction and manual pressure. His bowels were evacuated daily, manually.

He was well rehabilitated at a spinal injury unit and was supplied with both a self-propelling wheelchair and a Ministry of Health motorized tricycle. Over the next few years, many efforts were made to get him back to work. He went to an Industrial Rehabilitation Unit and plans were made for him to undergo training. On each occasion, some problems arose: he developed a small pressure sore, or he had abdominal symptoms attributable to urinary infection. Eventually he complained of giddiness and headaches associated with fainting attacks. He described attacks of loss of consciousness and although no objective evidence was obtained he was regarded as possibly having had an epileptic seizure and his motorized tricycle was withdrawn.

He the nattended a hospital occupational therapy unit two or three times a week for diversional activities. His wife treated him almost like a child, doing most things for him. For example, she lifted him in and out of his chair, although he was quite able to transfer independently. At the request of his general practitioner and the occupational therapist he was admitted to the Disabled Living Unit to reassess the possibility of him being trained for work. There was no doubt that he was physically able to be trained for work and to care for himself.

On each occasion that the possibility of training or employment was discussed, he raised some objection, or he had attacks of headaches or abdominal pain or the sore on his hip broke down.

The crux of the social situation lay in the fact that his employers, although they disclaimed any responsibility for his accident, had provided him with a rent-free house. They also carried out certain alterations to the house to make it more convenient for wheelchair usage. By implication, if he obtained remunerative employment, he would have to find his own accommodation or move into a local authority house in a different area, moving away from his own and his wife's friends and relations. Thus, there was a considerable disincentive for resettlement. However, through his hobbies he was able to earn pocket money, as a welcome addition to his sickness benefit and industrial injury insurance.

MYELOMENINGOCOELE

The high incidence of the congenital deformity of myelomeningocoele, coupled with the increased chance of survival which current surgical techniques have brought to the children who suffer from this disease, have made the long-term management of such children a multifaceted problem of major importance.

Meningocoeles are covered with normal skin and are not associated with paralyses, but these constitute only 5 per cent of the externally visible spinal lesions.

Myelomeningocoeles are treated by early closure by surgical procedures directed towards preservation of the neural plaque. Infection and desiccation are the two immediate dangers and adequate early skin cover is the surgical aim.

Myelomeningocoele occurs in about 3 of every 1,000 live births and about 2,000 new patients with this abnormality survive each year in the United Kingdom. The development of a ventriculo-atrial shunt, using a Spitz Holter or Pudenz Heyer valve, converts the accompanying hydrocephalus into a treatable condition. The next stage is to control the urinary incontinence and manage the residual paralyses.

These children present as 5 problems: (1) myelomeningocoele; (2) hydrocephalus; (3) locomotor paralyses or pareses; (4) urinary-tract problems, incontinence and infection; and (5) social and welfare management, particularly education.

Once a child has been accepted for treatment, there is a total commitment for care in all aspects. The prognosis and management in each case is dictated by the level at which the neurological lesion occurs in the spinal cord. Since this lesion is not equivalent to a complete transection at one particular segmental level, there may be some parts of the cord below the main lesion which are still functioning. The total clinical picture may thus be a confused one of upper and lower motor neurone dysfunction.

Abnormality of vertebral body structure may produce severe kyphosis in some children. Surgical correction of this by wedge osteotomy is justifiable in the presence of complete paralysis of the lower limbs and sphincters.

Hydrocephalus occurs in about four-fifths of the children with myelomeningocoele, and is usually treated by the insertion of a ventriculo-atrial shunt. Such a procedure has various hazards, infection or dislodgement of the valve and disconnection of the atrial end of the tube being among the most common. This disconnection tends to occur when growth of the child makes the tube too short for its purpose. Prophyllactic lengthening of the tube is therefore required until there is evidence that hydrocephalus has been arrested.

The urinary tract in a child with myelomeningcocoele presents the same basic problems of management as the urinary tract of a paraplegic adult, complicated by the miniature structure of the organs concerned. Within the first few years of life the neurogenic bladder will have produced back pressure in the upper urinary tract of 30 per cent of the children with this disability, and by the age of 5 years at least 60 per cent of the children will be suffering from recurrent urinary infections.

When incontinence of urine is present in boys, it is usually managed by the provision of a perineal appliance and portable urinal. In girls, between the age of 4 and 7 years, incontinence is treated by the surgical creation of urinary diversion unless the development of back pressure in the upper urinary tract necessitates earlier intervention.

The locomotor disorders are largely paralytic in origin and these may either derive from muscle imbalance or from flail joints. The great majority of foot deformities are equinovarus or equinovarus-cavus. These are best treated by manipulation during the first few weeks, the correct position being held by strapping. If correction cannot be maintained, then soft tissue release may be needed to overcome fixed deformity. When there is normal muscle power, tendon transplants can be considered. When spastic muscle is causing the imbalance, surgical procedures involving only soft tissues are usually unsuccessful, and bone surgery will probably be required as the child grows older.

Dislocation of the hip occurs in about half of these children and is secondary to muscular paralysis. The dislocation may be present at birth or soon after, but with lower spinal lesions, the subluxation or dislocation may not develop until months or years have elapsed. Dislocations due to imbalance are unlikely to respond to prolonged splintage. For the high lesions with bilateral flail legs the dislocations may be best left alone; but for the commoner lesions at the 3rd or 4th lumbar segments, iliopsoas transfers are currently widely employed. When successful, such iliopsoas transfers will slowly correct vertical or valgus femoral neck deformities in young children. Persistent valgus deformities of the hips may require osteotomy later. The leg operations are best performed before diversion of the urinary tract is undertaken because of the problem of managing incontinence while the child is in a hip spica.

When severe spinal deformity is present, spinal fusion with the use of Harrington rods may be the only way to prevent eventual gross deformity of the trunk with the inevitable abdominal compression and respiratory embarrassment which accompany it.

Due to anaesthesia and osteoporosis, fractures are frequent; but provided adequate care is exercised, the young children remain remarkably free from pressure sores during treatment in spite of considerable instrumentation and immobilization with bandages, splints or plasters. Calipers, braces and walking-aids all play their part in achieving mobility for these children, and when necessary, are introduced during the second year of life unless walking has been achieved without them.

But for the very few children who cannot achieve walking at all,

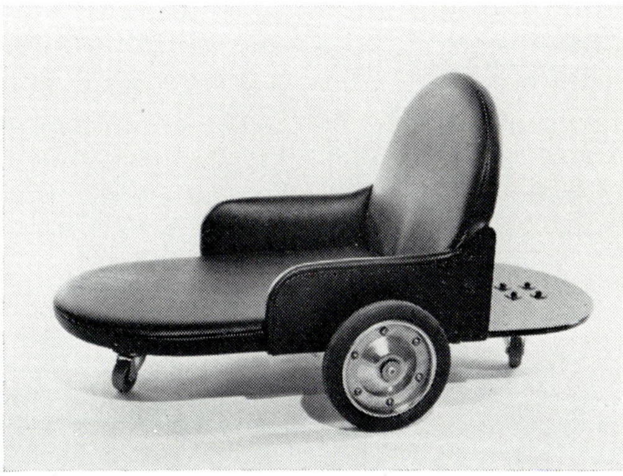

Figure 3.2. A simple wheelchair suitable for a small child with spina bifida or paralysed lower limbs

special small wheelchairs should be provided before they are a year old, so that the children can achieve their mobility by propelling the chairs with their hands, which they would normally achieve by propelling their bodies with their feet at the same age. Such chairs should be provided until the children are large enough to propel the standard size of child's wheelchair. *Figure 3.2* illustrates a simple wheelchair made from wood with 8 in (20 cm) castor wheels and $1\frac{1}{2}$ in (3·75 cm) furniture castors. The seat is padded with 1 in (2·5 cm) polyurethane foam and covered with rexine. This chair is suitable for small children, aged between 12 months and 3 years and is based on a design from Chailey Heritage Children's Hospital and School.

For chairbound children, regular physiotherapy is needed to prevent the development of the flexion deformities of the hips and knees which are all too commonly seen. Since this physiotherapy must not only be regularly but frequently given if it is to be successful, it is better that parents are instructed and made responsible for its administration in the home, rather than physiotherapists providing infrequent treatments during time-consuming out-patient attendances.

With the high survival rate of children with myelomeningocoele, long-term planning for care and education must be accepted as a part of the responsibility of the rehabilitation team, and must be initiated at an early age. At least half of the children are likely to attend normal schools, and most of the remainder will be able to attend schools for the physically handicapped. The majority will have marked physical handicaps, but with urinary appliances for the boys and ileal-conduit diversion for the girls, continence should not present an insuperable problem and the children should be socially acceptable. Many will need to use a wheelchair for at least some activities, even if only for speed of travel from classroom to classroom.

But it is not the need for the use of a wheelchair, but the presence or absence of the ability to transfer rapidly between wheelchair and seat, or wheelchair and other transport, coupled with the presence of absence of the ability to gain access to and use the toilets independently, which will determine what type of school a child can attend, and what success he will have in his attendance.

TETRAPLEGIA

During the past 25 years, the incidence of lesions of the cervical spine has steadily increased, and so has the survival rate of patients with such lesions. Most of the lesions are traumatic in origin, following road-traffic or sporting accidents. Currently, the ratio of tetraplegics to paraplegics admitted to spinal injury units is about 1 : 4 and is approaching 1 : 3.

The management of tetraplegia has several distinct phases; the first or acute phase, lasting from several weeks to several months, then the second phase of establishing a satisfactory care and maintenance regime, followed by the third phase of resettlement in a domestic environment. This may be in the patient's own home or in a special hostel or institution, and may not start for many months after the original episode; it will depend on the completeness or incompleteness of the lesion, the presence or absence of complications, the availability of suitable accommodation and assistance. More than most other severely disabled, the tetraplegic will depend on appliances and permanent available assistance.

The immediate management is directed towards the following:

(1) Prevention of additional neurological deficit.

(2) Meticulous care of the bladder, in particular, the prevention of the introduction of infection.

(3) The avoidance of pressure sores.

(4) The prevention of limb contractures, particularly elbow, wrist or finger.

(5) Planning and encouraging the restoration of relative independence as early as possible.

And to these ends, the early care is in 4 main parts:

(*a*) First aid for other injuries
(*b*) Management of the spinal injury
(*c*) Management of the bladder
(*d*) Management of the respiratory system

Early care

The nature of the first 2 parts of early care is determined by the distribution and severity of the spinal and associated injuries. For the management of the bladder, the most successful regimen seems to consist of non-interference for 24 hours, then intermittent catheterization under strictly sterile conditions every 8–10 hours, resorting to an indwelling catheter as a late measure if an automatic bladder does not supervene.

Although tetraplegics represent only about a third of the admissions to spinal injury units, they absorb a relatively high proportion of the resources available.

Tetraplegics can work and enjoy life in a properly equipped and conducted hostel, but are far more likely than other severely disabled patients to deteriorate physically and mentally if discharged to an unsuitable home or institution.

The prognosis for a patient with tetraplegia depends partly on the severity of the initial spinal lesion, that is, its level and whether it is complete or incomplete, partly on the availability of intensive specialized care immediately after the onset of the tetraplegia, and partly on the facilities which exist for long-term supervision.

Most deaths occur within the first few months, usually from chest complications. Deaths from respiratory failure occur most frequently in lesions at C5/6 or higher. Ventilation for these patients is almost entirely diaphragmatic, sometimes the vital capacity may fall below 1 litre. Respiration is often further depressed by the injudicious use of drugs, and paralysis of the respiratory muscles prevents the patients from coughing. Over-transfusion, aspiration pheumonia and frank pneumonitis may also occur.

Pressure sores

Pressure sores, if allowed to develop early, may contribute to early death; they are also a potent factor in later death. Tetraplegics with complete lesions are more likely to develop sores early, while incomplete lesions are associated with a better general prognosis.

The prevention of pressure sores in the tetraplegic is the time-consuming responsibility of the nursing staff, and all pressure sores are theoretically preventable. Frequent turning by nurses or by mechanical or electrical beds, general care of the skin, the use of alternating pressure-pads or the use of sheepskins are some of the methods available for preventing the occurrence of pressure sores and are thus essential for maintaining the existence of the tetraplegic.

Bladder regimen

Tetraplegics have the same problem of the neurogenic bladder as paraplegics, but with additional disadvantages. Tetraplegics are relatively immobile and, even if mobile are often unable to transfer on to toilet or commode. With their total loss of vesical sensation, overdistension of the bladder can easily occur, and they are usually unable to exert any manual or abdominal pressure on the fundus to stimulate reflex evacuation. Also because of upper-limb involvement, they are unable to manipulate urinals and incontinence appliances or to carry out self-catheterization. Thus, in higher spinal lesions the aim of treatment is to produce an automatic bladder, which if successful, usually leaves little residual urine.

Recurrent infection of the bladder, bladder distension, ureteric reflux, and dilation of the upper urinary tract are common complications. The reflux of infected urine producing acute pyelonephritis is commonly produced by a blocked catheter or acute retention. Reflux can also be induced during bladder irrigation if care is not taken to avoid rapid or excess filling of the bladder. Calculi, hydronephrosis, chronic renal failure or renal amyloidosis are late complications.

Many early deaths among tetraplegics could be prevented by the greater availability, and earlier institution of intensive care, particularly intensive respiratory care, with a freer use of mechanical ventilation. Corresponding improvement in the over-all mortality among tetraplegics could be brought about by improved domestic and institutional care, involving scrupulous day-to-day supervision, and frequent comprehensive urological reviews.

Bowels

Bowel function, usually well organized in the Spinal Injuries Centre, is too often neglected at home. The importance of maintaining the established regime is not appreciated sufficiently, and the bowel if neglected becomes rapidly overloaded, producing secondary effects on respiratory and urinary systems. Pressure on the diaphragm by the overloaded bowel further diminishes respiratory excursion, while pressure on the bladder predisposes to ureteric reflux.

Constipation

Constipation in the tetraplegics is secondary to the spasticity of the neurogenic bowel, and is relatively simply managed once the attendants understand the problems and accept the need for an appropriate regular regimen.

Contractures

Other problems of tetraplegics assume importance as survival extends beyond the immediate acute phase. Limb contractures will handicap independence, but their development can be prevented by gentle passive movements and by maintaining functional positions by splinting. Both procedures carry risks. Splinting of insensitive limbs can too easily cause pressure sores, and over-zealous passive movements may cause myositis ossificans and thus further restrict available movements.

Osteoporosis

Osteoporosis is common in the paralysed limbs rendering them liable to fractures during treatment or activity. The involvement of trunk muscles makes balance difficult and young tetraplegics are likely to develop scoliosis.

Vertigo

Many high-lesion tetraplegics suffer from vertigo and fainting when they are sat up. This tendency can be reduced by the use of strong abdominal binders or corsets and the condition tends to improve with time.

Those who care for tetraplegic patients should be instructed in transfer techniques designed to avoid sudden changes from the horizontal to the vertical position. If vertigo or faintness do occur, the elevation of the legs usually relieves the symptoms rapidly, particularly if the head of the patient is simultaneously lowered.

Mechanical aids

Tetraplegic patients with severe upper-limb involvement will require mechanical and electronic devices which can be operated by residual movements of a finger, mouth or head. Such devices can be designed to control their environment, for example, lights, heating, alarm system, telephone, radio, television. The appliances can be extended to operate electrically-powered wheelchairs, tape recorders, and typewriters, so that not only can these patients obtain some degree of independence in their home or hostel, but some have already achieved independent employment (*see* Chapter 8).

TABLE 3.1

Functional Goals in Tetraplegia

Level of spinal cord lesion	*Key muscle control*	*Functional goals*
C5	Neck Upper trapezius	Control electronic device with head switches or 'suck-blow' pneumatic switches. Control electrical wheelchair with mouthstick. Certain activities (*e.g.* feeding) using ball-bearing arm-supports, and externally-powered hand splints.
C6	Shoulder muscles Elbow flexors	Control electronic device with head switches or 'suck-blow' pneumatic switches. Use two-handed grip. Turn self in bed with overhead arm-slings. Transfer to and from bed with assistance. Propel wheelchair with hand rim projections. Self-feeding with externally-powered hand splints or clip-on aids. Dress upper trunk, brush teeth.
C7	Wrist extensors Supinators	Use two-handed grip. Transfer to and from bed and car without assistance. Transfer to commode chair with assistance. Transfer to commode chair with assistance. Propel wheelchair with hand-rim projections. Self-care (feeding, shaving, hair, dressing, writing and skin inspection) using wrist-driven flexor-hinge hand splints where prehension is required. Drive car with hand controls.
C8	Elbow extensors Weak hand	Transfer independently from bed to chair and toilet. Propel wheelchair without standard hand-rims; get wheelchair in and out of car. Independent in all self-care without hand splints except possibly urinal and self-catheterization. Household activities from wheelchair.
T1–T8	Hand muscles	Wheelchair independence, including transfer to and from toilet and bath. Therapeutic standing with calipers. Self-care of catheter or urinary appliance.

Functional aims

At each level of spinal cord lesion there are muscle groups which may be trained and which determine the maximum level of functional capability. Thus for each level it is possible to indicate the functional goals of the rehabilitation programme (*see* Table 3.1).

Domestic resettlement is relatively straightforward for the married man who has a wife to look after him, but is far more difficult for single men, and for women whether married or single. While the parents of the tetraplegic patient are young enough and fit enough to cope with the physical and mental strain of caring for such a severe disability, home care is possible, but eventually it becomes essential for such a patient to be cared for in an institution.

M.M.L. No. 420 born 1944 male

Diagnosis: Fracture C6/7/8

In 1963 the patient was involved in a motor-cycle accident which resulted in tetraplegia due to fractures of the 6th, 7th, and 8th cervical vertebrae. He was treated in a Spinal Injuries Unit and then eventually returned home in 1964, some 11 months after the accident.

He attended a rehabilitation unit as an out-patient and returned to the Spinal Injuries Unit at intervals for urinary check-up.

He was referred to the Disabled Living Unit in 1966, because he was still dependent on his family for many aspects of personal care, and although apparently well-motivated, was becoming depressed and frustrated by the poor prospect of his regaining work. He was admitted in March 1966 and was found to have complete loss of power and sensation below C7, strong upper arms and powerful wrist dorsiflexion, but his hands were flail. He was able to self-propel his wheelchair, and having been an enthusiastic judo exponent before the accident, had continued the exercises and activities which he had been taught at the Spinal Injuries Unit.

Although apparently well organized, he was still very dependent upon his family and was unable to get in and out of bed himself. He had trouble with his calipers and his urinal. His writing was very slow and poor and both he and his family were sure that he would not be able to obtain realistic work. Apart from his exercises, some archery and writing practice, he had no other interest or hobby.

He was admitted initially for one week, and although suspicious of new ideas, soon found that he was able to achieve added independence, particularly in transferring, and was very keen to try flexor-hinger splints. The therapists' discharge report for this initial admission was as follows:

Reason for admission

Assessment for increased independence.

Wheelchair

Has a self-propelling adult Everest and Jennings wheelchair which seems satisfactory. A hard-based sheepskin cushion was ordered for him to enable him to transfer sideways with a sliding board.

Appliances

Assessed for flexor hinge splints and is to come back to have these made. Two very strong wrists.

Walking

Has calipers, which he wears over his trousers as the knee locking-device makes them too big to go underneath. They are also too long and should be altered before he is readmitted.

Transfers

Bed; chair. Has a very high hospital bed with swinging monkey-pole at home, supplied by the Spinal Injury Unit. Was found to be able to transfer sideways from a hard-based cushion and with a sliding board, if the bed was at the same height as chair. Practised this while here; medical social worker to write to local authority about getting the bed changed. (*See also* Nursing toilet.)

Personal care

Washing.—Can only wash face, hands and arms.

Bath.—To go into this on his return.

Dressings.—Can manage clothes over his head. When he has got his splints, to sort out buttons, trousers and urinal.

Eating

Again, when he has got splints he will probably be able to cut food up. Otherwise, already independent.

Household

Does not apply, although appeared interested in kitchen activities.

Physiotherapy

Passive movements for arms particularly. Walking in calipers, cannot manage very far as calipers so heavy. Difficulty to stand because of height (6 ft 4 in, 193 cm), but can help considerably with strong triceps.

Job assessment

Was a manufacturing jeweller. Job was largely done by hand and he says he would require at least 4 dexterous fingers on each hand to go back to it. Firm have not kept in touch with him after first 3 months, but he could possibly return to them in some capacity if able to use hands more efficiently. He has evidently thought a good deal about a future job and accepted the fact that he might have to be employed in some other sort of work, and has considered telephone operator or such-like.

Nursing toilet

Has an incontinence urinal (condom-type) which was adequate. He could not put it on himself but had an adapted tap and could with difficulty empty it himself. He drank fairly well, but in spite of this and being on antibiotics, the urine was often thick and offensive. He had recently had a check-up at the Spinal Injury Unit. He had very definite ideas about his bowels, and liked to have 5 Senakot every third night and 2 Dulcolax suppositories the following morning, with disastrous consequences. The number of Senakots was reduced to 3, and 2 glycerine suppositories given with quite adequate results.

He was very pleased when the height of the bed was adjusted and he found he could transfer on a sliding board with very little help. At home, he is got out of bed at about 8.00 a.m. and has to sit in his chair until about 8.00 p.m. (when the male nurse returns). He had a ripple mattress, but tried sleeping on a sheepskin and liked it. His skin was in good condition but he was over-apprehensive about getting sores.

His calipers were not satisfactory as they had a cumbersome knee-locking device which made them too big to go under his trousers. Furthermore, they interfered with his urinal, intermittently restricting the flow of urine into the bag.

Summary of assessment

He has definite views on his care, seems intelligent and willing to try anything that would give him increased independence. He is approximately 6 ft 4 in (93 cm) tall, and although his father is of the same stature, would like to be independent of his parents' care. At first he was very dubious about making any change in his routine but as he found that there were things he could do for himself, he became less suspicious and more co-operative. He was readmitted 6 weeks after first admission for manufacture of flexor-hinge splints and remained in the unit for 4 weeks.

Therapist's discharge report after first admission

Appliances

Flexor-hinge splints were made for both hands. He could use them for eating, picking up and holding objects and manipulating pencils, typing sticks, tools, and so on.

Walking

Walked daily in parallel bars. Improved considerably both in distance and in strength of arms, and therefore, able to lift himself better.

Transfers

Chair to bed.—He was able to transfer sideways with a sliding board on seats and into a car, and so on, as long as the height was correct; but this was felt to be better kept for necessary occasions and to keep his monkey-pole on the bed as sliding might be liable to dislodge his urinal or rub him.

Washing and dressing.—He was able to manage his top half, but it took tremendous amount of energy and left him literally panting, also very slow. It was possible, but if he was going to work, his energy would be better saved for this and activities during the day. His height and the weight of his legs were great disadvantages and made it almost impossible for him to get anything over his feet, *e.g.*, trousers, socks, shoes. He might eventually do so with a lot of effort and practice (Moccasin-type shoes). His trousers had long zips put into the inside seams, so that he could undo them and put his calipers on under his trousers. If there was ever real need for him to be completely independent in dressing himself, the outside seams of the trousers could have zips inserted from top to bottom, with the band fastening at both sides, so that the trousers can open out completely and be laid on the chair before he sits down on them. It was suggested that he had heavier weight material for his trousers, at least in the winter, as he says his corduroy ones only last 3 months and changing zips every 3 months seems a lot of work.

Rating

Could eat without any splints, but these gave him a firmer grip on the knife and spoon, and he could cut food up. This needs further practice.

Drinking

Was better without splints—at the moment anyway.

Assessment of splints and activities

Tried various activities connected with a sedentary job.

Writing.—Used right splint; needs a lot of practice as yet but a good start and leaves other hand free.

Typing.—Had never used a typewriter.

Use of telephone directory.—Good and reasonably quick wearing right-hand splint.

Use of telephone.—Wearing both splints, was able to pick up and hold receiver and dial numbers at normal speed with a dialling stick held in other hand. For this, he sat very upright in his chair, avoiding the need to lean one or other arm on the table as he usually does when leaning over a working surface.

Filing of cards.—Using right splint; slow, fairly accurate.

Use of guillotine staplers.—Better without splints for anything requiring push or pull, but not much grip. Slow but accurate in centring page to be stapled.

Other activities

Use of screwdriver.—Plugs, screwing into, again slow, but quite possible and seemed to gain some satisfaction in the fact that he could do it if necessary.

Picking up.—Picking up matches, pens, sticks, papers, utensils; very good. Has not tried heavy articles.

Archery.—Practised target archery which he had originally learned at the spinal Injury Unit. He could not use his splint for this.

Gardening.—The patient became quite interested in gardening though he did not have much time to do it. He tried various long-handled hoes and cultivators using both his splints, not very successfully. He also tried some light potting which he managed fairly well.

Comprehension test.—Concentrated hard and good answers.

Summary

Can put own splints on, given time. Had not worn them for more than 2 hours at a time on discharge. Needs gradual increasing hardening of hands, and a lot of practice in use. He will find out if and when he needs both and what activities he does best with which splint.

Seemed likely to continue to work hard at all subjects of his rehabilitation and is in a good area for jobs. His general activities and thought-processes are slow, but reasonably intelligent and one feels that his previous job has necessitated his working very accurately.

He was readmitted 3 months later for a further check-up and now was using the splints well and had developed a keen interest in gardening. Nine months later (April 1967) he was readmitted for alteration to the flexor-hinge splints. He was now so active that he was wearing the splints continuously, but was finding some difficulty in propelling his wheelchair with the splints on. The parallelogram linkage was, therefore, transferred to the dorsum to clear the palm, and the splints no longer impeded his wheelchair propelling. By now, he had contacted his old employers and was awaiting interview regarding re-employment in a secretarial capacity.

In September 1967, he was readmitted so that new splints could be made, as the original ones had worn out! He was now working a 34-hour week and his only major problem related to outdoor transport. His size presented considerable technical difficulties as he could not get in and out of standard invalid tricycles and he was having to use an open electric tricycle which was unsuitable for travelling to work in inclement weather, and he was having to use a taxi service organized by the local authority. By 1968, he was driving his own adapted car.

Comments

This case history illustrates many interesting features. At first, with every possible facility and forward planning from the Spinal Injuries Unit, he had not achieved a level of independence even in transferring in and out of bed, which was within his capability. He had not been able to achieve a sufficiently high level of functional competence to make him contemplate returning to work, and indeed, he had had no realistic assessment or advice concerning work.

However, as a man of considerable drive and motivation, he was prepared to try different methods and techniques when he was convinced that they might be of advantage to him. He is an excellent example of a good flexor-hinge splint user and has achieved considerable competence in writing and manipulating small tools and appliances.

A further interesting feature in this patient's rehabilitation is the value of a creative hobby. Gardening techniques were introduced to him as a training exercise for using flexor-hinge splints. He was given the task of taking and striking cuttings and puting rooted cuttings. These activities involved manipulating tools and gripping objects of various sizes, weights and textures. From these training exercises, he developed a real interest in gardening and eventually obtained his own greenhouse and has become quite a competent greenhouse gardener. This interest in a creative hobby helped considerably in developing his manipulative skill and his endurance, leading to his return to work—a successful social adjustment (*see Figure 3.3*).

Here again, this case history is of interest because although contact had been lost with his employers and not maintained during his hospitalization or rehabilitation, they were ready to help and have

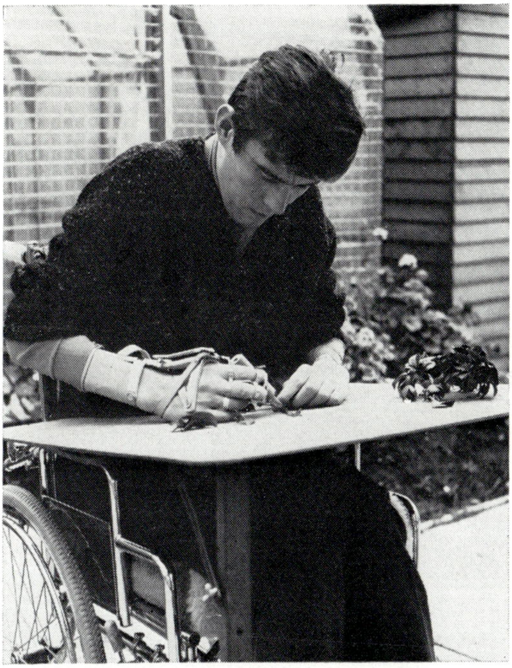

Figure 3.3. Patient No. 420 working in a greenhouse using a table on the wheelchair and taking cuttings using his flexor-hinge splint

him back in a different capacity when he contacted them and demonstrated his competence. Earlier and continuing contact with his employers might have speeded this return to work and reduced the patient's worries about possible employment. Finally, this case again illustrates the need for continued reassessment of severely disabled people, and the step-by-step reorganization of their activities.

PROGRESSIVE NEUROLOGICAL AND MUSCULAR DISORDERS

Chronic neurological disorders present one of the major groups of management problems with which hospitals, rehabilitation units, local authorities and general practitioners are faced. Most acute disorders of the nervous system are relatively mild; for example, neuropathy of various causes, migraine, epilepsy. The severe disorders may have an acute onset—a stroke or head injury—but many have a slow and insidious onset, for example motor neurone disease, multiple sclerosis. Others are familial or hereditary in nature: congenital diplegia, Friedrich's ataxia or Wilson's disease. These disorders give rise to a continuous disability—cerebral diplegia, for example—or may have a fluctuating downhill course, such as multiple sclerosis, or may exhibit a remorseless deterioration, such as motor neurone disease.

The general management of patients with these disorders must be related to the nature of the causative disorder and its known prognosis, as well as to the functional disability which it entails. The patient's personality, and the family circumstances are of paramount importance when planning for the future, because the patient's attitude, and the family's attitude and social background will determine the extent and nature of the rehabilitation which should be attempted. Thus the rehabilitation may need to be directed towards retaining or regaining maximum activity for the patient, or towards the provision of his general comfort, or towards supporting the family.

Caring for such severely handicapped patients imposes a great physical and emotional strain on the immediate family and relatives, when long-term hospitalization is not possible. Children can be catered for in day nurseries or play-centres for a few hours a day, later attending a residential or day-school for the physically handicapped. In some areas, local authorities have diversional workshops where disabled patients can meet, and perhaps can earn some pocket-money at diversional craft occupational therapy. Such attendance, even if only possible once or twice a week, can provide much-needed relief for the relatives and other supporters who often do not realize under what stresses they live.

The management of the family is often as important as the management of the patient. One chronically disabled member can destroy the normal family relationships and for this reason the relatives must be helped to understand the disability, its natural history and its vicissitudes. They must be helped to accept the inevitable outcome philosophically; a realistic appraisal is not a callous one. Once the family can approach the disability in a realistic fashion, plans can be made for supportive services, and energy is not dissipated on attempts to rehabilitate beyond the realms of possibility.

Broadly, the effects of neurological disease can be described as:

(1) affecting voluntary movement, either by weakness, or by altering muscle tone, or by associated involuntary movements (this will

determine functional ability to achieve independence and to utilize aids and appliances); (2) affecting sensation, by reducing sensory capability, or by distorting sensation, or by producing pain; (3) affecting the intellect or behaviour of the patient, either by loss of intellect (dementia) or by distorting normal behaviour (aggression) or by the loss of insight (euphoria) or dysphoria (as is so common in patients with multiple sclerosis), or by general deterioration in intellectual status as often occurs after cerebrovascular accidents.

Each of these disabilities presents its problems but when two or more co-exist, the functional disability and the problems of management are increased out of all proportion. A chronic physical disorder involving any system of the body tends to produce a significant reactionary psychological disorder, often depressive in character, but in the presence of a chronic neurological disorder, an associated personality defect will often constitute an insoluble social problem.

The slowly advancing disorders, such as peroneal muscular atrophy, cause less social and financial disturbances than disorders of sudden onset such as poliomyelitis or cerebrovascular accidents, because their slow development allows time for the patient and family to adjust their attitude and lives to the disability. The episodic disorders allow for periods of relative normality, and the intermittent interference with normal life can, to some extent, be planned for. However, it is the diseases with remorseless deterioration, such as Parkinsonism and multiple sclerosis and motor neurone disease which present the greatest problems of adjustment both to patient and family. Motor neurone disease and Parkinson's disease are distressing for the family to observe, and little can be done to help a patient with the former condition other than to provide for his maximum comfort, and to ease the family's nursing problem.

Recent work on the treatment of Parkinson's disease, however, both surgical and medical, has given hope for at least a temporary arrest in the progress of the condition. Untreated, its management involves largely supportive care for patient and family.

In multiple sclerosis, the distress caused to the family by the patient's physical deterioration is paralleled or even exceeded by the distress occasioned by the personality change with which the disease is commonly associated.

MULTIPLE SCLEROSIS

Multiple sclerosis is characterized by the dissemination of its episodes of neurological dysfunction both in time and space. It is a disease of remissions and exacerbations which are consistently inconsistent.

However, there are 3 main patterns of the disease which can be recognized, and which help to assess the prognosis:

(1) The spinal form, presenting as a spastic paraplegic or variable severity, is usually slowly progressive, without remission and without spatial dissemination (the episodes involving different areas of the nervous system or recurring in the same area).

(2) The cerebral form is particularly characterized by visual disturbances, ataxia and widespread spasticity and weakness. An initial attack may be followed by a series of attacks, or by partial or complete remissions of long duration. Some patients are left with an increasing disability after each attack, whereas others may have a complete remission.

(3) In the most frequently occurring cerebrospinal form, the general pattern is that the initial attacks are followed by remission, and then after several years and several exacerbations the disease enters a phase of steady deterioration.

There is a tendency for all patients to become steadily worse after the first 5 years of the disease, either in a relatively benign fashion or with an inexorable progression of symptoms. Therefore it is possible to predict the likely future of patients who have been closely followed-up over the first 5 years, and when this is possible, the general management can be planned accordingly.

Dysfunction of the bladder occurs in about three-quarters of all patients with multiple sclerosis and is a presenting feature in a few. But many patients deny difficulties in spite of obvious indications of incontinence. Complete retention is rare, and usually only occurs as a transient episode in the young patient with the early spinal form of the disease. The commonest problems are incomplete emptying of the bladder with consequent infection, urgency of micturition, frequency and incontinence. The symptoms are often worse in the upright position, and the patient's other physical disorders make it difficult for him to cope with urination quickly before incontinence occurs. The symptoms are often variable and multiple. Treatment is largely directed towards the management of the incontinence and the frequent renal infections which occur. Spasms of leg muscles and abdominal muscles may precipitate micturition and reduction in these may help reduce the tendency to become incontinent. If, however, incontinence exists, it may be controlled in male patients by wearing portable urinals. These are usually reasonably satisfactory if care is taken in obtaining and applying suitable types. It is preferable, whenever possible, that patients should be seen, measured and fitted by experienced technicians, who specialize in such work.

As mentioned earlier, no suitable appliance exists for the control of incontinence in females. An indwelling catheter with appropriate antibiotic cover is usually the only way to manage the incontinent female patient. Surgical reconstruction has some advantages and there is currently considerable research and development in progress which is directed towards controlling the sphincters by electrical stimulation. Such techniques are not yet generally available.

Intellectual deterioration occurs in about two-thirds of patients with multiple sclerosis. The predominant symptoms are loss of memory for events over the previous few years, and an impairment in conceptual thinking usually expressed as a euphoria or loss of insight, particularly in relation to the causative disability; but the changes may range from mild loss of memory to profound dementia.

As the physical disability progresses, so the intellectual impairment proceeds. Those patients with the spinal form of the disease are less likely to have an alteration in mental status than those with obvious cerebral involvement.

The implications of the intellectual impairment are immense. The characteristic cheerful complacency of the patient with multiple sclerosis is an unreasonable cheerfulness and is often misinterpreted as a high morale. On deeper investigation, the patients may be found to be depressed. The euphoria and loss of insight not only make the patients difficult to understand and to manage, but also unable or unwilling to learn new things. Thus they cannot learn to use trick movements, to use gadgets, or to co-operate in the usual techniques of overcoming physical disability. They frequently persist in an unwarranted belief that a remission or a cure will occur in the near future. Realistic rehabilitation is most difficult, and the relatives and social workers have to shoulder a complex burden.

M.M.L. No. 1120 born 1913 female

Diagnosis: Multiple sclerosis

History

When aged 42 years, this woman awoke one morning with loss of power and sensation in the right arm. There was considerable recovery over the following 6 weeks. However, both legs then began to get weaker, her balance deteriorated and she developed spasticity in both legs. By the age of 48 years, she could no longer walk more than a few steps and could only manage these by holding onto furniture. She had become virtually wheelchair-bound and was admitted to our Disabled Living Unit for advice on the organization of her personal care and housework from a wheelchair.

Social state

She is married with two children. Her husband is an agricultural worker, leaving home early in the morning, returning mid-morning for a meal, and then leaving her again until evening. Her son is married and lives 4 miles away. The daughter is 18 years of age and lives at home, but is out at work all day.

Their house is a semi-detached council house with 3 bedrooms upstairs, a living-room, kitchen and small bathroom downstairs. The only toilet is outside. At the time of her admission, her house was scheduled for 'modernization' in 2 years time. The local authority welfare department had meanwhile installed a commode in the bathroom, and had also made a ramp from the back door to the outside concrete path. This she was frightened to use alone.

On examination, there was weakness, spasticity and incoordination of all limbs. The spasm was particularly severe in the lower limbs and it was impossible to obtain extension of the hip or extension of the knees. She could stand up, if helped up. By holding on to furniture or a walking frame, she could shuffle a few steps backwards but not forwards.

Personal care

She was able to wash her face, neck and arms, and at home she did this at the kitchen sink, there being no wash-basin in the bathroom. She did not use the bath as she had considerable difficulty in getting in and out, and in any case, there was no running hot water. She could dress her top half but was unable to put on corset, stockings or shoes. She had considerable difficulty with pants.

Toilet

At home she used the commode in the bathroom. Apparently, she wheeled herself into the bathroom and then got out of her chair, shuffling backwards to the toilet with the assistance of a walking-aid. She managed to readjust her clothing while leaning against the large hot-water boiler which is installed in the bathroom, finally shuffling back on to the wheelchair.

Domestic organization

The patient apparently cooked her husband's mid-morning meal, usually fried eggs and bacon. She had a home help 5 days a week; 2 days from 9.30 a.m. to 1 p.m. and 3 days from 11 a.m. to 1 p.m. The home-help coped with the housework and prepared the evening meal ready to be warmed-up when the family came home. The patient's husband, daughter and home-help coped with all necessary household organization.

Performance in Unit

The patient was quite cheerful and completely adamant that she was independent for toilet and personal care. She declared that she always prepared and cooked her husband's meals. However, while in the Disabled Living Unit, she was manifestly not independent. It took her 20 minutes to peel a potato using the same equipment which she had at home. She did not bring her own wheelchair with her (a standard Ministry of Health Model 8G) and so was provided with an identical model: however, she maintained that, because it was not her own, it was different enough to prevent her getting up from it. When her own chair arrived, less than a week later, she declared that she had got so stiff from lack of practice that she could not get in and out of her own chair any more. Throughout her stay in the Unit, she made no effort at all to go to the toilet independently, to use the assessment kitchen, or to initiate any activity of daily living. In spite of the fact that the staff were all engaged in attempting to assess her capabilities, she maintained that it was because they did everything for her that she was getting worse.

Comment

Although a pleasant, quiet and apparently co-operative and well-orientated woman, it was only when she was continually under observation, that it became clear that her statements regarding her independence were quite unrealistic, although apparently made in all good faith. It was the lack of insight into her own disability which was the greatest barrier to helping her.

This case history illustrates how valuable visits to a patient's home can be as a means of acquainting the assessing therapist with the conditions which prevail there. It also emphasizes the need for close collaboration between the hospital staff and the domiciliary personnel who are in frequent touch with home conditions. Lastly, it illustrates the need for continuous observation in a Disabled Living Unit to confirm or disprove the claims of independence made by patients with possible intellectual impairment.

MOTOR NEURONE DISEASE

Degeneration of motor cells and the corticospinal tracts characteristically affects men between 40 and 50 years of age. The disease runs a steadily progressive course lasting from 1 to 10 years, depending upon the clinical variant. There is no specific treatment, but much can be done to provide help both for the patient and for the family throughout the duration of the illness.

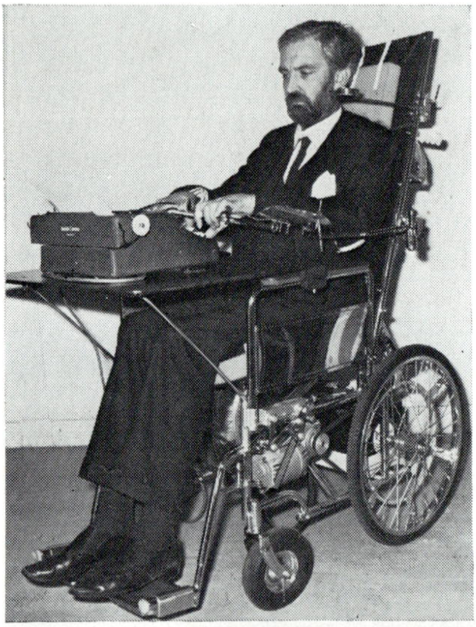

Figure 3.4. Patient No. 662 seated in an electrically-powered indoor chair using an electric typewriter by means of ball-bearing arm supports with T-bar extension and typing stick

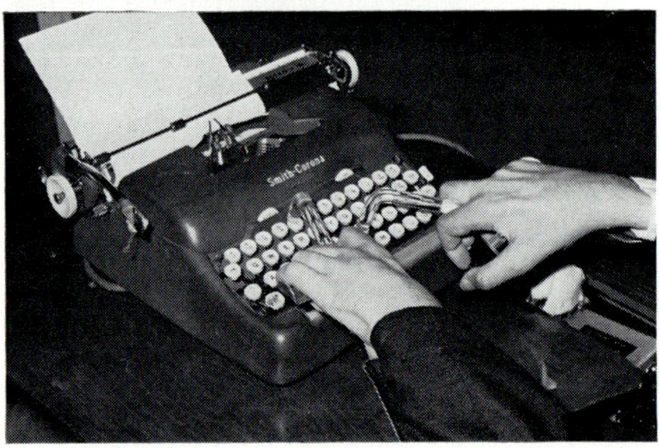

The case history No. 662 illustrates how complex aids and appliances can keep a very disabled man at work. In this instance the disease was motor neurone disease, but the techniques used here may be utilized in many chronic progressive neurological and muscular disorders.

M.M.L. No. 662 born 1927 male

Diagnosis: Motor neurone disease

At the age of 38 years, this man began to develop signs of motor neurone disease, having an increasing weakness of all muscle groups.

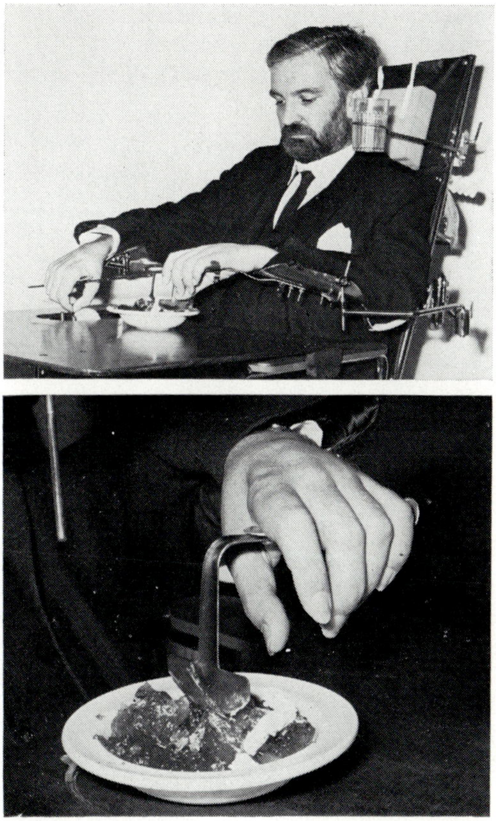

Figure 3.5. Eating with ball-bearing arm supports using spork and pusher

Within 2 years of the onset of symptoms and signs, he was unable to sit unsupported; but when stood, could take a few steps.

He was an intelligent man with full insight into his clinical condition. Although completely dependent for dressing, washing, toilet and transfers, he was still able to undertake certain activities related to his work, particularly counselling the disabled; he communicated with them by tape-recorder and letter.

He had been lent a standard Powerdrive electrically-powered indoor chair by his own hospital, and on referral to the Disabled Living Unit he was issued with a reclining Powerdrive chair which gave more support to his back and shoulders.

Mobile arm-supports were fitted to the chair with standard proximal and distal arms, standard arm-troughs and offset swivels. He could type using an electric typewriter and a typing stick (*Figure 3.4*).

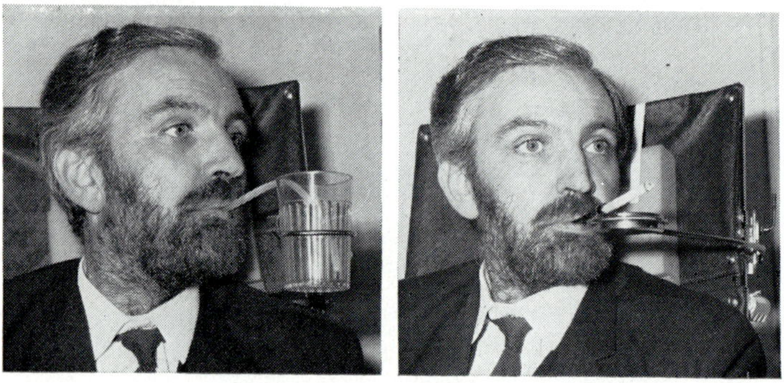

Figure 3.6. Drinking and smoking by bracket attached to wheelchair headrest

An extra arm trough and T-bar was supplied for the right side support, with a supinator and spork to assist feeding. Eating was accomplished by using the T-bar and spork in the right hand and the 'pusher' in the left (*Figure 3.5*). A glass-holder, ash-tray and cigarette-lighter could be attached to the headrest so that he could be independent for drinking or smoking (*Figure 3.6*).

The control box of the wheelchair was slightly adapted to make it easier for him to operate the controls.

This somewhat complex equipment enabled this most determined man to keep active intellectually and to continue making a professional contribution until a few weeks before his death, a year after the equipment was supplied.

MUSCULAR DYSTROPHY

The life span of children with muscular dystrophy appears to be increasing, partly because intercurrent infections can be treated with antibiotics and partly because with medical, social and welfare services, they are, in general, better cared-for at home and in institutions.

The commonest form of dystrophy is pseudo-hypertrophic muscular dystrophy, which usually manifests itself in early childhood (about 3 years of age), by a wide-based abnormal gait, an inability to run as fast as other children, a tendency to fall over, and tiredness. The children usually remain walking until they are 8 or 9 years of age, and then, unless they are fitted with calipers, and spinal braces, they rapidly become wheelchair-bound. Most of them are usually completely wheelchair-bound by 11 years of age.

Comprehensive training and the employment of bracing may enable the children to continue walking and keep out of a wheelchair for a year or two longer than they otherwise could; but such training is complex and restricting for many other activities, and there is no evidence that it makes any difference to the long-term outcome of the disease.

One of the major problems is the development of a collapsing scoliosis or lordosis. This tends to become severe, causing discomfort and ultimately causing impairment of pulmonary and cardiac functions. Once the collapse begins, it is inexorable. Full Milwaukee braces may control the scoliosis for a while, but such braces are in themselves uncomfortable and poorly tolerated. With progressive muscular weakness, collapse eventually occurs in spite of comprehensive bracing.

A less efficient but more comfortable spinal support can be achieved by means of appropriate pads, placed against the back, side and seat of the wheelchair (*see* Chapter 6).

Flexion contractures almost invariably develop at the hips, knees and ankles soon after the child becomes wheelchair-bound. They can be delayed or minimized by a programme of active stretching and periods of prone lying. But stretching soon becomes painful and prone lying involves additional manoeuvres to take the child out of his chair and return him to it.

Many parents are loathe to cause the child pain by stretching the tight contractures, and frequent lifting in and out of the chair for this purpose is unacceptable to both parents and patient. Night splints are another measure which in theory prevent and correct these deformities. But the children with muscular dystrophy are often uneasy sleepers, require frequent turning or attention for micturition and the splints are an added discomfort and complication, which, if supplied, are usually soon discarded. If the flexion contractures become severe, hamstring or Achilles tendon tenotomies may make nursing, sleeping and sitting in a wheelchair more comfortable.

Mobile arm-supports (*see* Chapter 7) are often of considerable value to children with muscular dystrophy, as the shoulder girdle and upper arm muscles may become severely affected early in the course of the disease, while the hands remain functional for many years. Mobile arm-supports require the trunk to be stabilized for maximum function to be achieved, and thus form an appropriate combination with the side pads for supporting the collapsing spine. But the mobile arm-supports may be rejected as the child deteriorates and tends to transfer more weight on to them, thus detracting from their efficiency. Furthermore, the child needs help to set and adjust the supports, and desks and tables all have to be at the same critical height for the optimal function of the arm supports. This may be possible to arrange in the child's own home, but in an institution or school for the physically handicapped, the difficulties of using these appliances are often too great for them to be given full opportunity.

As the children soon lose power to propel the wheelchair, an electrically-powered indoor chair is a most effective means of retaining independent mobility. Because shoulder-girdle muscles are involved, a powered chair with a two-handed steering column is often the most appropriate type. This steering mechanism is suitable for ball-bearing arm supports, whereas the other types available are not. For those unable to control these chairs, a simple joystick control can be fitted to the Powerdrive chair or microswitch controls adapted for the A.C. Epic with power steering (*see* Chapter 6).

Thus powered indoor chairs fitted with side pads and mobile arm-supports have become standard equipment for children with muscular dystrophy when they become wheelchair bound.

It is relevant at this juncture to refer to education and home life. A severely disabled child can be a great strain on a family and the strain of attempting to continue a realistic education and suitable hobbies for him can stretch a family to breaking-point. Furthermore, the average house has insufficient range for an electrically-powered indoor chair. Clearly, if the child can have a full, integrated life at home, without affecting the parents' own health or that of their other children, then this may be preferable; but special residential schools for the handicapped can give these severely disabled children an interesting and active life until very late on in the disease.

Although these comments may seem to be negative, this only reflects the inexorable progress of so many of the conditions. Comfortable wheelchairs with side pads, electrically-propelled wheelchairs, mobile arm-supports and the other aids and appliances can nevertheless help both patients and family over many years. Many of the younger patients have some 6 or more years of wheelchair life, and those patients in the older age-groups often survive to 50 years of age. Measures to provide comfort, mobility and assistance of hand function are more than worthwhile. The parents and relatives who have to watch the steady deterioration are also helped by repeated assessments and reappraisals of activities and aids.

In patients with limb-girdle type muscular dystrophy or facio-scapulahumeral dystrophy, the disease takes a more benign course and although the patient may have become wheelchair-bound in adolescence or even earlier, he may well live for many years. These patients present as problems of mobility, in the first instance, and then as problems of handling. Many tend to grow fat, although others become extremely thin. Lifting may be a particular problem in handling certain patients, and for them hoisting is usually the solution. For those who have the will to remain independent, much can be done with aids and appliances, and case history No. 106 is an excellent example of what a determined man can accomplish in the face of severe and increasing disability.

M.M.L. No. 106 born 1937 male

Diagnosis: Muscular dystrophy

At the age of 2 years, this patient was noted to be falling frequently and was soon diagnosed as suffering from muscular dystrophy. He managed to attend a normal infants school, and was soon transferred to a private school. By the age of 12 years, he was confined to a wheelchair. He was then admitted to a school for handicapped children, and on leaving it at the age of 16 years, he had a 6-month course in Accounts and Costing at a Training Centre. On leaving the Centre, he was unable to obtain employment because of his disability and as his mother's health was failing, he was admitted to a residential home at the age of 17 years. After he had been resident at the home for 10 years, he was admitted to the Disabled Living Unit for reassessment of his ability to achieve independence.

This admission (in 1964) was largely accomplished at his own instigation. When first admitted he was struggling to propel himself in a standard wheelchair and the first step was to provide him with an electrically-propelled indoor chair and standard mobile arm-supports and T-bar. Once he achieved independence of mobility and the ability to use his hands without fatigue, there was no holding him. With an electric hoist and some help he clearly demonstrated that he had both the will and the capability to achieve domestic independence.

The welfare officer of his local authority took a considerable personal interest and the council eventually housed him in an adapted bungalow. The adaptations were worked out in detail in the flat of the Disabled Living Unit and in 1965 he set up independently in this bungalow.

He had an electric elevating bed with an electric hoist over it tracking across a room to a commode. A home-help came in each morning to help him get up and dress and the district nurse visited

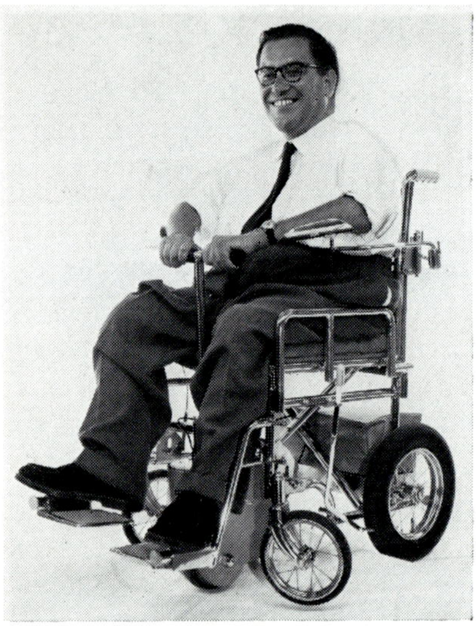

Figure 3.7. Patient No. 106 with muscular dystrophy using an electrically-powered indoor chair with mobile arm-supports and T-bar. (Reproduced by kind permission of the Editor, 'Orthopaedics': Oxford)

regularly for bathing and general check up. A local men's club undertook, on a rota basis, to come in every evening and help him to bed.

He had various adaptations of his own design made in the house, which were installed by friends or the local authority. These included adaptations to the lavatory, wash-basins, bed-tables, telephone extensions and loud-speakers, and adaptations to his typewriter. He was able to type, telephone, wash, shave and undertake minor domestic chores. But the major triumph was that within a year, he was so busy with real work that he was earning a surprising amount of money and filled every day with activity. He acted as a telephone-switchboard operator for two general practitioners; he was also the booking agent for two driving schools; he acted as a marketing agent for various sales organizations; he was actively involved in the local Boy Scouts troop; he was an active and enthusiastic radio 'ham' and in his spare time he typed manuscripts for an author.

He was readmitted to the Disabled Living Unit nearly a dozen times over 3 years for short periods for alterations or adaptations to his equipment, or to solve a new problem which had arisen. But as he achieved more independence, and accrued more activities, and work into his daily routine, he became happier and more contented than he had ever been previously in his life.

Inevitably he must deteriorate and his independence is limited; but while it lasts he is making a definite contribution to his local community, he has achieved a personal ambition, and he is an inspiration to many who come in contact with him.

M.M.L. No. 46 born 1957 male

Diagnosis: Muscular dystrophy

At the age of 3 years it was noticed that this boy was walking badly and by the age of 4 years a diagnosis of pseudohypertrophic muscular dystrophy was made. By the time he was 6 years of age, he could not get up off the floor, and by the time he was 8 years of age he could no longer walk and was using a wheelchair.

Soon he was developing a collapsing scoliosis which was partially controlled by lateral padding, and by the age of 9 years he was too weak to propel himself other than for short distances on flat smooth floors. He became very withdrawn and depressed, and his only interests were his pet animals, including dog, cat, guinea-pigs and rabbits.

He was provided with an electrically-powered indoor chair with a fitted tray. The electrically-powered chair helped to change his mood considerably, and the independence of mobility was accompanied by an improvement in his general personality.

At home, there were many architectural problems due to restricted space, and to the fact that the bathroom was upstairs and the downstairs lavatory was inaccessible in a wheelchair. The possibility of rehousing was discussed on several occasions and the local authority were sympathetic. However, the move would have entailed leaving the neighbourhood where he had friends; but what was more important, it would have meant leaving a garden which he could negotiate in his powered chair and which had been adapted to house his pets. These were such an important aspect of his life that the family had organized a local nature study group to meet in their house. Consequently, the family were prepared to put up with the extra work and inconvenience in order to maintain the patient's happiness and morale.

Although there was continued deterioration, at the age of 12 years he was still leading a very full life mainly centred around his pets and nature study. But he was entirely dependent upon his family, except for the use of the electric indoor chair and partial independence for feeding.

Comment

This case history illustrates the great value of independent mobility provided by electrically-propelled indoor chairs, and also the value of an interesting hobby for a severely disabled child. It emphasizes the need to assess all aspects of the problems in the individual patient's circumstances and also the fact that the solution to problems may often have to be compromises. In addition, it illustrates that the family's acceptance of the disability must be followed by re-integration of the disability into total family life, if the child and the family are to continue to live happily together.

RHEUMATOID ARTHRITIS

Rheumatoid arthritis is a common disease affecting patients of both sexes and all ages, its peak incidence occurring during middle age. Although population surveys are bedevilled by problems of diagnostic criteria, and involve complex laboratory investigation, there is considerable evidence that in the Western world the disease is present in 2–3 per cent of the adult population.

Although rheumatoid arthritis is a progressive disease with no known cure, its prognosis is frequently better than is generally realized. Often it is mild and self-limiting, appearing in middle life, and leaving 60 per cent of the affected patients socially and economically independent, although with some impairment of function.

As the rheumatoid patient gets older, however, degenerative changes take place in the already damaged joints, and the elderly arthritic frequently presents the complex picture of rheumatoid arthritis with an overlying osteoarthritis, with symptoms, signs and deformities of both conditions. The late effects of the disease may therefore be severely disabling. Planning a treatment programme for a patient with rheumatoid arthritis thus presents a continuously changing challenge.

The severely crippled rheumatoid arthritic requires complete clinical and functional assessment. The patient must be treated adequately: even though deformities are already established, neglect of the simple principles underlying the general management of rheumatoid arthritis will only lead to further deterioration. A clear general regimen of treatment must be established before it is possible to make constructive recommendations for future management.

particularly in relation to alteration of domestic routine and the planning of reconstructive surgery.

Rheumatoid arthritis is a systemic disease, predominantly involving joints, but also involving loss of weight, development of a moderate anaemia, disturbances of peripheral circulation, undue fatigue and generalized morning stiffness. The persistence of pain and general malaise tends to make such patients mildly depressed and reluctant to undertake activities likely to precipitate further pain. It is because rheumatoid arthritis is so common, and because it is a progressive systemic disease that the general management and rehabilitation of the patients who suffer from it, cannot be separated from the day-to-day clinical care.

Treatment of rheumatoid arthritis consists of a judicious admixture of complete rest; joint immobilization (splints); physical therapy, palliative or active (joint mobilization); analgesic drugs; suppressive drugs; prophyllactic surgery; reconstructive surgery; and social resettlement.

During acute exacerbation of the disease, periods of complete bedrest are most effective providing due care is taken to prevent unnecessary functional deterioration. The value of rest decreases and the problems of maintaining joint function increases as the disease progresses. Thus in the early stages it is often difficult to persuade the young or middle-aged patient to accede to a period of controlled bedrest supplemented by correct splintage or gentle maintaining and mobilizing physiotherapy, at a time when they would most benefit from such a regimen. Later, as deformities progress, the older patients often too easily resort to bedrest, and are reluctant to maintain joint mobility or to wear splints, exacerbating by such conduct the natural tendency for the development of crippling joint deformities.

Local treatment

Heat can be applied by electrical pads or by radiant heat-lamps or by poultices, by wax baths or hot water. Heat has no curative effect but only suffices to produce a feeling of well-being and may allay pain. Occasionally, heat exacerbates the pain and icepacks are more effective.

Splints

An active rheumatoid joint can be immobilized for several weeks without leading to permanent stiffness. If the joint is adequately supported the muscles acting across it can be exercised isometrically without exacerbating the joint symptoms, and a combination of splintage and static exercises leads to settling of joint symptoms without consequent muscle wasting or joint softness. Firm splintage can be achieved with plaster of Paris. More prolonged splintage is best provided by plastic or fibre-glass splints made up from casts taken from the limb. Night splints can be made of plaster of Paris or expanded polystyrene (Plastazote). The splint can be held in position by a crepe bandage or Velcro bandages in preference to straps which are often difficult for the rheumatoid patient to manage. Serial plasters or serial plastic splints may be used to correct deformities of joints which are in an unfavourable position.

Exercises

Static exercises in plaster have been mentioned, but as the acute inflammatory condition in the joints settles, gentle non-weight-bearing movements help to regain mobility, progressing to movements against gradually increasing resistance. The level of resistance is determined by symptoms, and exercise should not produce joint pain.

General exercises, including deep-breathing, arm, leg and trunk movements are often of great value to even the most severely disabled patients and encourage them to progress to independent activities. Quadriceps-setting exercises for the knees, dorsiflexion of the wrists and the extension of the hands and fingers make up the most important group of such exercises and should constitute an essential part of the daily programme of every patient with rheumatoid arthritis.

Hydrotherapy

Active exercises in warm water have long been established as a means of treatment for rheumatoid arthritis. The heyday of the spa is now past, but hydrotherapy should be available in all centres where rheumatic diseases are treated. Warm water provides the ideal medium for obtaining the relaxation of muscles and for the performance of weight-relieved exercises or resisted exercises. It not only relaxes the muscles, but also the patients; and walking re-education can be introduced even for those with severe involvement of the lower limbs.

Local injection

The injection of hydrocortisone or predisone into painful joints, or into tender peri-articular soft tissues has its value, but repeated intra-articular injection may be associated with accelerated destruction of joint tissues. Injection into and around the carpal tunnel can ease the symptoms of medial nerve compression, but surgical decompression is more lastingly effective.

Drug treatment

Analgesics

The control of pain is an important feature of the management and therapy of rheumatoid arthritis, but analgesic drugs should be integrated with local physical measures. It is essential to establish an adequate dosage-level of suitable drugs for each patient, and this treatment should not be lightly altered. Patients should be instructed clearly that the dosage should be maintained and not reduced as symptoms wane; reduction in dosage may well precipitate an exacerbation of symptoms. If one drug is effective in the relief of pain it should be continued indefinitely. If, however, it is only partially effective and not toxic, then another analgesic should be added. Only if the analgesic proves toxic or ineffective should it be completely replaced by another drug.

Aspirin.—Aspirin is still the drug of choice in the general management of rheumatoid arthritis; but it should always be exhibited in maximum tolerable doses or in such doses as control the symptoms. Rarely should the dose be less than 30 gr (2 g) per day and often the dose will be 60–150 gr (4 g–10 g) per day. Soluble calcium aspirin may have less gastrointestinal irritant properties than other analgesics, but there is little evidence to support this. Enteric-coated aspirin does have a reduced irritant effect, and polyoxoaluminium salicylate (Palaprin) (containing 600 mg per tablet) has the advantage of reducing the number of tablets needed to be taken daily.

Phenylbutazone and oxyphenbutazone (*Butazolidine and Tanderil*).—These are usually the second choice of analgesics for rheumatoid arthritis although they have a greater application in acute gout and ankylosing spondylitis. Their potential toxicity although remote is real, and the toxic effects (gastrointestinal symptoms or blood dyscrasias) occur early rather than later. However, trouble rarely occurs if the daily dose is restricted to 300 mg daily.

Indomethacin.—Another second-line analgesic in rheumatoid arthritis is indomethacin, which has been advised for those who have gastrointestinal symptoms. Indomethacin suppositories (100 mg) have an invaluable use when nights are disturbed by pain, or morning stiffness is a troublesome symptom; but complications of gastric intolerance and proctitis are not uncommon.

Suppressive drugs

This book is not a suitable forum to discuss the advantages and disadvantages of the more powerful drugs available to suppress rheumatoid arthritis. Gold, chloroquine, prednisone, prednisilone and adrenocorticotrophic hormone (ACTH) all have their place. By the time the rheumatoid arthritic has reached the stage of severe disability, most will have been tried and a commitment established. Prednisone and prednisilone remain the drugs of choice in treating the severe progressive uncontrolled case. The optimum dose is usually between 5 and 10 mg a day. The use of 1 mg tablets allows flexibility of dosage; 2 mg 3 times a day and 4 mg last thing at night is a commonly suitable regimen.

For those patients severely crippled with deformities, the institution of steroid therapy may occasionally be justified if there is a real chance that it might lead to the raising of the patient's functional level of activity in order to restore personal or social independence. However, if surgical procedures are planned, the complication of steroid therapy during surgery and in the post-operative phase may well warrant postponement of the introduction of these drugs into the patient's medication.

Not infrequently, some of the problems of the severe rheumatoid cripple are attributable to prolonged steroid therapy, for example, peptic ulceration, exacerbation of hypertension, exacerbation of co-existing tuberculosis lesions, osteoporosis and vertebral collapse particularly in post-menopausal women, delayed union of fractures or delayed healing after surgical procedures.

Anaemia

The anaemia of rheumatoid arthritis is sometimes severe and may contribute significantly to the patient's disability. The anaemia is resistant to iron by mouth, but intravenous or intramuscular administration is usually followed by a good response.

The patient's iron requirements can be calculated approximately from the formula:

mg iron required = (15-patient's haemoglobin in grams/100 ml) × bodyweight in kg × 3

The entire requirement can be given as iron dextrose by an intravenous infusion over 8–10 hours, but this has little advantage over a transfusion of packed red cells and reactions to the infusion are not uncommon. Repeated small injections of 200–250 mg are usually preferred, the injection being given every few days or so until the required dose (usually about 1 g) has been given.

Surgical procedures

Since rheumatoid arthritis is a progressive disease with multiple joint involvement, the surgical procedures used in its treatment are also likely to be multiple. For this reason, the attitude of mind with which a patient accepts operative treatment and the prolonged post-operative physiotherapy which it entails is of the utmost importance.

It is essential that the patient be given a clear picture of the probable consequences of conservative treatment, and a cautious estimate of the improvement which may be expected from surgical intervention. Failure to appreciate the effects which immobilization of a joint may have on the various activities of daily living may be responsible for post-operative disappointment and resentment, and may cause a patient to refuse subsequent offers of surgical treatment. Likewise a failure to understand that deformity may recur and pain may persist after surgery, because of the nature of the disease, and not because of inadequate surgical technique, may cause mistrust and depression.

The most careful explanation will not counteract the great effect that the personality of the patient will have upon the quality of the end result, but even the most inadequate personality can be helped considerably by the administration of adequate pre-operative and post-operative analgesics. It does much to establish the correct attitude of restrained optimism if the first operation performed is a simple one, from which a good functional result, or a painless joint may be confidently expected. When a positive gain from surgery has been established, a patient is more likely to co-operate and collaborate with further surgical procedures which might be of greater clinical and prophyllactic benefit (for example, synovectomy or debridement) even though they require a more demanding post-operative regimen of rehabilitation.

It is not necessary to await a natural remission of the disease before embarking on elective surgery, but yet the timing and order of possible operative procedures is critical. Thus, certain procedures may advantageously be combined, provided their sequence in the total rehabilitation of the patient permits it. Operations carried out on both arms or hands simultaneously can incapacitate a patient unnecessarily. Conversely, combining upper-limb with lower-limb surgery, or the performance of simultaneous bilateral lower-limb operations can materially reduce the total rehabilitation time. The need for arm function for crutch-walking during rehabilitation after lower-limb surgery may determine the operative sequence. Such additional stresses may help or hinder recovery of upper-limb function. Thus, surgical rehabilitation should be based on a detailed clinical, functional and personality assessment and should be integrated with the careful planning of pre-operative and post-operative rehabilitation and with resettlement management both in hospital and at home.

Upper-limb surgery

Upper-limb surgery is aimed at increasing mobility and dexterity. However, before embarking on a surgical programme, it is wise to attempt to establish what the total functional level of the limb is likely to be, for in a progressive disease this is more important than the specific functional level of any one joint. For example, arthrodesis of the wrist is often advocated, and has the advantage of producing a stable painless joint and improved hand function in consequence. But in the presence of active disease of shoulder and elbow, mobility at the wrist may be the only movement which allows the patient to feed himself and for this reason he may understandably refuse operation. A period of trial in a lightweight splint may help to establish the advantages or disadvantages of the procedure. Surgery of the rheumatoid hand is now the subject of considerable study. Synovectomy and joint decompression are offered early to prevent or delay the development of deformity. As deformities develop, tendon repair and joint reconstruction can preserve active function, and for the severely disrupted hand, stabilization (arthrodesis) of some joints may restore active grip.

Lower-limb surgery

Operations on the lower limb of severely disabled rheumatoid arthritics are largely confined to arthrodesis of the larger joints aimed at achieving walking or standing stability, or arthroplasties performed to enable the patient to sit and transfer from chair to bed and toilet in comfort. Unfortunately, it is often impossible to satisfy both requirements. Patients who are well satisfied by bilateral knee arthrodesis while they remain mobile will find two stiff knees a serious handicap when deterioration of their hips and general condition forces them to adopt a wheelchair mode of life. Replacement of joints by internal prostheses offers much hope for both relief of pain and mobility, but this work is still in its early stages of development.

Case history No. 99 illustrates how assessment, rehabilitation, appliances and surgery can combine to achieve a marked benefit for the severe rheumatoid cripple.

M.M.L. No. 99 born 1925 female

Diagnosis: Rheumatoid arthritis

At the age of 22 years, this woman developed acute rheumatoid arthritis which by the age of 25 years had left her with severe deformities in many joints. When admitted to the Disabled Living Unit in 1964, her movements were as follows:

Cervical spine	fixed
Jaws	mouth opens 1 cm only, no lateral movement of jaws
Shoulders	less than 40 degrees abduction and 30 degrees flexion in both shoulders
Elbows	fixed at right-angles
Wrists	less than 10 degrees pronation or supination from neutral position
Hands	metacarpophalangeal joints mostly fixed proximal intophalangeal joints—swan-neck deformities
Legs	a few degrees of movement only at hips, knees, ankles and toes. Fixed flexion deformities at hips and knees of 90 degrees

The patient had been cared for by her mother until the mother died suddenly. She lived at home and was then on her own all day. The district nurse called every day to get her up into her chair (standard general-purpose wheelchair). A home-help attended three mornings a week. Her sister came in every evening to give her a bedpan and put her to bed.

After considerable training with aids to daily living, assessment indicated that even with aids and appliances she was still unable to continue living independently, but that with improvement in elbow range and hand grip, she might well become more independent.

The proximal interphalangeal joints of the index, middle, ring and little fingers of the left hand were arthrodesed in flexion and the distal interphalangeal joint of the index finger was also arthrodesed. Some months later, the right hand was operated on and then an excision arthroplasty was performed on the right elbow.

During the post-operative phase, rehabilitation was directed towards maintaining mobility in the right elbow and towards training her to use aids and appliances to cope with daily living activities from her electric wheelchair. With various simple aids and an electric hoist in the right surroundings, she was almost entirely independent (*Figure 3.8*).

Her own house was quite unsuitable because of inaccessibility and circulation problems, but the local authority agreed to rehouse her in the same area. An electric hoist was installed in the bedroom and minor adaptations for cooking were installed in the kitchen.

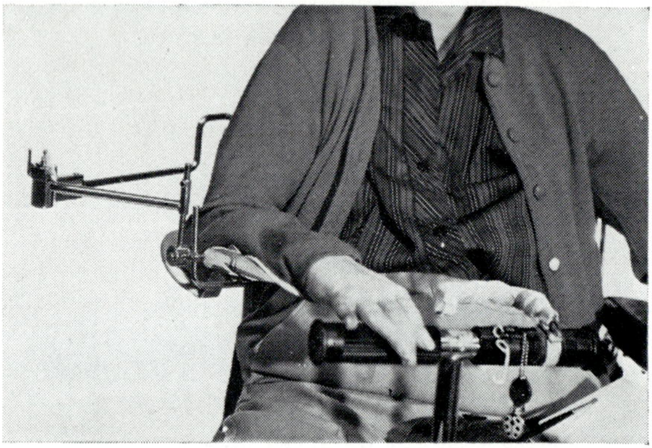

(*a*)

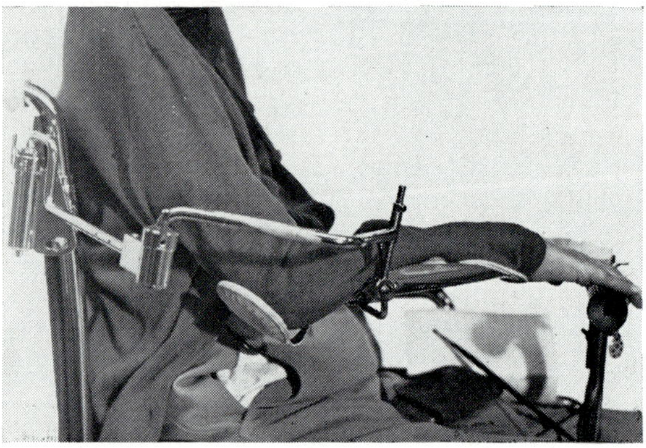

(*b*)

Figure 3.8. Patient No. 99 with rheumatoid arthritis using ball-bearing arm supports on an electrically-powered indoor chair

(*a*) *front view indicating functional position of hand;* (*b*) *side view showing support given to forearm*

With the combination of surgery, rehabilitation, rehousing, provision of aids and appliances, and support for heavy domestic work, she has remained living independently for over 4 years. She paints, undertakes some housework, prepares and cooks all her own meals, is learning Spanish, and is planning to take on a part-time job at home.

STILL'S DISEASE

Still's disease is a relatively uncommon disease but represents a potent source of severe disability in young adults, although recent advances in treatment have improved its prognosis. Although Still's disease presents in many ways, the outstanding clinical feature is a chronic polyarthritis developing in childhood. In more than half of these children the outcome is not particularly disabling. The arthritis becomes inactive and the residual deformity depends on many factors, in particular, the care with which the acute phase was supervised. Some patients, however, have many joints involved and are left with multiple deformities and ankylosis. Those who required corticosteroids may have failed to grow in stature and remained sexually immature.

The aim of treatment is to carry the patient through the active period of the disease until remission occurs, so that permanent deformities are avoided as far as possible. Physiotherapy is based on active exercises maintaining muscle power and joint range. Hydrotherapy is of particular benefit to these patients. The active treatment should be interspersed with rest in splints for the affected joints to ensure a good functional position—that is, knees straight, wrists straight and ankles at right-angles, and elbows slightly flexed. Work splints are sometimes indicated when one or two joints persist in being painful and it is necessary to maintain the joint in a position of function during activity. Bedrest is only indicated for severe generalized symptoms.

An adequate dosage of aspirin is still the safest form of medication, corticosteroids being occasionally required to control severe systemic disease. With an active and supporting regimen, the majority of patients are able to lead reasonably normal adult lives. In nearly two-thirds of the adults who have had Still's disease in childhood, the disease remains inactive and deformity rather than activity is the usual reason for whatever incapacity occurs. Flexion contractures of the hips and knees, often associated with pes equina, are potent barriers to adequate walking. Ankylosis of the elbows and stiffness of the wrists are considerable handicaps for most activities of daily living. Case history No. 168 (*see* Chapter 6) and No. 655 (*see* Chapter 4) illustrate some of the problems.

HAEMOPHILIA

There are about 3,000 haemophiliacs in the United Kingdom, and although they make up one of the smallest groups of children with physical handicaps, they present special problems of management which likewise demands close co-operation between hospital, school, social and welfare service.

The prompt management of acute bleeds by immediate admission to appropriate units can reduce long-term disability. The continuance of school facilities in the hospitals and treatment centres can reduce the effect of loss of school hours. Comprehensive management of this calibre necessitates a round-the-clock collaboration of such a degree between treatment centres, school and patient that there is considerable argument in favour of special residential schools for haemophiliacs, sited near to special treatment centres.

For the adult haemophiliac the greatest problem is finding and keeping suitable employment. This is partly due to fear and lack of understanding of the problem by the prospective employer, partly due to problem of transport, and partly due to lack of education and training consequent upon multiple protracted admissions to hospital during childhood and early adolescence.

Haemarthroses usually first occurs in the second or third year of life, as the child becomes more active and agile. The weight-bearing joints, particularly the knees, are most frequently involved. The knees probably account for about half of all haemarthroses in haemophilia, and the ankles for about one-third.

Recurrent bleeding into joints leads to destruction of the articular cartilage. Intra-articular adhesions and capsular fibrosis lead to restriction of movement, and ultimately the gross destruction of the joint and the severe fibrosis leads to fixity and deformity. Minor traumata are probably the cause of many haemarthroses.

In later life, the elbows constitute about 20 per cent of the joints affected. Circumstantial evidence indicates that the use of unsuitable motorized transport may be a potent factor associated with the increased frequency of bleeds in these joints.

Fixed flexion deformity of the knees is a frequent and crippling deformity, and if it is of long-standing and associated with joint destruction and subluxation, complete correction may not be achieved. Hip flexion deformities may also occur, although haemarthroses of the hip joints are relatively rare. Intramuscular haemorrhage may involve the iliacus and calf muscles. The latter leads to equinus deformity of the foot.

With the recent advanced in the knowledge of blood-clotting mechanisms, the treatment of the effects of haemophilia has been greatly improved, and many haemorrhages can now be arrested early. Likewise such knowledge has made orthopaedic correction of deformities possible. Even so, haemophiliacs continue to constitute a problem of management to a Disabled Living Unit with their potential and actual deformities.

The major problem which presents is often the provision of adequate transport, whether indoor or outdoor. Great care is needed in the choice of wheelchair and outside vehicle, so that undue trauma can be avoided during transfers, and further trauma attributable to the structure and the operation of the vehicles prevented. Thus outdoor mechanized transport should have minimal controls, easily operated steering, and no potentially harmful projections within reach of the driver.

Small motor-cars with automatic transmission, safety belts and padded fascia are preferable to the standard invalid vehicles. Structurally more suitable, they are also mechanically more reliable and easier to have repaired in an emergency than the usual invalid tricycles, since many garages are reluctant or have not the facilities to undertake repairs and maintenance of the latter vehicles. Furthermore, as haemophilia is not considered a barrier to marriage, many haemophiliacs are family men, and a car enables them to travel with their families, whereas an invalid tricycle does not. The additional provisions of heating and defrosting apparatus and softer upholstery are further advantages which make the provision of a car a desirable alternative.

Even if the mechanical problems are sometimes over-emphasized by the patients, the pain and capricious nature of the disease engenders a corrosive fear, and unless the patients have confidence in their vehicles and confidence in their ability to reach the expert centres, then their range of activity is necessarily limited. Outside the special centres help is uncertain, and therefore secondary deformities from haemarthroses which are repeated and inadequately treated become far more likely. A haemophiliac is already so limited in the activities which he may follow that it seems unjustifiable to limit drastically the area in which he may enjoy them, by failing to provide him with efficient and reliable transport.

AMPUTATION

Each year there are about 4,000–5,000 primary amputations performed in the United Kingdom. The total number of amputees currently alive in the United Kingdom number about 100,000. The majority of amputations are carried out in the elderly for peripheral vascular disease. Approximately 60 per cent of all amputees are over the age of 60 years, and the ratio of lower-limb to upper-limb amputations is greater than 10:1.

Amputations following injuries account for about 20 per cent of amputees and these tend to occur in the younger age-groups, while tumours account for about 6 per cent and tend to occur in the young and middle-aged. Congenital malformations represent about 6 per cent of amputees.

The single amputation of a lower limb in a young person should not constitute a severe disability unless there is a long delay in providing the artificial limb. It is only patients with short or badly-scarred stumps who may give rise to difficulties of rehabilitation.

Upper limb amputations may give rise to special problems if they are performed after a protracted period of disability such as that following a brachial plexus lesion or poliomyelitis. If the decision to operate is long delayed, the patient will already have adapted to being functionally one-handed and training him to use an artificial limb is often unsuccessful. The artificial arm is either not used at all, or else only as a cosmetic appliance or a simple prop. However, early amputation, coupled with a short period of intensive rehabilitation immediately after early fitting of a prosthesis leads to excellent functional results.

Severe disability

Amputees need to be considered under the general heading of the severely disabled in two general groups. Firstly, the elderly patients who, because of the underlying peripheral vascular lesions have bilateral lower-limb amputations and secondly, the children born with multiple congenital limb deformities.

With advancing surgical techniques for the conservation of limbs, amputation frequently has come to be regarded as an ablative procedure, and an indication of failure of other methods of management. But it should always be regarded as a constructive procedure leading to artificial-limb fitting and a return to active function.

Liaison between vascular surgeon, prosthetist and rehabilitation department is often not as close as it should be. Too often, amputation is still regarded as mutilation rather than as a positive technique to restore competent function. The prosthetist is frequently presented with a stump unsuitable for current artificial limbs, instead of a stump which is the result of pre-operative consultation leading to advance decisions and preparation of an appropriate prosthesis. It is partly because of the separation of the limb-fitting service from the hospital service, partly because of delays in referral, manufacture and fitting of the prostheses, and partly because of the lack of adequate facilities and interest in the rehabilitation of the elderly amputee, that a high proportion of these patients never use their artificial limbs in an optimal fashion and a considerable proportion of them do not use the limbs at all.

The first few days and weeks after the supply of the initial appliance are critical, and whenever possible this critical period of rehabilitation should be undertaken in an intensive manner in appropriate hospital accommodation; either day-hospital or in-patient hostel accommodation. Carefully graduated training with firm guidance is necessary to encourage the elderly patient to work through the initial stage of discomfort and to establish confidence in his ability to walk again.

The current trends towards multi-component prefabricated (modular) systems of prosthetic construction should streamline the limb-fitting service and should allow for much decentralization of fitting and training centres and therefore lead to easier rehabilitation of these patients. This, together with closer co-operation between physiotherapist and the limb fitters, should ultimately ensure that the amputee who does not accept and use an artificial limb, becomes an increasingly rare exception.

Elderly patients have special problems. Their muscles are weak, joints in the other leg and in the arms are often arthritic. Their balance may be faulty, their general condition poor, and their ability to tolerate exercise an activity considerably reduced. They are often easily disheartened and may already have had considerable hospitalization and suffered disappointments after previous arterial surgery. For all these reasons, their rehabilitation must be gentle, realistic and graduated to targets which are within their comprehension and ability to achieve. This process devolves upon the physiotherapist who must be given adequate facilities and time to achieve the results which they know are attainable. It is relevant to remember that when amputation of one lower limb has been performed because of ischaemia in an elderly patient, it is the circulatory competence of his other lower limb which determines the rate, level and duration of his ability to walk again.

An elderly amputee with angina while in bed, dyspnoea at rest, uncontrollable postural oedema, lack of sitting balance, or the presence of several other diseases, such as renal failure, should not be considered for prosthetic management. Flexion contractures can render prosthetic management virtually impossible. An elderly patient's mental state can do likewise and is always an important factor in determining the acceptance and use of a prosthesis. Senility, severely defective eye-sight and hearing, and poor motivation, renders prosthetic rehabilitation impossible.

Pre-operative management

Elderly patients who are awaiting amputation may be helped considerably by adequate pre-operative management. This should include a thorough clinical examination with active treatment of any abnormal conditions which this uncovers. It should also include certain basic pathological investigations such as haemoglobin, blood film, chest radiography and urinalysis, together with any further tests specifically indicated by the clinical findings. Apart from the direct management of the vascular insufficiency, preparation for the actual amputation should be aimed at producing optimal posture, strength and general condition in patient and stump alike.

To use a lower-limb prosthesis to its best advantage, a hip free from flexion contracture, and capable of strong active abduction and extension is essential. This applies to above-knee and below-knee amputations, and in the latter case, the possession of full active knee extension is also necessary.

In the pre-operative management designed to promote these conditions in the joints, the hospital bed should have a firm mattress, preferably with fracture boards, to prevent hip flexion contractures developing, and physiotherapy should be directed towards reducing any contractures which are present by stretching and prone lying. Power of the hip extensors and abductors can be improved by exercises and in some patients, direct training in 'amputee walking' can be given by using a pre-prosthetic pylon for short walking training periods.

Treatment of the patient's general condition should be directed in particular towards the improvement of trunk posture by means of exercises to strengthen the spinal extensors and shoulders, the eradication of chest infection and the improvement of respiratory excursion, and the improvement of the strength and range of movement of the upper limbs and the contralateral lower limb. The muscles of the pectoral girdle and of the arm itself should be strengthened in preparation for the extra work which they will have to do in transferring, using crutches and propelling wheelchairs. Extra work will also be permanently required of the muscles of the pelvic girdle and leg on the side opposite to the limb awaiting amputation, and exercises to promote their strength should take equal precedence with those for the latter limb.

A period of two weeks on this type of regimen can make a considerable general improvement and make prosthetic management easier and more likely to succeed. Even those patients restricted to bed can be given mobility training in bed, by means of simple apparatus to push up on the firm, hardbased bed.

Immediate and early post-operative fitting

Post-operatively, it is more important to rehabilitate the patient than the stump, but any discussion of this period of care has become intertwined with the advantages and disadvantages of different types of amputations and different methods of prosthetic management. Much is being written about early post-operative fitting of prostheses and immediate post-operative fitting, and it is difficult to analyse all the factors involved. However, whether the patient is being treated in the traditional fashion, or is having immediate or early fitting of a prosthesis, the first 4–6 weeks after amputation are critical, for the eventual successful employment of the prosthesis concerned.

The 3 major aims of management immediately post-operatively are (1) to promote stump healing, (2) to promote mobility and power in the stump, and (3) to promote general clinical rehabilitation.

Traditional conical stumps require careful pressure bandaging, but even with meticulous surgery and intensive post-operative management, a considerable amount of oedema in the stump is almost inevitable. Careful bandaging must be continued for weeks after operation, and this introduces a considerable problem for those elderly patients who are unable to bandage their stumps without assistance. Indeed, ideal stump bandaging cannot be carried out in the traditional manner by the patient alone, even if young and otherwise able, but needs co-operation between patient and an experienced stump bandager.

Immediate post-operative fitting

Traditionally, the two common sites for lower limb amputation are 10–12 in below the greater trochanter and 5–6 in below the knee. The conventional stumps are conically shaped, this being achieved at operation by dividing the muscle about 1 in above the skin incision, to prevent adherence to the scar, and shaping the bone ends. As far as below-knee stumps are concerned, the fibula is cut about 1 in shorter than the tibia. Stump shaping is further continued by rigorous bandaging techniques.

In recent years, the trend has been towards total surface contact for above-knee prostheses, and for the use of patellar-tendon-bearing below-knee appliances, suction sockets and early post-operative fitting. The surgical techniques used to provide the fleshy stumps suitable for such techniques and appliances, involve long skin flaps tailored to the requirements of the individual stumps. The muscles are divided distally and overlapped. Bone ends are covered with a periosteal flap; nerve trunks are divided well proximally and their ends buried in muscle. Meticulous haemostasis is a *sine qua non*. Such techniques produce rather thick bulbous stumps but are reputed to engender less stump pain, less trouble with phantom limbs and better post-operative healing.

Rigid bandaging is possible in the case of amputation surgery because the wound is terminal and thus pressure on the wound does not produce constriction of the blood supply, yet it adequately controls post-operative oedema. Providing adequate pressure is maintained consistently over the distal end, oedema of the stump is minimal, healing of the wound is more rapid and certain than stumps produced by the traditional operative and post-operative techniques.

From the success of firm pressure bandaging on the stump in the immediate post-operative stage, arose the idea of a rigid post-operative dressing, to which some form of temporary pylon could be attached. Techniques were evolved to allow for the application of such a rigid dressing in the form of a plaster of Paris cast, with facilities for adding a temporary pylon. Patients for whom such techniques are used may be stood out of bed at 24 hours, providing end pressure is maintained, and the temporary pylon is then aligned. The first partial weight-bearing standing is introduced at about 3–4 days. By the time the sutures are ready for removal, the patient can be standing and walking short distances. At about 14 days post-operative, the cast (rigid dressing) is removed, the stitches taken out, and a second rigid dressing (either plaster of Paris or plastic) applied with a temporary pylon attached. Providing there are no other problems, the patient can be discharged from hospital 28 days post-operatively, walking with his pylon.

The critical factors in this procedure are the surgical techniques, the application of the initial plaster and the first plaster change. Patients for this type of management must be carefully selected in terms of their clinical, mental and domestic situation. Having made the selection, and prepared the patient with pre-operative physiotherapy, it is necessary to set up a complicated organization with special equipment to undertake the initial application of the plaster, and to prepare for the immediate prosthetic fitting. Although these procedures have been widely used in some centres in America, they are still undergoing clinical trials in the United Kingdom, and their early and long-term effects have not been fully evaluated.

Early post-operative fitting

Providing there is close collaboration between the surgeons, the limb-fitting service and the rehabilitation team, present experience indicates that traditional management with pylons can match the results of immediate post-operative fitting when similar facilities and organization are available in both cases.

Lower limbs

Early fitting of traditional pylons will speed the absorption of stump oedema more efficiently than stump bandaging. In many patients so fitted, there is no reason why they should not start their rehabilitation in a pylon 2–3 weeks after amputation, provided that the amputation scar is completely healed. This procedure can obtain end-results comparable to those achieved by immediate post-operative fitting of temporary prostheses.

Upper limbs

The same concept of early prosthetic fitment can also be applied to upper-limb amputees, fitting simple plastic or plaster sockets equipped with a variety of interchangeable attachments to train the upper-limb amputee to retain upper-limb function. These can be applied as soon as the stump wound has healed.

Rehabilitation of the elderly amputee

Selection for prosthetic management entails careful consideration of the general condition of the patient and of the probable condition of the stump to be produced by amputation. The elderly amputee with vascular disease has an average life-expectancy of 3–5 years. Many have suffered from circulatory insufficiency for some years before amputation or may have had previous vascular surgery. Prolonged bedrest may have encouraged flexion contractures at the hip. Long-standing vascular lesions with progressive ischaemia may have induced a high level of toxaemia and a poor general clinical condition. However, these patients often make a dramatic recovery after amputation and reassessment of their progress at regular intervals is essential if an accurate estimate of the effects of operation is to be obtained (*see* case history No. 373, page 106).

Mental deterioration associated with arteriosclerosis, general senility or previous cerebrovascular accidents are contra-indications to prosthetic management, although a pre-existing hemiplegia is not in itself a contra-indication.

The preliminary assessment of a patient for whom amputation is considered should be clinical, functional and domestic. The clinical assessment will determine the feasibility of prosthetic management and the likely outcome.

The functional assessment should establish the probable level of physical competence which may be expected to be present following amputation.

Domestic assessment should facilitate resettlement of the amputee in his home surroundings, by indicating what alterations are needed in the structure of the home to enable the patient to attain maximal independence, and by enabling his family and local welfare services to make these alterations and organize adequate help before his discharge from hospital. For example, if a patient has an above-knee amputation, she may need to use a wheelchair to reach the toilet during the night, when she is not wearing her prosthesis. Can a wheelchair be manoeuvred into the toilet? Is she likely to be able to get from wheelchair to toilet? Is it necessary to instal a commode, or can more permanent arrangements be made?

M.M.L. No. 373 born 1912 female

Diagnosis: Above-knee amputation

This woman had had varicose ulcers of her left leg for nearly a year and then the leg suddenly became swollen and cold. Four days later, she was admitted to hospital in a state of severe collapse.

The left foot showed signs of early gangrene with swelling and blistering. She was sweating profusely, she was drowsy, toxic, and was found to have a systolic blood pressure of only 65 mm Hg and an unrecordable diastolic pressure. Her temperature was 101·8° F (38·8° C) and the blood urea was 218 mg/100 ml (normal: 20–40 mg/100 ml). Within 24 hours the blood urea was 268 mg/100 ml; the patient became comatose and anuric. An above-knee amputation was carried out as an emergency on the patient with pre-operative and post-operative intravenous cortisone cover. Three days later, she regained consciousness and began to pass urine.

The amputation stump had to be revised 2 weeks later. By this time, she was still disorientated and had developed sacral bedsores. Six weeks after admission, she had improved sufficiently in general health for the possibility of rehabilitation and limb-fitting to be considered. However, she was anaemic, she still had a large sacral bedsore and was still unable to concentrate on exercise for very long without becoming tired. The anaemia was treated by transfusion of packed cells and she was nursed on a sheepskin. The sacral sore then began to heal and she was measured for a pylon.

She was admitted to the Disabled Living Unit for walking training when the pylon was ready, 3 months after the amputation. After 2 weeks' training, she was able to go home, using the pylon and a walking-frame. She attended the local hospital physiotherapy department for continued supervision. A permanent limb was provided 4 months later, and she was able to use this, at first with a pair of quadruped sticks and later with ordinary walking-sticks.

Comment

This lady was desperately ill, with the classical features of gangrene. She had a stormy illness and protracted post-operative convalecsence after the emergency amputation. However, through careful nursing, and intensive rehabilitation as an in-patient, she eventually made a good recovery and became proficient in the use of her lower-limb prosthesis.

Above-knee amputation in the elderly

After an above-knee amputation an elderly patient is initially provided with a temporary prosthesis (pylon). These may have sockets made of plaster of Paris, plastic, or more usually, metal, and to these sockets are fitted simple wooden supports and a block foot; a caliper-type knee-lock can be fitted to facilitate sitting down. Such appliances are light and easy to produce and therefore relatively cheap. In theory, such appliances can be fitted within a week or two of amputation. The patient therefore rapidly becomes mobile during the few weeks in which the stump requires to settle down to its final shape and size. This initial period of shrinkage and walking re-education are most important and delays in supplying or fitting can determine the patient's acceptance or rejection of the final prosthesis.

Many elderly patients fitted with a satisfactory pylon are reluctant to exchange it for a definitive limb, which is heavier and 'more difficult' to use. When given a definitive artificial limb, they are reluctant to introduce free knee movement. Thus, the only advantages which the definitive limb offers are cosmetic in nature and many patients sacrifice this advantage for the lightness, comfort and stability of the pylon.

Current developments are towards the development of appliances which combine the best of both approaches. Prefabrication and the use of multi-component (modular) constructional systems permit early fitting of a light, stable appliance. The prefabricated multi-component nature allows easy interchange of sockets as the stump changes in volume and shape. The modular construction includes a system of simple alignment correction, and knee movement and cosmetic covers which can be added later.

Through knee or transcondylar amputation

Some surgeons favour amputation through the knee or through the femoral condyles. A simple knee disarticulation has the attraction of being a simple, quick operation giving little trauma to the patient. Both these operations have the advantage of producing better end bearing stumps than the traditional above-knee stump. However, they are the prosthetist's nightmare as they have none of the advantages of a traditional above-knee or below-knee stump. The knee joint has been sacrificed and the stump is so long that there is no facility for providing a simple knee mechanism within the prosthesis.

These stumps are sometimes termed as 'surgeon's stumps', whereas fleshy 10–12 in (25–30 cm) myoplastic above-knee stumps are 'prosthetist's stumps'.

Management of bilateral amputation of the lower limbs

Bilateral amputation following multiple injuries are relatively uncommon and rehabilitation may be long and complex, but the final functional end result is often excellent, as illustrated by case history LB.

LB born 1920 male

Diagnosis: Multiple injuries

While serving in the Royal Air Force as a pilot, this man was involved in an aircraft crash, in which he sustained (1) traumatic amputation of the left leg; (2) closed head injury with loss of consciousness for several days; (3) compound comminuted fracture of right ankle; (4) Montegia fracture of the left forearm; (5) fractured pelvis with sacrioiliac dislocation and separation of symphysis pubis.

The left leg was traumatically avulsed at the knee and the injury converted to an above-knee amputation on admission to hospital.

The pelvic fractures involved the right pubic ramus and the dislocation of both sacroiliac joints, and a separation of the public symphisis of 4 in (10 cm).

He had a closed head injury and was unconscious for several days. The right ankle sustained a severe compound fracture dislocation, but this was treated conservatively although it became severely infected He spent some 5 months in hospital undergoing treatment for the fractures and the infection. This required extensive soft-tissue surgery, sequestrectomies and skin grafting. Eventually, when the wounds had almost healed and he was transferred to a rehabilitation unit.

At this time, the right leg was immobilized in plaster of Paris with a large window over the unhealed aspect of the ankle. The above-knee stump was in good condition and the pelvis, although widely separated at the symphysis, gave little trouble. Rehabilitation was difficult because the combination of a long-leg plaster, an above-knee amputation and an unstable fracture of the left arm made any form of ambulation with crutches difficult.

The first step in the rehabilitation of this patient was the supply of an above-knee prosthesis. As soon as he could stand and walk using the prosthesis and a walking plaster, the degree of separation of the symphysis pubis began to decrease. However, as rehabilitation proceeded, the use of crutches and sticks placed an increasing strain upon the disunited fracture of the ulna, and each attempt to introduce weight-bearing on the right leg was followed by increasing pain in the right ankle.

The right ankle was operated on again in an attempt to obtain healing and the fracture of the ulna was also treated by open reduction and insertion of a bone graft. Rehabilitation continued on conservative lines until it was clear that weight-bearing on the right ankle was unlikely to be successful even after arthrodesis. An elective below-knee amputation was then carried out 18 months after the original injury.

Three months later, he was walking satisfactorily, using a walking-stick only over rough ground, and returned to ground duties with the Royal Air Force. Shortly after this, he left the Royal Air Force and trained as a schoolmaster.

Comment

This patient illustrated the functional recovery which is possible after considerable severe multiple injuries. The case history also illustrates the value of careful reappraisal and rehabilitation during the various stages of recovery and between surgical procedures. Furthermore, the atmosphere of an active rehabilitation unit helped to maintain the patient's morale and motivation when he was faced with severe injuries, a great deal of pain and long-term prospects of considerably reduced activity and circumstances. The final successful outcome was helped by the fact that in this case, the patient was able to adapt to one prosthesis before his second amputation.

Bilateral amputation of the lower limb

The rehabilitation of simultaneous bilateral above-knee amputations require a different approach. The patients are usually first fitted with very short pylons (rocker pylons), which are only about 7 in (18 cm) long. These short pylons enable the patient to become ambulant, gain confidence and balance. Such appliances also have an assessment value, as patients who are unable to cope with them will certainly be unable to cope with full-length artificial legs, and a wheelchair existence can be planned forthwith.

Longer pylons are introduced as the patient gains confidence. Finally, full-length pylons can be used before graduating to two definitive limbs. One of the important exercises during this phase is practice in falling and in getting up again. Confidence in his ability to cope with these situations considerably helps the patients to return to full functional activity. Elderly bilateral amputees may become ambulant on pylon rockers but be unable to cope with the heavier articulated limbs. Even this independent mobility is of functional and psychological value.

All bilateral above-knee amputees will require a wheelchair even if they are able to use pylons or legs. During intercurrent illness or intervals in which the prostheses are damaged and cannot be worn, visits to the toilet at night must be achieved on stumps if a wheelchair is not available.

Without a wheelchair, the activity of a bilateral amputee may be severely limited by the geography of his garden path and the streets near his home. For those patients for whom powered outdoor transport is not desirable, a wheelchair immediately increases the range of activity, and makes the possibilities of re-employment more realistic.

The choice of wheelchairs is important, since the centre of gravity of a bilateral amputee seated in a wheelchair is very different from that of a normal person. Ordinary wheelchairs are liable to tip backwards when going up a slight slope, or even when at rest if the patient leans back suddenly. This makes it necessary to provide a special amputee chair, with the rear wheels set some 4–6 in (10–15 cm) further back than usual. And since the advantages and disadvantages of front- and rear-wheel propulsion are equally applicable to bilateral amputees, the most suitable chair for their use is a folding rear-wheel hand-propelling chair, with the rear-wheel axle set back (*see* Chapter 6).

If the patient never uses artificial limbs, then footrests should not be fitted as they only get in the way; if the patient uses pylons or legs, then the footrests are necessary but should be capable of swinging outwards, to enable the patient to get in and out of the chair without risk of catching the limbs against the footrests. Bilateral artificial legs add considerably to the patient's sitting width and this point should be carefully checked before ordering the final chair. Such patients often fall into one of the special categories qualifying for powered outdoor transport, and problems arise here because the proper amputee chair, being slightly longer than usual, is more difficult to get into the Ministry of Health invalid tricycle than a standard wheelchair.

Because of the difficult problems involved with maintaining mobility, a domiciliary assessment is essential and particular attention should be directed towards accessibility of the toilet, both for walking using the artificial legs and also by wheelchairs. Bed heights, chair heights, toilet-seat heights are all critical for transfers, and may vary for those occasions when using the limbs and those when using a wheelchair. Bathing is often very tricky and may require specially constructed bath seats to enable patients to transfer from wheelchairs to the bath and out again. Accessibility of the house (steps, and so on) availability of space for garaging the invalid tricycle, wheelchair manoeuvreability all need checking.

Case history No. 901 illustrates many of the problems described.

M.M.L. No. 901 born 1919 male

Diagnosis: Bilateral above-knee amputation

Due to an accident at work (heavy industry), this man sustained severe crush injuries to both legs requiring bilateral above-knee amputations. Six weeks after admission to hospital, he was transferred to the Disabled Living Unit to start training for the use of artificial limbs. Stump training and independence training were started, short pylons followed and then longer pylons of almost full length were introduced.

He was very apprehensive at first and it took considerable patience to build up his confidence. Without the continuous supervision and encouragement of a residential unit, it is doubtful whether he would ever have graduated beyond this stage.

He was given a double amputee wheelchair since both the stumps were very short and he tended to overbalance backwards in a standard wheelchair. Three months after the accident, once he was confident on his pylons, he returned home and daily attended the local physiotherapy department for practice in walking and in getting the pylons on and off. The definitive limbs were supplied 2 months later (5 months after the original injury) and he was, therefore, readmitted for a further period of in-patient rehabilitation. Over a period of several weeks, he became confident and competent at putting on and taking off the artificial legs and walking with them. He was issued with a Ministry of Health invalid tricycle and was ready to return to full employment.

Within a year of the original accident, he was back in full-time work with his original employers, in a sedentary clerical capacity.

Comment

Bilateral above-knee amputation is a severe physical disability. It required considerable effort and courage to overcome the problem of using two artificial limbs. Certainly, in this instance, it is very doubtful whether the patient would have managed to do so without admission to a residential unit where considerable time and encouragement was devoted towards helping him overcome his fears and lack of confidence.

CHILDREN WITH MULTIPLE CONGENITAL LIMB DEFORMITIES

Introduction

The incidence of multiple congenital limb deformities is very small, and those children who survive are usually seen and treated in orthopaedic hospitals and limb-fitting centres, often managing to live full lives, even bringing up a family or achieving academic success.

It was not until thalidomide was manufactured and prescribed as an effective sedative in early pregnancy that the incidence of multiple congenital limb deformities rose to significant proportions. The need to help the children with these deformities became suddenly and dramatically apparent, and acted as a catalyst to the study of the congenital amputee. Since then, a great deal of work has been done in various centres, particularly in those countries in which thalidomide was originally widely used. The importance of such work is difficult to evaluate, because of the overlying social and psychological implications of guilt of parents and community, and because of the undecided issues of allotment of blame and compensation.

No agreement has been reached yet on the appropriate prosthetic and rehabilitation programme for these children. The need for complex powered devices is relatively small, their technology is sophisticated and expensive and their application very limited. Yet the development of ideas and techniques which has followed research into their manufacture and use has been immense. It has forged links between clinical and engineering departments, clarifying and emphasizing their mutual need of each other, and establishing the advantages and accelerated advances of research projects pursued along closely integrated lines.

Thalidomide deformities

In the United Kingdom, approximately 400 children were born with deformities attributed to the administration of thalidomide to their mothers during the early weeks of pregnancy. Of these 400 children, 230–300 survived. Approximately 25 per cent of the survivors have limb deformities of sufficient severity to require particular prosthetic management, and a further 33 per cent require help from other aids and appliances.

Typically, the limb deformities involve 2 or 4 limbs. Many children have both upper limbs affected, and a few have all 4 limbs affected. None are recorded with abnormal legs in the presence of normal arms. Many children have associated abnormalities of soft tissues and bone, particularly of the eyes, ears and vertebral column.

Non-thalidomide deformities

Congenital limb deformities not attributable to thalidomide arise from time to time in association with exposure to certain types of infection, to radiation or to Feratogenic drugs administered to the mother in the early days of pregnancy. There is also a familial tendency to produce children with congenital abnormalities. But for the majority of the congenital deformities of limbs, the causative agent is unknown.

Management of children with multiple congenital limb deformities

The management of children with multiple congenital limb deformities varies with the type and severity of the deformities, depending on whether the deformities are in the upper limbs, the lower limbs or all 4 limbs. Management also depends on the child's personality and environment. Broadly speaking, the management should consider:

(1) The teaching and encouragement of compensatory movements and activities of the child's own body.

(2) The surgical correction of shape, size and position of the abnormal limbs, and of the stability of the deformed joints.

(3) The provision of supplementary or substitution appliances or prostheses.

(4) The supply of corrective appliances.

(5) The encouragement of an attitude of acceptance of the disability and a determination to achieve a superiority through academic, craft or artistic expertise.

(6) The support of the family's morale by the provision of a

definite centre which assumes the over-all responsibility for correlation of all the various aspects of the disabled child's care, and to which the family can appeal for advice and guidance.

(7) The integration of the disabled child into the most normal environment with which the disabilities are compatible, ensuring normal schooling and the maximum degree of independence at the earliest possible moment.

It is evident that the management of a child with multiple congenital limb deformities demands the closest co-operation between all those concerned in his care. The surgeon, physician, psychologist and prosthetist must integrate their treatments, and combine their skills if the child is not to spend unnecessary time in and between hospitals. Furthermore, close liaison with the school and local authorities will ensure that hospital attendances do not unnecessarily disrupt the educational programme.

Such management can only follow careful assessment at regular intervals. The assessment must be partly clinical, partly radiological and partly functional. Clinical and radiological review is needed to search for other congenital abnormalities. Functional assessment must be in realistic terms, and must integrate the parents, teachers and the children themselves in establishing current and future problems.

Many of these children do not need surgical or prosthetic intervention initially. Some do not need it at all. But as all children grow older and develop, their activities, interests and environment change, and at any stage a need for surgical correction, provision of an appliance or psychological assistance may become evident.

Teaching of compensatory movements and use of child's own body

If a child can use one part of his body to compensate for the deficiencies of another, he will choose to do this rather than accept a mechanical appliance supplied for the purpose. Children with normal lower limbs, and small or absent upper limbs, can usually learn to supplement the function of their arms by acquiring extra skill in their use of their feet and legs. Conversely, children with absent or phocomelic lower limbs are never able to use their upper limbs to compensate for their lower-limb deformities.

In the first group, therefore, training in the use of the feet should be started early, and should be as deliberate as any other form of training. Provided that the natural revulsion which parents and relatives feel can be overcome, children can be quickly trained to dress, feed, wash and cope with toilet activities, using only their feet.

Social acceptance depends more on dexterity than appearance, and the moment that a child can be independent of parental help, he is free to join in with the activities of normal children. Children admire skill. Although swift to observe differences and to criticize,

Figure 3.9. (a) Spoon and spork with cruciate handle; ((b) spoon in use; (b) reproduced by kind permission of the Editor, 'Occupational Therapy')

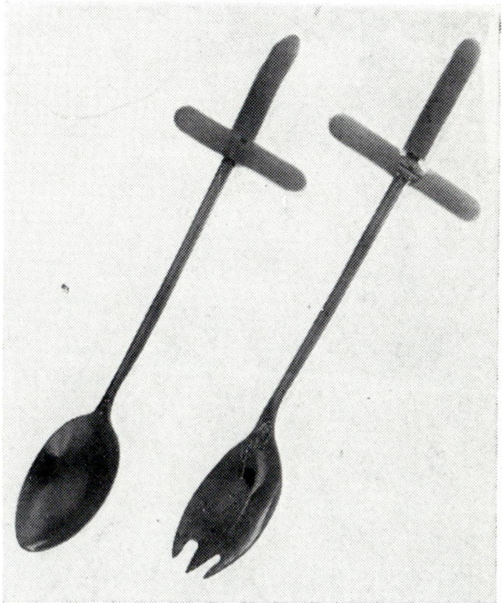

(*a*)

(*b*)

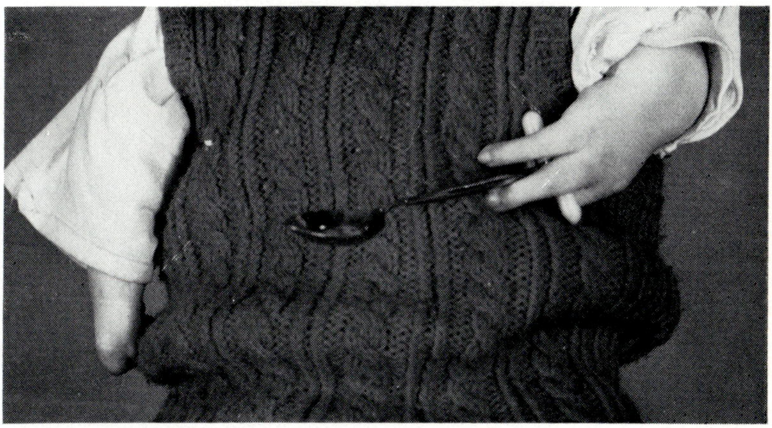

they will balance possibly hurtful remarks on the absence of hands and arms, with gratifying comments on the skill of feet and legs.

Children with absence or deformities of upper limbs learn a variety of grips, using shoulder tip and cheek, shoulder tip and mandible, teeth and lips. They also use their trunk position to balance themselves, becoming adept in the distribution of their weight on the

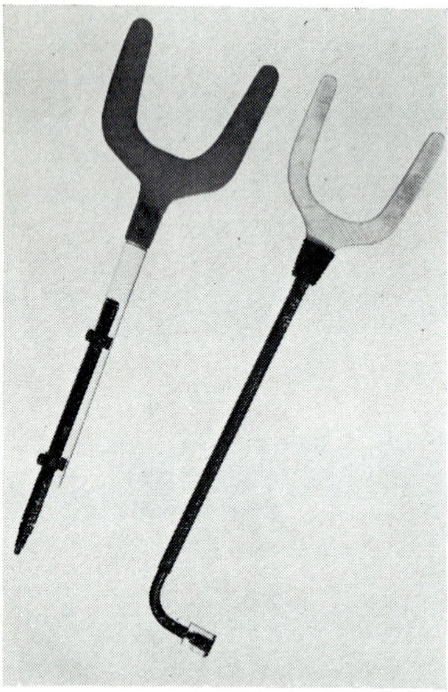

(*a*)

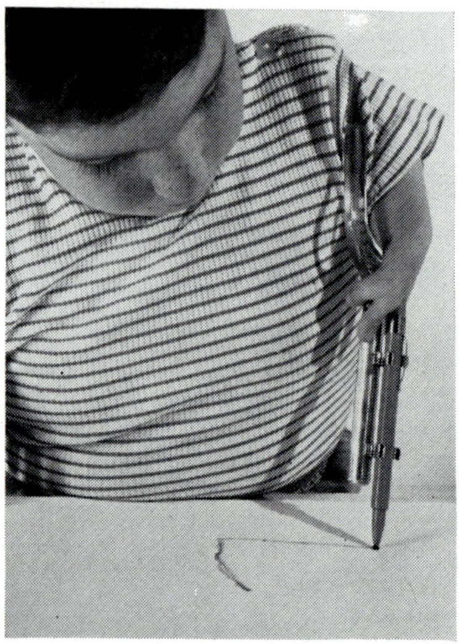

(*b*)

Figure 3.10. (a) Typing stick and pencil holder with horseshoe handle; (b) pencil holder in use

hips or feet. For the child with absent arms, all experience of texture and manipulation which usually comes through the hands, must come through the corresponding use of the feet. Such a child should therefore be allowed to run barefoot whenever possible.

Feeding with the feet is often more efficient than feeding with

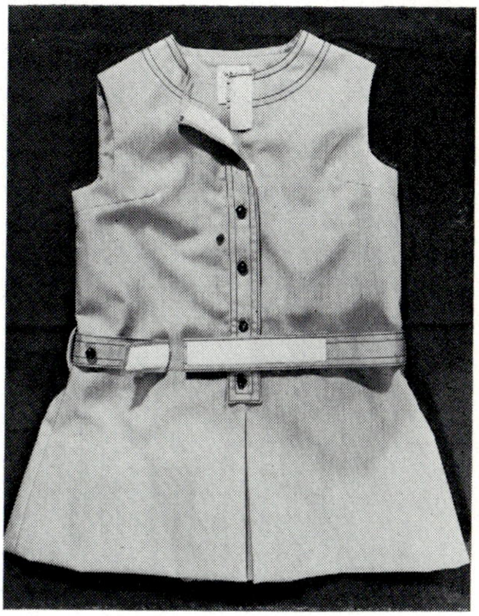

(*a*)

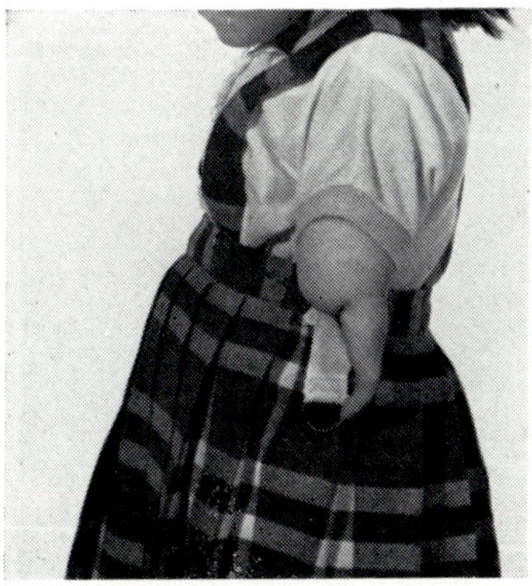

(*b*)

Figure 3.11. (*a*) *Off-the-peg dress with fastenings replaced by Velcro;* (*b*) *D-ring attached to webbing enables this pattern to open the side-vents which are fastened by Velcro; tapes prevent the vent from opening too far*

phocomelic arms provided with aids or appliances. For amelic children, it is not only more efficient but essential. In the presence of phocomelic arms, the nature of the problems which present depend upon the length and mobility of the upper limb remnants, and the available grip. Spoons or spoons with fork ends (sporks), either fitted with a swivel or shaped to a child's needs, are the commonest aids supplied. The addition of a cruciate handle to such an aid makes it suitable for children with two or three digits but no thumbs (*Figures 3.9, 3.10*).

When foot feeding is used, the relative heights of chair and table may need adjustment. A non-slip plate-mat, and a plate-guard are also helpful, and a hard-based, foam-filled, moquette-covered cushion makes an ideal surface for the foot-feeder to sit on. Foot feeding is not always socially acceptable in public eating-places, but when trousers are worn instead of mini-skirts, and when a quiet table at the side of the room is chosen, there can be little cause for complaint.

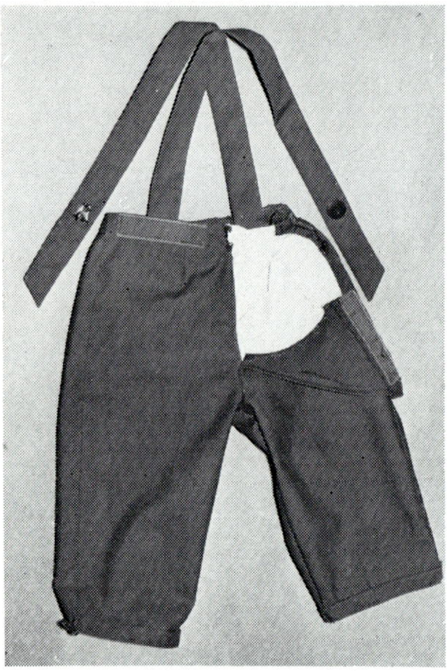

Figure 3.12. Trousers adapted for toilet independence, the legs are wider to accommodate prostheses, the waist is elasticated and Velcro used for all fastenings

Dressing with the feet is a more complicated process. Much of our clothing seems designed to defeat attempts to take it off or put it on. But with skilful adaptations, particularly regarding fastenings and openings, and with careful selection of design, it is possible to compile a wardrobe from which an amelic child may dress itself independently. Many articles may be 'off the peg', when advice is available to recommend necessary alterations; but often home-made clothes purpose-designed, are cheaper, better-made and more effective (*Figure 3.11*).

For girls, pinafore dresses and cloaks are particularly suitable, and for girls and boys alike, long trousers are ideal for covering calipers, and for allowing modesty and mobility to co-exist in the use of the legs. A front flap, or cod-piece in the trousers helps to simplify toilet regimen (*Figure 3.12*). Tightly-fitting pants and trousers are to be avoided, since loosely-fitting ones can be more easily pushed down with a toilet stick, or pulled down with the feet, using specially fixed loops. Pulling them up again is more difficult Sometimes the feet

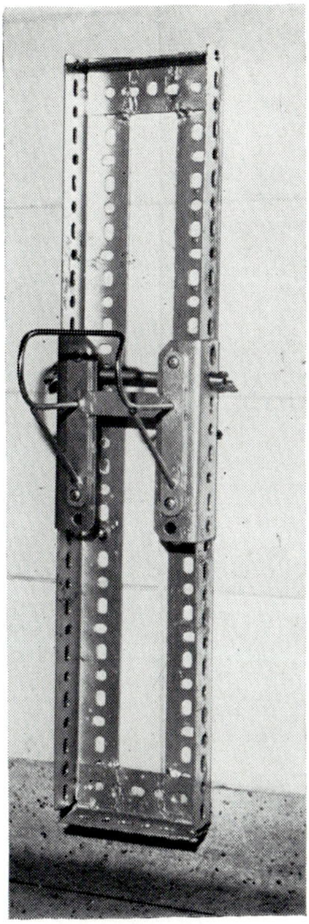

(*a*)

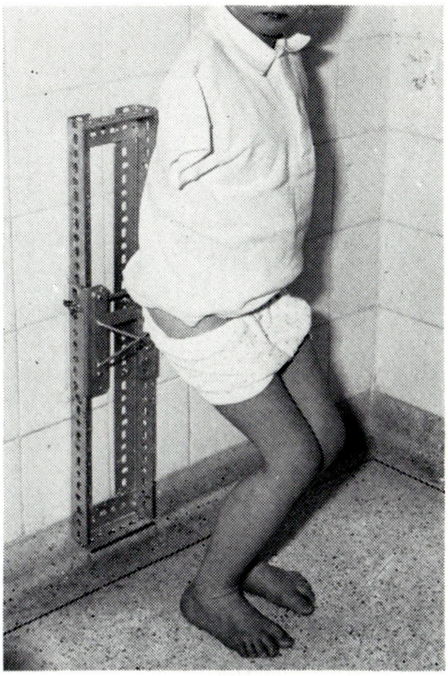

(*b*)

Figure 3.13.

(*a*) *A simple adjustable-height pant puller-upper;* (*b*) *a child with no arms using this device.* (*Reproduced by kind permission of the Editor, 'Occupational Therapy'*)

can cope. Sometimes a well-fixed hook on the wall is more helpful (*Figure 3.13*).

Socks with a separate compartment for the big toe keep the feet warm without impairing the grasp between big toe and second toe. Foot-users need careful selection of socks and shoes and the importance of avoiding secondary toe malformation from badly-shaped, ill-fitting footwear cannot be over-emphasized. For the child with amelia or short phocomelia of the upper limbs, the preservation of the feet in perfect functional condition is vital. Indoors, shoes should be chosen which can be taken off easily, but which do not slip off accidentally; 'flip-flop' sandals come into this category.

Managing the acts of micturition and defaecation with the attendant activities of undressing and dressing and perineal cleansing is a continual problem for the physically handicapped. Boys and girls with absence or severe reduction deformities of the upper limb can be

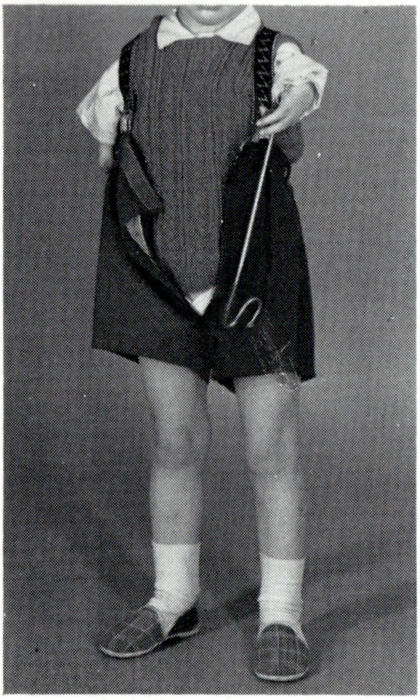

Figure 3.14. A small boy using a toilet stick. Note Velcro fastening on trousers.

trained to micturate standing astride a boat-shaped urinal or a stand of appropriate height.

Defaecation is better carried out while seated on a normal toilet seat, either on top of a superimposed frame surrounding a small central aperture, or else mounted on a low lavatory pedestal.

When phocomelic hands or useful digits are present, a toilet stick may be used for managing trousers in boys and girls, and for supporting the penis in boys (*Figure 3.14*). It may be used to assist perineal cleansing with toilet paper.

When children have upper-limb amelia, they can still be independent for toilet, if they learn to use their feet. Perineal cleanliness can usually be achieved by the sitting-on-the-heel technique with toilet paper, towels or other cleansing material being spread on the heel.

Attention to the diet and bowel habits is essential if the child is to attend normal school. The daily production of a soft, well-formed stool at a constant time, in a place where all facilities are optimal for independent defaecation, is the aim for such children. Regularity and rhythm and the production of conditioned reflexes can do a great deal to substitute for physical disability. A child who is certain of following a rhythm of activities which will lead to the passing of a daily stool before leaving home each morning, will be able to face a school day confident that he will not have to seek assistance from teachers or friends.

Some of the difficulties which exist for the child with upper-limb deformities also beset the child with deformities of the lower limbs. Dressing, washing, feeding and perineal cleansing do not usually present problems in the presence of normal or near- normal upper limbs. It is the locomotion involved in reaching the toilet and getting on and off which may be the barrier to personal independence in a child with severe lower-limb deformities.

Upper-limb prostheses

The provision of upper-limb prostheses is usually considered when there are rudimentary arms present of such length that small objects cannot be grasped bimanually, and when neither arm is able to reach the mouth for feeding purposes.

Prostheses of different types and complexity are fitted as the child grows and its intellect develops. In an attempt to follow normal behavioural patterns, simple, bilateral, cosmetic or 'pat-a-cake' prostheses are fitted at about 9 months, to accustom the child to wearing an appliance, and possibly to assist the development of sitting balance.

Active grip is introduced at about one year, but substituting prostheses in which paired, terminal hooks are operated either by cables which the child controls by body movement, or by power which he operates by switches. The power may be supplied by compressed gas, or else by electricity from a small portable battery.

Other movements, such as wrist rotation, are introduced as the child becomes capable of mastering the controls and the sequence of their use.

Experience has shown that although some children become adept in the use of upper-limb prostheses, they are rarely able to tolerate the prostheses for more than short periods at any one time. Furthermore, they tend at some of the various stages of their development to reject the prostheses. Children, like all other disabled patients, will usually prefer to use their own bodies whenever possible, rather than sophisticated devices designed to perform the same function. Over their bodies they have immediate and self-monitored control, which can often command and manipulate simple aids to add to its reach, increase its range of direct effect, and increase its mobility.

Lower-limb prostheses

The normal development of a child follows a constant pattern, in which movement complexes are acquired in a definite sequence. Thus sitting, standing, and walking are expressions of development, and each in turn makes further development possible. In all these processes, the vertical positioning of the spine is an important factor. The prostheses supplied for a child with congenital lower-limb deformities should enable him to correspond with, as far as possible, the movements of the lower limbs and position of the trunk at each stage of development of the normal child.

The usual basic orthopaedic principles of correcting deformities may be applied, and the techniques used may influence the design of the walking appliances supplied. The height will often depend on the child's competence and confidence, but should always be that which will give the child as near natural height as its body trunk size determines.

Prostheses for upper and lower limbs

Reduction deformities of all 4 limbs imposes a considerable physical and intellectual strain on a small child. The physical manoeuvres necessary to walk with bilateral lower-limb appliances are often considerably restricted by the presence of upper-limb appliances. The child's activities and needs have to be balanced and training-programmes phased to allow him to obtain practice with both sets of appliances separately and together. In some, upper-limb appliances are an aid to balance, whereas in others, they are a severe impediment.

Training

Adapted clothing, aids to daily living and training activities must be planned to fit with the child's normal expected development, and independent activities should, wherever possible, match the accepted stepping-stones of child's development. Once schooling starts, training in the use of an appropriate appliance should be part of formalized education in the school surroundings, and this demands close collaboration between therapists and teachers. The teacher does not need to be particularly orientated towards the physically handicaped. Children with limb deformities usually do better at normal schools than at schools for the physically handicapped unless they have all 4 limbs severely involved. Very often a normal school near home is more appropriate for a handicapped child than a school for the physically handicapped located further away, providing the child is not penalized by unsuitable classroom furniture, nor unduly physically fatigued. Each alteration either in clinical status or prosthetic status will reflect on the over-all pattern. Furthermore, as the child develops, its own personality will change; thus any prosthetic or training programme must be flexible. Continued reassessment is essential, and objective records of writing and the performance of other pre-arranged tasks which can be timed, or for which some degree of accuracy can be charted, are of more value than a clinical impression or answers to a questionnaire.

Acceptance and rejection of appliances

Acceptance and rejection of these appliances depend on 4 major factors.

(1) The mechanical efficiency of the appliance.

(2) The relative efficiency of the appliance compared to the child's own competence.

(3) Parental acceptance.

(4) School acceptance.

As has been earlier said, children with multiple congenital limb deformities achieve remarkable levels of manipulative skills using their residual upper limbs, chin, shoulder tip, feet and mouth. The wearing of an upper-limb prosthesis frequently hampers these skills, while only providing a much cruder form of function. For children with absent or deformed legs, almost any form of lower-limb appliance gives them an immediate advantage either in standing, achieving reasonable height and, as a bonus, walking short distances. The almost complete acceptance of lower-limb appliances from an early age indicates that if an appliance fulfils a real need, even if inefficiently, the appliance will be accepted.

In general, patients must obtain an immediate advantage from an appliance for it to be accepted. The immediate post-fitting phase is of great importance. If the appliance looks unfinished, if the technicians have to fiddle with the fittings, if it is uncomfortable or scratchy, if the mother's face registers horror at the appearance, the child will often react by rejecting the appliance. If the antagonistic features outweigh the advantages, then acceptance is unlikely, or at best partial and more a matter of deference to authority, or part of a game, rather than a true integration of the appliance into the body image. For full acceptance, the advantage gained must outweigh all the antagonistic factors. If this occurs quickly, the child will persist through further stages of fitting, training and redevelopment.

Cosmesis is often a motivating force in acceptance of any appliance, and can occasionally extend to a pathological acceptance, the child insisting on wearing an artificial limb of no functional value.

Education

As the children grow older, education in its widest sense assumes a greater importance and it is incumbent on therapists to keep pace with the children's progress at school, and close liaison between

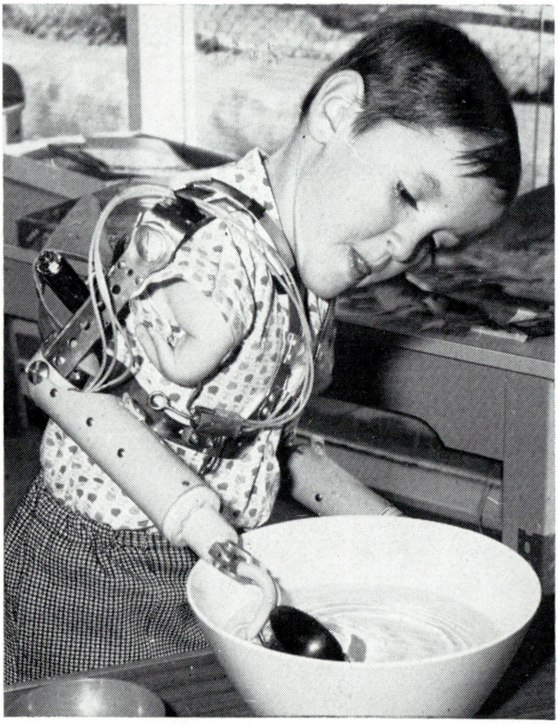

Figure 3.15. An upper limb gas-powered appliance. Trunk movements compensate for lack of arm movements

school, hospital, and welfare services is essential at this stage. All children want to write, draw and paint. Simple writing aids can readily be devised to suit the individual child, when necessary.

The upper-limb amelic will learn to draw with mouth, feet, or prostheses. In the latter case, the prosthesis often provides little more than a means of reaching out and holding the writing appliance. The manipulation is mainly achieved by trunk movements. *Figure 3.15* shows a small boy wearing an upper-limb gas-powered appliance comprising a metal-frame jacket; friction elbow joint; double-acting wrist rotators; right gas-powered hook; left gas-powered hand.

Undoubtedly, much time and effort can be wasted in teaching

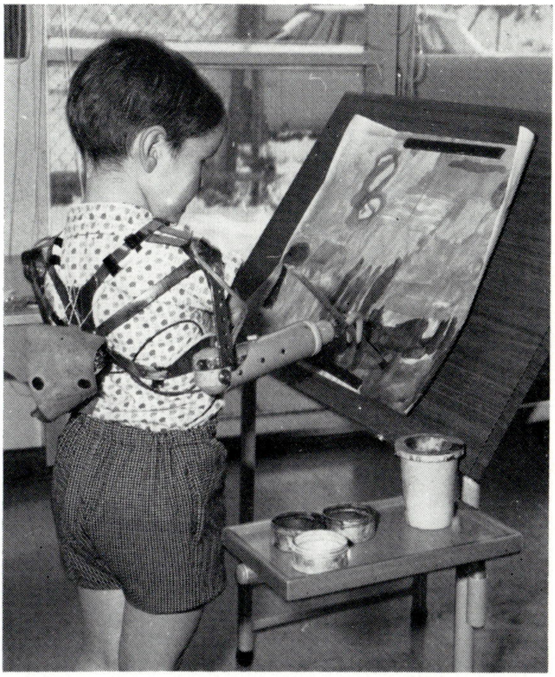

Figure 3.16. A tilting desk with side tray and non-spill water container (Reproduced by kind permission of the Editor, 'Occupational Therapy')

the severely disabled to write when the use of mechanical aids such as an electric typewriter, an electric adding machine and teaching machines produce the same end-results more efficiently and more quickly with less expenditure of effort and frustration.

However, self-expression is essential in the early stages and considerable ingenuity may be needed to produce acceptable results. A suitable desk which is adjustable in height and angle has metal under its Formica surface, thus magnets can be used to stabilize paper and book. It has a small tray also at the side for paints, pencils and suchlike (*Figure 3.16*).

Case history No. 332 illustrates the remarkable independence of a child with 4 congenital amputations who was independent except for feeding when first admitted. This independence was achieved by simple aids. The other case history in this section illustrates the independence which a child with upper limb amelia can achieve.

M.M.L. No. 332 born 1954 male

Diagnosis: Multiple congenital abnormalities

This boy was born with congenital abnormalities of all 4 limbs. He has a below-knee congenital amputation of the right leg and a deformed left foot with syndactyly. He has worn a below-knee conventional prosthesis since early childhood and walked well. The

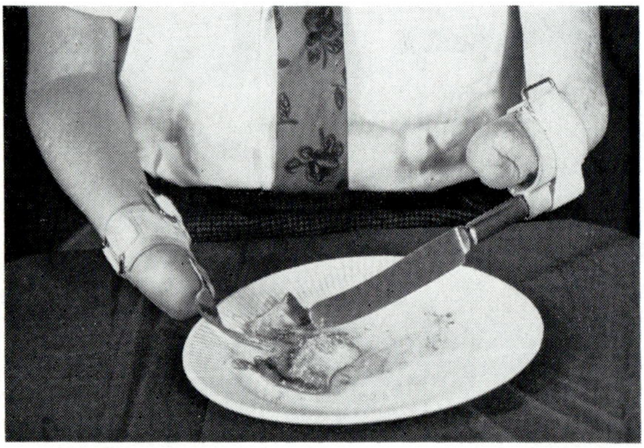

Figure 3.17(a). Patient No. 332 using simple aids to control knife and fork

right arm has a congenital amputation at the level of the wrist and the left arm had a congenital amputation at the elbow. All his clothing was adapted using Velcro or zips with long tags for fastening instead of buttons.

He was independent except for the ability to use a knife and fork.

Although he was supplied with conventional upper limb prostheses, he rarely wore them as they impeded his activities in all spheres. He preferred to use his stumps and a simple leather cuff or a writing aid, according to his need.

As he had a small, mobile, below-elbow fragment in the left arm, an attempt was made to give him a longer below-elbow stump by means of a bone graft and a skin graft. Eventually a below-elbow stump of nearly 3 inches in length was produced. This proved to be very mobile and useful for him, but it was not stable enough to risk fitting a conventional below-elbow prosthesis. Instead, simple cuff

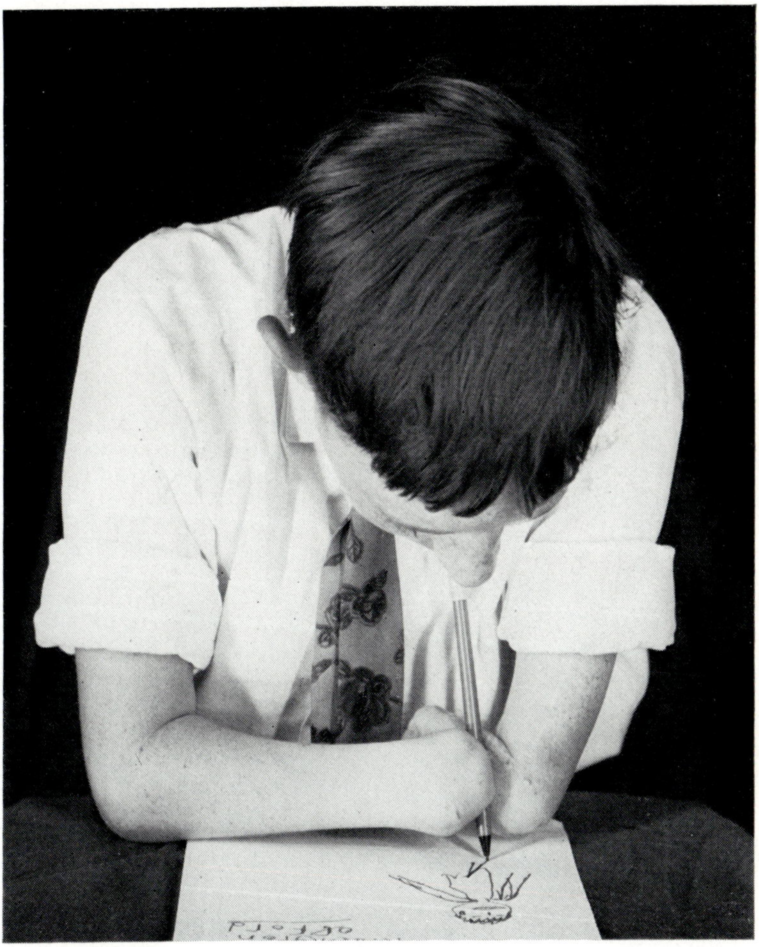

Figure 3.17(b). Right through wrist stump and left below-elbow stump to control a pencil

appliances were supplied and allowed him to use cutlery in a natural bimanual fashion. With D-rings and Velcro, he was able to apply and remove the appliances himself. He was now completely independent (*Figure 3.17*).

M.M.L. No. C32 born 1962 male

Diagnosis: Upper-limb amelia

This boy was born with absent upper limbs, associated with thalidomide. He attended the Disabled Living Unit regularly for the fitting of artificial limbs, starting with a simple powered 'pat-a-cake'

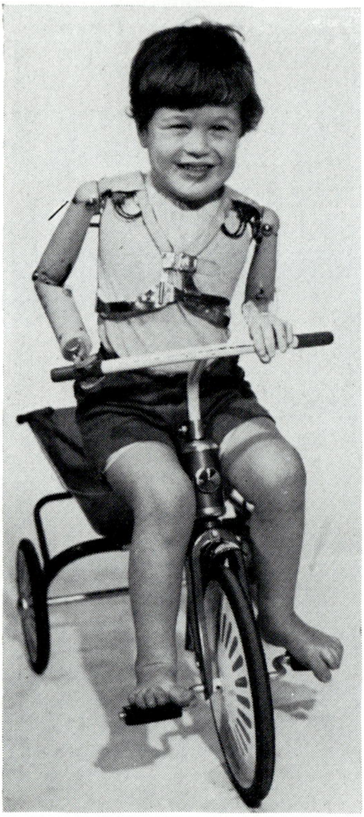

Figure 3.18. Patient No. C32 aged $4\frac{1}{2}$ years using gas-powered artificial arms for riding a tricycle

appliance when about a year old. From this, he graduated to gas-powered artificial arms with a wrist rotation movement, and an active powered hook or hand. He used the arms for writing and drawing and riding a tricycle (*Figure 3.18*). He started attending a nursery school at 3 years of age and then was admitted to a normal primary school at the age of 5 years.

He was always more adept with his feet than with his powered arms which he undoubtedly found a nuisance under many circumstances. However, by continually finding activities which he enjoyed and could accomplish only with the arms, he continued to use them and practiced with them for about 2 hours each day. One of his great interests is gardening, and he can use rakes and watering appliances with the arms; also he can wheel a wheelbarrow. He uses his feet for potting plants and holds other tools with his chin.

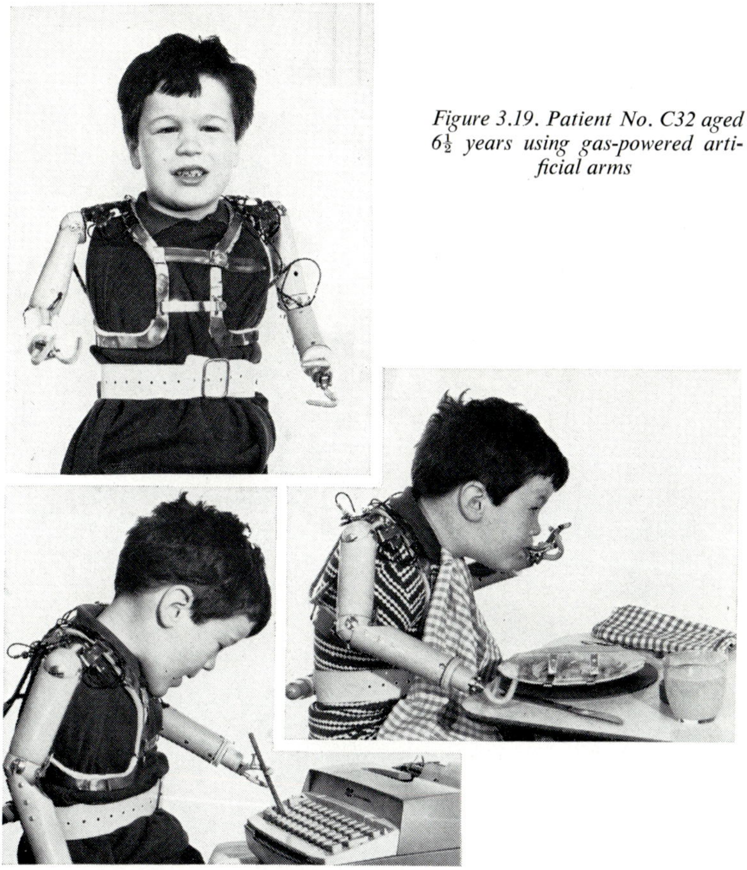

Figure 3.19. Patient No. C32 aged 6½ years using gas-powered artificial arms

School was an important step. When he started there was some natural reluctance on the part of the staff to accept responsibility for such an apparently severely handicapped child. However, visits to the Unit to see him being trained to use both feet and powered arms and the review of a film of his progress, convinced the teachers that he was indeed remarkably independent. He had been quite

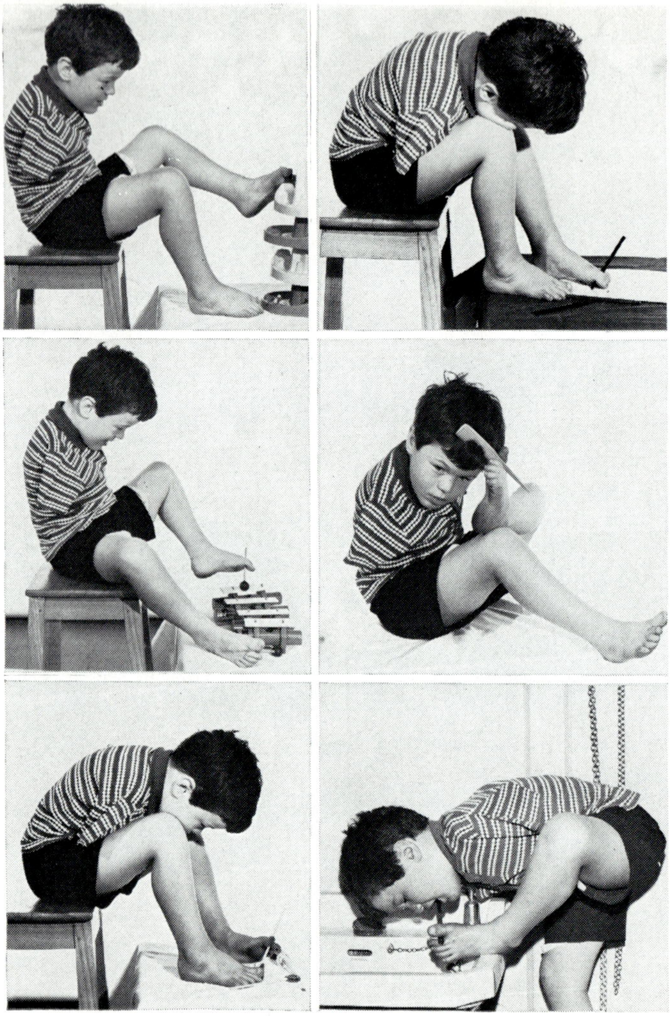

Figure 3.20. Patient No. C32 aged 6½ years using his feet

See p. 131 for Figure 3.20 continued

independent for dressing (with adaptations to his trousers and underclothes) for a year or so, and he was rapidly accepted and integrated into the school. (*Figures 3.19* and *3.20*).

It is noticeable to all concerned that there is a continual conflict between his natural preference to be without the powered arms, to

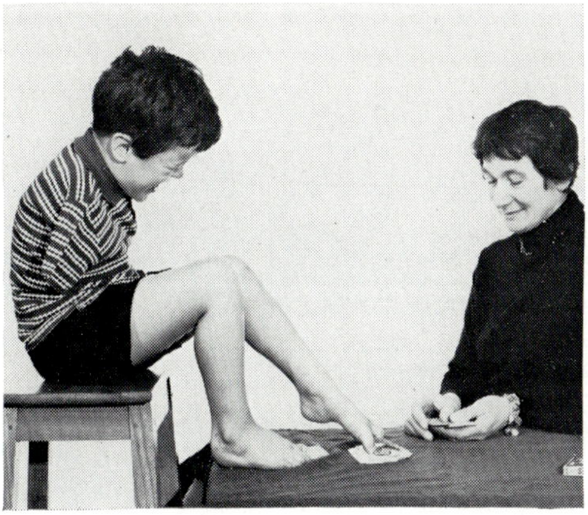

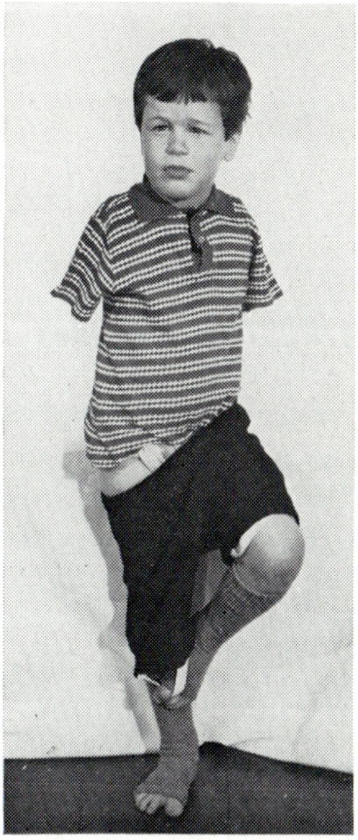

Figure 3.20 continued—Patient No. C32 aged 6½ years using his feet

use his feet or mouth to get direct contact and control, and the need to keep him in practice with artificial arms, without forcing a total rejection. By skilful and patient encouragement at school and at home, a balance is being maintained, so that when further advances are made with the design of powered limbs, or he needs the artificial limbs for specific activities, he will have the necessary skill available to manipulate them.

4—General Care and Nursing Problems

INTRODUCTION

The severely disabled are often difficult to manage both physically and psychologically. The chronic nature of their disability makes it even more difficult to assess the significance of changes in symptoms and signs. Many of their problems may appear to be of a minor nature compared with their main disability. Furthermore, most severely disabled are being cared for at home or in institutions which provide only general care, and the time, experience and facilities for sorting out some of the problems may not be readily available.

They present many problems of general care, nursing and physical management. A disability interacts upon another function and often the patient appears to present a vicious circle of problems. It is, therefore, important to establish good simple management routines wherever possible within the patient's own control. Even more relevant for the severely disabled, each therapeutic attack must be carefully assessed for its possible effect on other functions and great care taken to avoid unnecessary iatrogenic dysfunction particularly of the circulatory, respiratory, gastrointestinal, urogenital and nervous systems.

For example, many disabled are anaemic. In some instances (for example, rheumatoid arthritis), anaemia is part of the pathology of the underlying disability, but most severely disabled are taking analgesics and the majority of these have been implicated in the causation of anaemia through multiple haemorrhages into the gastrointestinal tract. Furthermore, many severely disabled patients are not able to look after themselves adequately and cannot buy, prepare, cook or eat a sufficiently nutritious diet.

Most wheelchair-bound patients develop postural oedema of the ankles, and many of them are unnecessarily provided with diuretics. It is not infrequent that mild attacks of potassium insufficiency ensue and produce weakness which may be ascribed to the patient's major diability. Nausea, anorexia and weakness may also follow digitalis intoxication and remain unnoticed in a patient with weakness due to other causes.

It is apparent that the difficulties in diagnosis arise because in a patient already severely physically disabled with a locomotor disorder, there is a multiplicity of possible causes for their symptoms. They may arise from the underlying disorder, from the therapy applied for that disorder or from unrelated disorders.

This chapter attempts to describe some of the problems of the severely disabled which are amenable to relatively simple measures.

PAIN

Many of the severely disabled suffer no pain, but pain may be part of the physical disability (rheumatoid arthritis) or a product of increasing physical deformity (backache of scoliosis in muscular dystrophy).

When physical movements are severely restricted, common muscular aches and pains cannot be worked off and may assume an exaggerated importance to the patient. Furthermore, it is frequently difficult or inconvenient for the severely disabled to obtain help or advice. Assistance is not available for affecting a change of position, attendance at a surgery may be physically impossible and a doctor's call be considered unwarranted. The chronically disabled are often reluctant to bother the doctor lest they be labelled 'chronic' or 'difficult', and so minor disabilities are lost in the problems of the major disability. Thus, warning signs of impending trouble may be missed.

A man aged 40 years with poliomyelitis was severely disabled and confined to a wheelchair. His legs were virtually flail and his shoulder girdle weak. He worked full-time as a graduate scientist but for several years had complained of increasing backache. His general practitioner had ascribed this to his poor posture associated with a kyphoscoliosis. However, the pain persisted and was beginning to interfere with his work. When admitted to the Disabled Living Unit for complete functional assessment, radiography revealed a hitherto unsuspected ankylosing spondylitis. Normal physical examination for this condition was impossible, and the characteristic morning pain easing off during the day with activity was not present as his only activity was minimal wheelchair propelling. Phenylbutazone 100 mg 3 times a day relieved all symptoms in a matter of days and he was then maintained symptom-free on 100 mg twice a day.

A woman aged 27 years with severe deformities and joint stiffness from juvenile rheumatoid arthritis complained of persistent and increasing pain in the right buttock while sitting in her wheelchair. This had been variously ascribed to sciatica, recurrence of active arthritis and incipient pressure sores. She obtained no relief from sitting on a sheepskin or a soft sorbo-rubber cushion. Her fixity and inability to alter her position in her chair had led to increasing discomfort and inability to work or concentrate because of the pain in her buttock. After a trial injection of hydrocortisone into the tender area, producing dramatic relief of pain, surgical exploration was considered warranted, and a large bursa was removed with permanent relief of symptoms.

Pain in rheumatoid arthritis poses many problems and the expectation of pain on joint activity is a potent source of physical disability. The patient is reluctant to attempt activities which are likely to cause pain. Adequate regular medication with aspirin, indomethacin, or phenylbutazone coupled with simple splinting, may reduce pain on activity and enable functional assessment and rehabilitation to proceed. Assessment without adequate preliminary treatment will give a false measure of the patient's likely capabilities. It is only upon the foundation of adequate general medication and conservative management that realistic plans for independence can be made, and the need for surgical intervention determined.

A middle-aged lady had considerable pain in her shoulders and arms in spite of adequate prolonged medication. The symptoms were found to be directly related to her method of getting in and out of chairs which involved pushing and pulling. Full assessment of her activities and possible alternatives in the context of adequate general care and medication dictated a surgical plan for the relief of symptoms; synovectomy of the left shoulder and excision arthroplasty of the left elbow to achieve one mobile arm for feeding and personal care and stabilization of the right arm to facilitate pushing and pulling for her transfers.

This illustrates many of the problems of pain in severe disability; the physical handicap determines certain patterns of activity which cannot be altered, whereas for the non-disabled alternative patterns can be found. If these activities are the source of pain, other remedies have to be sought. The patient may have to change from walking with aids and appliances to using a wheelchair, or from a self-propelled wheelchair to an electrically propelled indoor chair. Alternatively, it may take major surgical intervention to provide the solution. For example, many patients with widespread muscular weakness develop a collapsing scoliosis with consequent impairment of respiratory function, disturbance of digestion and backache.

Perhaps more of these patients should be submitted to spinal fusion, even if the disability is progressive, as a means of preventing intractable pain and inevitable dysfunction of several systems.

INDIGESTION

Many severely disabled patients suffer from indigestion. The symptoms are often associated with marked deformity (such as scoliosis), weakness or paralysis of the abdominal musculature, or paralysis of the diaphragm. Asymmetry or muscle imbalance appear to be important aetiological factors whether from weakness or from spasticity. In some patients the symptoms are related to dietary indiscretion or the unsuitable diets which the severely disabled often indulge in, but often the symptoms are associated with oesophageal reflux. Discomfort or heartburn after meals may be present, but the typical postural relationship of the pain may be more difficult to elicit than in the physically able.

However, pain occurring when lying down or when straining to propel a wheelchair (similar to the bending forward position of the able-bodied) may indicate the nature of the condition. Some severely disabled become markedly overweight, another aetiological factor in producing oesophageal reflux and hiatus herniation.

The physical background of this cause of indigestion is other aggravating factors. Many severely disabled are taking drugs which are known gastric irritants; salicylates and butazolidine and indomethacin in particular. Furthermore, the chronically disabled are so used to tablet taking that many do not bother to crush their tablets or to take them with milk or during meals, in spite of repeated instructions.

Spasticity or spasms such as are present in many neurological lesions add to the frequency of increased intra-abdominal pressure in an uncontrolled fashion. Coughing and vomiting are other potent causes of raised intra-abdominal pressure. Thus, the severely disabled should always be advised to take their analgesics with milk, and to avoid obesity. Those with symptoms may well gain relief from simple measures such as milk drinks with antacids between meals (suitable ones are available as mixtures with dried whole milk in tablet form).

Aluminium hydroxide gel or magnesium trisilicate after meals often relieve the post-prandial indigestion. The severely disabled frequently have to pay more attention to their bowels than the able-bodied; aluminium hydroxide tends to produce some degree of constipation whereas magnesium trisilicate tends to produce loose motions. The antacid can therefore be chosen for its most suitable effect on the bowels.

A suspension of surface anaesthesia in an alkaline gel (Mucaine) taken before meals helps when acute oesophagitis is present. For patients with nausea and vomiting exacerbating the symptoms (for example post-operatively) then perphenazine or a similar tranquillizer is helpful. Severely disabled patients with oesophageal reflux who are subjected to surgical procedures are particularly prone to acute indigestion in the post-operative period.

M.M.L. No. 1036 born 1950 male

Diagnosis: Poliomyelitis

This young man had a generalized attack of acute anterior poliomyelitis with respiratory involvement at the age of 4 years. He was left with widespread muscle weakness and wasting involving all 4 limbs; but particularly his legs, and also his trunk. He lives a wheelchair life and has worn a spinal support since childhood. He was referred to the Disabled Living Unit at the age of 18 years, particularly for advice on hoisting and to attempt to increase his personal independence prior to planning further education and training for work.

He had a severe kyphoscoliosis and his vital capacity was 600 ml while sitting upright and 700 ml lying down.

While in the Unit, it became clear that he was suffering from quite severe indigestion, with vomiting, each morning. Inquiry revealed that these symptoms had been present for many months and he had increasing attacks of heartburn. Barium swallow revealed that the oesophagus was slightly dilated and there was a reflex from the stomach.

Symptoms did not respond to antacids, but when the head end of his bed was raised, so that he was sleeping in a half-reclining position, the symptoms rapidly disappeared. Twelve months later he was still symptom-free.

COLD FEET

Many of the severely disabled who spend much of their time in the sitting position with their legs dependent and motionless, complain of cold, blue, swollen feet and ankles.

This set of symptoms can be distressing for a variety of reasons.

(1) When sensation is present, both coldness and swelling of the tissues can separately cause discomfort and even pain.

(2) Whether or not sensation is present, but particularly if it is

deficient or absent, minor traumata to the skin of the feet and ankles from the wheelchair and furniture are likely to cause abrasion and persistent ulceration.

(3) When the swelling is sufficiently great to prevent the wearing of shoes suitable for the purpose, standing becomes difficult or even impossible, calipers cannot be utilized, and the mobility needed for normal activities is reduced.

There are several contributory factors causing these symptoms, and it is by the control of these factors that the condition is best treated. The dependent posture and immobility of the legs and feet are the main synergistic conditions which diminish venous return, by increasing the effect of gravity and decreasing the assistance given by muscular activity to the circulation.

When respiratory insufficiency is present, and tissue hypoxia results, ankle oedema and cyanosis are further increased.

Lastly, any of the conditions producing such symptoms in an able person, such as cardiac or renal insufficiency, may equally well be present in a disabled person.

The most useful treatments of the condition are physical measures to counteract the precipitating physical factors. Thus, raising the foot of the bed by about 6 in (15 cm) at night, resting on the bed after lunch, elevating the legs for at least part of the day by use of elevating footrests if chairbound, or of footstools for both ambulant and wheelchair patients, all help to counteract the effects of prolonged dependence.

The regular exercise of any muscles in the leg and foot which remain active, however few or weak, and the use of the feet to assist in wheelchair propulsion (unless contra-indicated by some other circumstances) will increase venous return.

The use of tubular stretch bandages (Tubigrip), elastic stockings or elastic bandages, if applied before the patient gets out of bed, will limit the swelling by providing a mechanical resistance to its development. But few disabled patients have the strength or agility needed to apply the supports and their use is further limited by the fact that they may prevent the wearing of a normal shoe.

For those who, being chair-bound, do not need special shoes for standing or walking, sheepskin boots with long zips are probably more useful than bandaging, being more easily put on, and more effective in preventing heat loss and protecting the feet and legs from minor injuries.

General measures which can help prevent or minimize the development of cold, blue, swollen feet and ankles are weight control and regular deep breathing. Obesity further disables the patient by increasing the load which muscle action must move, and increasing the load on an often precarious cardiovascular system. Fat deposition in the abdomen further impedes circulation by increasing the intra-abdominal pressure and so obstructing both venous return from the lower limbs and the action of the diaphragm. By deep breathing exercises, diaphragmatic excursion and therefore venous return is facilitated.

Treatment of oedema of the legs by the use of a diuretic is usually contra-indicated in a disabled patient, unless an indwelling catheter or other incontinence appliances avoids the need for regular micturition, or the patient is sufficiently able to manage the frequent swift transfers necessary to reach urinal or toilet after the exhibition of the diuretic. If diuretics are given, it is important that regular serum potassium estimations be made, and potassium supplements given when necessary. Otherwise, fatigue and muscular weakness due to potassium deficiency may well be attributed to the progress of the disabling disease.

The usefulness of vasodilator drugs is difficult to evaluate. If and when arterial spasm is implicated in the production of the symptoms, tolazoline hydrochloride (Priscol) 25–50 mg 3 times a day, or isoxsuprine hydrochloride (Duvadilan) 10–20 mg 3 times a day may help in their prevention.

PRESSURE SORES

Pressure sores, whether superficial or deep, occur when external pressure obstructs the blood supply to the skin and underlying tissues to a degree sufficient to cause tissue death. They may occur in any patient who is confined to bed with an immobilizing disease, during drug-induced sleep, during prolonged purposeful immobilization, or during voluntary immobility, in fact in any patient who is unable to record or respond to the warning sensation of pain or discomfort which is induced by prolonged pressure on any part of the body, by effecting or requesting a change of posture.

Predisposing factors to the development of pressure-sores are senility, mental deterioration, confusion, poor general physical condition, unconsciousness, limitation of mobility and incontinence. Since these factors tend to coexist in geriatric patients, it is among the elderly that pressure sores are most often seen, particularly in patients with neurological rather than traumatic disorders.

The type of pressure sore which arises depends upon the state of the patient and the duration of the stimulus which produces it. Thus, superficial sores tend to develop from minor traumata, such as friction from rucked sheets or knocks against the wheelchairs or bed and from maceration of the skin from sweat or incontinence, whereas shearing forces over the sacrum and trochanter due to the body tending to slide down in bed or wheelchair may precipitate deep lesions.

Theoretically all pressure sores are preventable, as indicated by the low incidence of pressure sores in Spinal Injury Units, where prophyllactic treatment is intense and unremitting. Strict nursing routine with regular hourly or 2-hourly turning, use of turning beds or Stryker frames, strict attention to pressure areas, careful smoothing of sheets, bedclothes or underwear, prevention of maceration of the skin from incontinence or sweat, distribution of pressure about the skin by sheepskins or ripple mattresses are all important active measures in prevention. But the shortage of nursing staff and the lack of expensive equipment in many institutions caring for the severely disabled, makes it inevitable that a proportion of patients will develop pressure sores. To a certain extent this shortage may be mitigated by use of trained, non-nursing personnel to assist in regular turning, particularly at night, when prolonged periods of unrelieved pressure otherwise occur.

This regular alteration of position limits the actual duration of pressure on any one part. The amount of pressure may be limited by use of a bed-cradle or well padded foot-board to take the weight of the bedclothes. The distribution of pressure may be partly controlled by the use of sheepskin or ripple mattresses and cushions, with sheepskin bootees or ring pads of covered rolled foam applied to bony prominences.

Regular daily inspection of the skin of the seriously disabled is the responsibility initially of the nursing staff, and finally whenever possible, of the patient himself, so that redness, swelling, blistering, excoriation or other warning signs of skin damage may be rapidly treated and their cause eliminated.

It must be urged on patients, attendants and relatives alike that where serious disability exists, rehabilitation is as long-lasting as the disease responsible for the disability. And the measures for preventing the development of bed-sores can therefore never be discontinued, although some of them may be relaxed if and when there is some recovery of sensation or mobility.

The value of local applications in the prevention of pressure sores is not proven. Soap and water, or spirit and talcum powder, or zinc and oil-rich cream all have their advocates; but there is no statistical evidence that any of these treatments has any real effect. Talcum powder tends to block the pores. Spirit reduces the skin's natural oiliness. Perhaps one of the most important aspects of the traditional 'back' treatment regimen was its provision of a regular daily inspection of the skin areas at greatest risk, and a beneficial change of posture.

Medical sheepskins

Medical sheepskins have a wide use in the prevention and management of pressure sores, particularly for those severely disabled patients who are being cared for at home. The skins are specially selected, preferably from Merino or Merino-type sheep with dense fleece and soft springy wool. The fleece is left long at shearing and the skin retained intact. It is then tanned so that the final sheepskin contains chromic oxide to 4·5 per cent of the de-greased, de-wooled, oven-dried skin and the tanned leather should not shrink when immersed in boiling water for 1 minute. The skins are then usually dyed with neutral pre-metallized or acid-milling dyes which are fast to washing and perspiration. Finally, the wool is clipped to a uniform length of 1 in (2·54 cm).

Synthetic fleeces do not appear to have the same qualities of resilience and water absorption as the natural fleeces and are rarely as successful in the prevention of pressure sores.

Medical sheepskins can be used fleecy side uppermost for lying on or sitting on. The patient can lie directly on the wool, and it has been recommended that pressure sores be left open. The wool fibres distribute the patient's weight over a large area, thus reducing the tendency to produce localized pressure points. The sheepskin will absorb up to one-third of its own weight of water before it begins to feel moist. The deep pile allows air to circulate and helps to keep the patient's skin dry. The springiness of the fibres tends to eliminate abrasion if the patient turns or moves and the leather backing tends to prevent sitting patients from slipping down into a recumbent position.

There is no evidence that there is any particular risk to the patient of infection from the sheepskin itself. In fact, the contrary seems likely as the fibres are firmly adherent and tanning makes them resistant to bacterial invasion. Soiling from incontinent patients is a nuisance and entails frequent laundering but does not otherwise harm a good medical sheepskin. Laundering is important and should be done once a week or more frequently for patients who are sweating heavily or have open pressure sores. The method of laundering and cleansing is given in Appendix U.

A medical sheepskin can be used in bed for the patient to lie on or as a fitted cover for a cushion in a wheelchair. It is often simplest for the patient to transfer the same skin from bed to chair and vice versa. It is always advisable to supply two skins so that one can always be in use while the other is being laundered. Small fragments of the sheepskin make excellent protection for heels and elbows if these are prone to breakdown from pressure.

Treatment of established pressure sores

When pressure sores have occurred and have become established, specific measures of curative treatment must be added to the continued prophyllactic measures. This local treatment aims at the prevention of infection and the promotion of healing.

The most important factors in preventing infection are the use of a scrupulous non-touch technique for dressing the sore and the employment of mild antiseptics and dressings, which do not stick to and damage any granulation tissue present. Eusol, boric solution 4 per cent, Dakin's solution 8 per cent or gentian violet are variously recommended, but the antiseptic chosen should depend upon the sensitivity of the patient and the state of the surrounding skin at any one time.

In the promotion of healing, the general condition of the patient needs to be assessed, and any necessary treatment instigated. Anaemia and diabetes are two causes of delayed healing of pressure sores, and their existence, if suspected, may be easily confirmed by appropriate laboratory investigation. A blood transfusion, intramuscular injections of iron or oral iron, in conjunction with a high protein diet containing an adequate amount of the factors promoting haemopoiesis may be indicated as treatment for the anaemia. Institution of insulin therapy and a controlled diet will stabilize the blood-sugar of the diabetic patient and in both cases healing will be encouraged.

Should infection occur despite prophyllactic measures, the sore must be swabbed and any infecting organisms cultured. A course of systemic antibiotics is far more effective than an application of a local antibiotic in the treatment of such infection. When the sore is very deep a chronic osteomyelitis may develop, and in this instance, wide debridement, sequestrectomy and skin-grafting will probably be needed.

For those sores which are indolent and slow to heal, ultra-violet light may stimulate the production of granulation tissue and have a beneficial antibiotic effect. Ultra-violet probes in sinuses or undercut edges of sores may also be effective in the encouragement of healing, with or without cauterization of the sore edge by silver nitrate. Light frictional massage round the edge of the sore with lanolin or other bland creams may help reduce induration and assist revascularization.

SPASTICITY AND SPASMS

Present knowledge of the mechanism of spasticity is still incomplete, and much of the experimental work on animals cannot be directly applied to man. The clinical condition of spasticity is a variable feature depending on the level and the severity of the lesion in the spinal cord and is based on the two main reflex patterns determined by the functional organization within the spinal cord. The stretch reflexes which subserve the main posture and locomotor activities are dependent on afferent and efferent arcs quite separate from the general flexion reflex which subserves the withdrawal of a limb and its protection against injury. Recent work on the muscle spindle distinguishes between its sensitivity to active stretch (a dynamic or phasic sensitivity) and its sensitivity to maintained tension (a static sensitivity) and indicates that these sensitivities are conveyed separately by different groups of afferent fibres of varying size and conductivity.

The stretch reflex originates in the annulospinal ring of the muscle spindles which lie between and parallel to the main muscle fibres, and participate in their attachments and activities. These spindles are connected via large afferent fibres, through a monosynaptic loop to motor fibres innervating the main muscle fibres. Spindle afferents are inhibited by active muscle contraction and activated by passive stretch. Muscle shortening continues reflexly until it balances that of the spindle. The spindle sensitivity is controlled by the separate, so-called, gamma-loop system, controlled by the recticular formation and higher brain centres. The flexion reflex is a polysynaptic reflex essentially nociceptive in its response and controlled by secondary smaller afferent fibres with slower conduction rates (Group II fibres). These reflexes play an important role in walking, based on afferents from the sole of the foot, and, if the stimulus is of sufficient strength a co-ordinated withdrawal of the leg by flexion at hip and knee occurs, accompanied by a crossed extension response in the contralateral leg.

During walking there is integrated interplay between the polysynaptic movement reflexes and the monosynaptic postural reflexes, integrating sensory input from the skin, joints and sensory receptors in muscles. The interplay between these 2 groups of reflexes may be disturbed by local lesions, damage to the spinal cord or damage to the higher centres. In damage to the spinal cord short of complete transection, some of the vestibulospinal and reticulospinal tracts may escape injury, thus retaining some suprasegmental influence on the muscle spindles. In the patient with a complete cervical lesion, the interplay is totally disturbed and the stretch reflex is of spinal origins only, no central tone being left. The action of the stretch reflex is postponed until sufficient passive stretch is reached. In the paraplegics, slight stimulation may provoke a severe flexor reflex and marked flexion contractures often occur spontaneously.

Afferent stimuli from viscera, such as the bladder and from joints and tendons, and stimuli associated with infection or wounds, such as pressure sores can influence the interplay when there is partial or complete destruction of the cord.

Before embarking upon treatment of spasticity, it is necessary to eliminate the source of nociceptive stimuli such as an ingrowing toenail, infected bladder, pressure sores, haemorrhoids or even duodenal ulcers or gall-stones.

Drug treatment

Many drugs have been tried in the past in attempts to relieve spasticity with little effect, but diazepam (Valium), an analogue of chlordiazepoxide (Librium) has been widely used on an empirical basis over the past few years. It appears to act partly by releasing emotional tension and partly through a direct action on the polysynaptic reflexes. The usual regimen is to start the patient on 2 mg of diazepam 3–4 times a day, increasing the evening dose and the midday dose. The final regimen is often in the order of 16–24 mg at night and 6–8 mg at midday. Some authorities advise doses considerably higher than this, even as much as 200–300 mg; the dose being increased until the required effect is produced. Many patients doubt the value of the drug until it is withdrawn, and then they appreciate how much improvement there has been. But it is difficult to determine to what degree this improvement is attributable to the direct effect of the drug on spasticity and how much it depends upon the drug's tranquillizing properties.

Drug therapy is a most useful supplement to physiotherapy, and may indeed be essential to produce the conditions in which rehabilitation can be pursued.

The tight muscles producing flexion deformity must be stretched several times a day if contractures are to be prevented, and this stretching can sometimes only be accomplished if the muscles are well relaxed previously by drugs or by injections of local anaesthetic or by the application of ice packs.

Peripheral nerve and muscle injection

Spasticity of a muscle can be reduced by injecting local anaesthetic, phenol or absolute alcohol into the motor-point of the muscle or around the motor nerve supply of the muscle or by general infiltration of the muscle concerned.

Phenol can be used for selective peripheral-nerve blocks using 0·3–0·5 ml of 2 per cent aqueous phenol at motor points or 1–10 ml at peripheral nerve level. For muscle infiltration or motor-point injection 40–45 per cent alcohol can be used. Up to 4 injections in the same muscle at 2-weekly intervals can be given. The only untoward reaction recorded is an occasional episode of painless muscle oedema.

All motor points and peripheral-nerve injections should be preceded by injections of 1–2 per cent Xylocaine or procaine as a diagnostic test.

Muscle and peripheral-nerve injections are worth trying in hemiplegia, disseminated sclerosis, paraplegia, tetraplegia and cerebral palsy, as therapeutic measures or as diagnostic procedures prior to soft-tissue surgery.

Phenol or alcohol spinal blocks

The intrathecal injection of phenol or absolute alcohol is advocated by some centres for the relief of spasm. Intrathecal injection of 4–8 ml of absolute alcohol or diluted phenol (10–20 per cent) induces a toxic radiculitis involving mainly the cauda equina and results in degeneration of the nerve roots, more severe in the posterior than the anterior roots. It also induces a toxic-myelitis of the caudal part of the spinal cord and leptomeningeal fibrosis causing partial obliteration of the subarachnoid space. This preferential involvement of the posterior roots is possibly real and due to positioning of the patient during injection, or possibly apparent and due to a regrowth of nerve fibres from the anterior horn cells, thus mimicking a preferential lesion of posterior roots.

Anterior rhizotomy

Anterior rhizotomy is indicated as a measure to relieve spasticity only when more conservative measures have failed, when there is no chance of regaining voluntary control of leg muscles, and when the function of the bladder is already abnormal. The usual procedure in anterior rhizotomy is the bilateral division of the anterior nerve roots of T12–S1 via a laminectomy exposure. T10 and 11 are preserved since they innervate the lower abdominal muscles and their destruction may weaken the voluntary expulsion of urine.

Although this procedure will lead to improvement in all but very few of the severe cases, it does carry the risk of involvement of the control of the urinary bladder in about 10 per cent of patients treated.

PROBLEMS OF MICTURITION

The control and the performance of the act of micturition constitute two separate major problems to the severely disabled.

Performance of micturition

In our present-day society, a number of conditions must be fulfilled before it is socially permissable to micturate, and a further set of conditions must be fulfilled if a patient is to be socially and personally acceptable after micturition has taken place. For a disabled person the fulfilment of these conditions presents many difficulties, particularly as there is a desire in almost everyone to achieve this particular bodily function independently of outside assistance.

Certain disabilities may involve an inability to communicate (such as dysphasia following hemiplegia). Patients so affected require a system of selective communication such as a buzzer or card indicating the nature of the need; for example, whether for urinal, bedpan or help to the toilet, and its degree of urgency.

If the disability involves the upper limbs, difficulty may be experienced in adjusting clothing before and after micturition, cleansing the perineum, operating the toilet-plug or chain, getting on and off the toilet-seat, and in and out of the lavatory itself.

Lower-limb disablement primarily involves difficulty in the movement of the patient, whether ambulant or chair-bound, in and out of the toilet, and difficulty in his transfer to and from the toilet-seat. The transfer may be from the standing position to the seat, from wheelchair to seat or from hoist to seat; but in each case the difficulty is usually enhanced by architectural problems. Lavatories are almost inevitably the smallest rooms in a house, and are often reached by awkward corridors and narrow doors, difficult or even impossible for the admission of a wheelchair or hoist. The difficulty is increased even more when a lavatory is reached by an outside door, or situated in a separate building at the bottom of the garden, with at least one doorstep, as an additional obstacle.

In combined disability of upper and lower limbs, when the lower-limb disability is such that micturition is carried out from chair or bed to eliminate unnecessary transfers, sensory or muscular dysfunction in the upper limbs may prevent effective manipulation of urinal or clothes, and spasm or weakness of the lower limbs may prevent the approximation of the urinal to the perineum.

When weakness of the trunk or defective control of balancing mechanisms are present in a disabled patient, the actual ability to sit upright on commode, bedpan or toilet-seat may make assistance necessary.

Control of micturition

Finally, the actual act of micturition may be difficult to plan and accomplish. Thus, for example, paraplegic patients may find it necessary to stimulate micturition to occur by striking the abdomen, dilating or massaging the anal sphincter digitally, or scratching and pinching the adductor surfaces of the thighs. Certain postures facilitate the act of micturition, and many patients find it much easier to use a urinal while sitting in a chair, or a commode, than a bedpan while lying or sitting in bed.

The programming of patients' activities to enable them to micturate independently may be complex, time-consuming and tiring, and the introduction of appropriate drug therapy to correct the hypertonicity or hypotonicity of the bladder musculature often alleviates the distress. When the bladder is hypertonic in a continent patient and tends to contract frequently, the administration of 15 mg tablets of Probanthin twice a day or 15 mg at night often reduces the number of times at which the need to micturate is felt, and minimizes the frequency of use of the urinal or of transfers to the toilet. Conversely, when the bladder is hypotonic as in the terminal stages of muscular dystrophy, 25 mg tablets of Bathanecol three times a day will increase the frequency of micturition and decrease the long time-lag between attempting to micturate and being able to perform the act. Carbachol, nortryptyline and various other cholinergic or anti-cholinergic drugs all have their advocates for the treatment of different conditions of inbalance of the neuromuscular co-ordination of bladder action.

Even in the presence of normal bladder function, the necessity of performing fatiguing physical effort in order to achieve independent micturition, or of asking for assistance when independence is not possible, often leads patients to restrict their fluid intake deliberately, so as to reduce the frequency of micturition to a minimum. Such restriction increases the tendency of all disabled patients to develop stones in the kidney and infection in the urinary tract, but the provision of an increased fluid intake to counteract this tendency is refused despite a realization of the consequences.

The management of such patients is thus a delicate balance between helping them to retain their hard-won independence, and attempting to impose conditions which are bound to reduce their independence, their freedom, and sometimes their ability to continue an independent or partially independent mode of life. Toilet independence is frequently the stumbling-block which prevents return to work, attendance at training centres, and a satisfactory social life.

Two case histories illustrate these points:

(1) A young woman with severe paralysis following poliomyelitis (*see* case history No. 288, page 363) has to be hoisted on to her bed and on to a bedpan when she needs to micturate, as she cannot balance on a toilet-seat. She resents this dependence, feeling that she cannot impose upon the overworked staff of the residential home where she lives and has deliberately restricted her fluid since the onset of her disability and trained herself to micturate only twice daily. She now has calculi in both kidneys.

(2) Another young woman with severe paralysis following poliomyelitis complicated by Ehlers–Danlos syndrome (case history No. 54, page 35) can transfer from her powered chair onto a toilet-seat, but finds it a complicated and painful procedure. Nevertheless, she refuses help. She insists on retaining her independence in this activity, yet cannot tolerate the discomfort which it entails more than twice daily. She restricts her fluid intake accordingly, and although she has a chronic urinary infection with frequent febrile episodes needing chemotherapy or antibiotic treatment, she will not reverse her decision.

Retention

A further problem associated with micturition is the acute retention which sometimes occurs, in chair-bound disabled patients, particularly in males. Loss of power in the abdominal ancillary muscles of micturition, either from paralysis or disuse, together with neuromuscular disorders of the bladder, may precipitate this. More rarely retention may follow the development of paraphimosis or balanitis in uncircumcized males.

In the absence of an obstructing lesion such as an enlarged prostate or urinary stricture, regular provision of a urinal and seating the patient on a paraplegic cushion are helpful in preventing retention, with the prescription of appropriate drugs when indicated (for example, bethanecol, carbachol). General measures are directed at obtaining as much bodily mobility as possible, such as changing the sitting position, standing and walking for even a few paces each day if possible, and frequent turning in bed.

Other distressing symptoms occurring in seriously disabled chair-bound men are priapism and prostatism. These may occur independently of retention or else precede it. The pelvic congestion which is thought to be largely causative may be partly relieved by the measures mentioned above for the prevention of retention. In addition, particular care must be paid to the state and position of the penis after transfer or toilet activities. When a patient is unable to attend to his own toilet, his attendant should see that the penis lies normally between the thighs, and is not twisted or bent beneath thighs or underclothes, and that the foreskin is never left retracted. The use of a paraplegic cushion obviates the need to haul a patient forwards by his trousers to enable him to use a bottle while in his wheelchair, and further help to prevent malposition or trauma of the penis.

Infection

No absolutely effective method of preventing the occurrence of infection of the urinary tract in disabled people has yet been devised, and continuous prophyllactic measures against infection are essential.

Apart from the highest fluid intake consistent with convenience and continence, and the maximum amount of movement permitted by a patient's ability and commitments, external cleanliness appears to be an important factor in prevention.

Such practical measures as careful cleansing after defaecation, with the direction of the cleansing tissue or paper being always from front to back, and daily baths or perineal washing with hibitane are helpful in maintaining the cleanliness of the perineum and thereby diminishing a likely source of infection. Unfortunately, it is often the patients who are struggling to maintain their independence who have the greatest difficulty in maintaining perineal cleanliness. For them, regular checks by the district nurse, with weekly baths or blanket baths under supervision, may prove to be an acceptable compromise.

Regular testing of the urine of severely disabled patients is essential with review of kidney function at regular intervals by one controlling hospital providing a guide to over-all management of the urinary tract. Even so, the guidance is not absolute, since different centres advocate different ideas of management which alter as knowledge of the behaviour of the urinary tract in disabled people increases with their life-expectancy.

The finding of asymptomatic bacilluria is no longer considered an indication for immediate systematic treatment by antibiotics or chemotherapy. It is, however, an indication for further examination of a specimen of urine obtained with strictest precautions to prevent contamination from an inadequately prepared perineum. The occurrence of fever or symptoms of urinary infection such as frequency, dysuria, penile, suprapubic or loin pain, with malaise or rigours, demands rigorous treatment either by antibiotics or chemotherapy, controlled by the nature and sensitivity of the infecting organism. This treatment should be continued until symptoms of urinary infection have subsided, and a further specimen of urine is sterile on culture. In patients who are likely to become reinfected, long-term chemotherapy as prophyllaxis against reinfection is often indicated. Thus sulphonamides, nalidixic acid or hexamine mandelate have been successfully used as prophyllactic agents in low doses, in addition to their action in therapeutic doses for the treatment of acute infections.

When urinary infection occurs in incontinent patients using indwelling catheters or other urinary appliances, systemic treatment is often combined with bladder washouts once or twice weekly with boric acid, Hibitane or Noxyflex solution.

INCONTINENCE OF URINE

Men

A vast selection of apparatus exists which may be worn to control urinary incontinence. Basically, each consists of the same 3 parts.

(1) The perineal fitment or appliance which encloses the urethra and part of the penis.

(2) A delivery tube.

(3) A bag or reservoir into which the urine drains.

When an indwelling catheter is *in situ*, this takes the place of the perineal or penile fitment.

An incontinence appliance of whichever kind needs skill in fitting and care in handling, for unless it fits well, drains well, is properly strapped on and is in good condition, it will not function properly, and leakage or damming back of urine is likely to occur.

Adequate drainage may be difficult to obtain when a patient is seated in a wheelchair. If the urine bag is simply strapped to the thigh, it is likely that urine will not drain adequately; many severely disabled tend to slump in their chairs with the thighs horizontal, or with the knees at a higher level than the hips. The drainage tube from the urinal must lead downwards to the collecting-bag; a cutaway (paraplegic type) cushion (*see Figure 6.13*) may be the easiest solution to this problem, allowing the incontinence apparatus to lie in the space created in the cutaway portion of the wheelchair cushion. For a patient in bed, drainage is also a problem if the mattress is soft and he sinks into it until the bladder is below the level of the drainage tube as it passes over the edge of the bed. A firm mattress is essential, and the drainage tube should lead from the perineal fitment into either a plastic collecting-bag contained in a cage attached to the bed, or into a collecting-jar standing on the floor beside the bed.

Further problems arise in patients using calipers; manipulating a urinary appliance and long-leg calipers can be a very difficult procedure, the caliper tending to interfere with drainage, particularly when the patient sits down. Transferring while wearing a urinary appliance needs practice, as the straps, tubes and collecting-bags all become additional hazards in an already complex procedure.

Among the available apparatus, one of the most efficient portable male urinals involves the use of condoms (to which some patients have a definite objection). Before application, the condom is fitted over a plastic valve and connected by a plastic tube to a urine collecting bag. When the condom, valve and tube are connected, the closed end of the condom is pierced with a pin, giving free drainage of the urine. The condom is then rolled onto the penis, previously coated with skin adhesive applied to the base as near the pubic skin as possible. Shaving the pubic hair helps with the seal. The adhesive can easily be cleaned off with chlorhexidine 1·5 per cent and cetrimide 15 per cent solution. This apparatus is very efficient, and leakage rarely occurs except when the plastic tube gets twisted or blocked. Most men with some residual function in the hands will be able to manage these appliances, but those with high cervical lesions will need help. The condoms can be supplied through hospitals or through the general practitioners, after obtaining a certificate of exemption from the local medical executive council.

Women

There is no effective appliance available for the external control of incontinence in women, other than the indwelling catheter, and that, although initially effective, if used over a long period, inevitably brings its own problems. The urethra tends to enlarge, and thus catheters of progressively larger diameter are needed to prevent leakage occurring. Catheters with internal and external balloons may be needed to ensure complete freedom from leakage.

Some disabled women will be able to cope with their own catheterization, but it is better that this should be the responsibility of a doctor or nurse, so that the necessary strict sterile non-touch techniques may be adhered to.

Urinary appliances need frequent regular cleansing if they are to remain acceptable clinically and socially. A daily wash in soapy water and rinse out with hibitane will keep them clean and free from smell. There are disposable urine bags for some appliances, but although more hygienic, they have a smaller capacity. Removal of these bags, operating the stoppers and taps, and repositioning the tubes is often not possible for quadriplegics, but most paraplegics cope with the incontinence appliances quite adequately.

Children and women and indeed some men with intermittent incontinence are sometimes padded or given protective pants. While this may be the only available method to help them keep dry while travelling or during a social visit, such a method is to be discouraged except as a rare expedient. To be effective, the padding must be bulky and the pants non-porous. They present problems in disposal, they invariably smell and it is almost impossible to prevent the skin macerating and breaking down. Furthermore, maintaining a constant supply of disposable pads, or frequent laundering of the non-disposable pads is expensive.

Partial incontinence

For male patients with some control, the use of the traditional bottle-shaped urinal is probably the simplest method of managing micturition. With practice, a urinal can be used in a wheelchair or a motor-car. A patient can be left with several urinals to use, which can be emptied later when help is available or the circumstances are more convenient. A female urinal (St. Peter's boat) can be used successfully by many disabled women after sufficient practice, but a satisfactory swan-necked urinal is not currently commercially available. A cut-away paraplegic cushion in the wheelchair facilitates the use of the urinal, but such a cushion needs a hard base or else the sides of the cut-away part will collapse under the patient's weight (*see Figure 6.13*, page 229). Ideally, such a hard-based cushion should have a replaceable section fitting into its cutaway segment and the section may be pulled out to allow a bottle to be used and then replaced. Cushions with a permanent cut-out section can be uncomfortable and can in some circumstances induce pressure areas along the under border of the thighs due to the seam of the cut-out portion of the cushion.

Micturition is physiologically, psychologically and physically a complex procedure, and working out a simple practical routine for its performance by a severely disabled patient may be correspondingly difficult and demand time and patience from patient and attendant alike.

Without such a routine, a patient may fail to obtain that social acceptance and personal independence to which his own efforts and those of any unit concerned in his care must be aimed.

CONSTIPATION

Constipation means either infrequent defaecation or undue difficulty in defaecation, and is usually defined as 'a condition in which no residue of food taken during one day is excreted within the next 48 hours'. This is an arbitrary definition, since the frequency of defaecation in the normal person ranges from 5–14 times a week, and while some normal people regularly defaecate 3 times a day, others do so only 3 times a week.

The rhythm of defaecation adopted by any able individual is usually fairly constant, and depends partly on his own metabolism, partly on deliberately established habits, and partly on the demands of his daily activities. Within these latter 2 groups are included work, exercise, diet, involving both timing and content of meals, availability and architecture of the places of defaecation which he frequents, and his ability to go there whenever he feels the need to defaecate.

When a seriously disabling illness or injury occurs, these habits and activities alter radically. They are influenced by the extent and nature of the disability, the degree of immobility which it entails, and the quantity and timing of the assistance available to the patient; they are no longer directly determined by the patient's wish or convenience. It is most important that an alternative regimen of bowel action should be instigated as soon as possible after the onset of disability, and that active measures should be taken to combat the development of the constipation to which all physically disabled people are prone. Such measures involve the planning of a patient's external and internal rhythms, after a consideration of the specific effect of his particular disability on the action of his gut and on the achievement of controlled defaecation.

There are 3 major groups of disorders liable to cause constipation.

(1) Diseases affecting joint mobility, such as osteoarthritis, rheumatoid arthritis, where limitation of range of joint movement, with or without pain, will reduce a patient's ability to get to and from the lavatory and transfer to and from the toilet-seat, quickly and painlessly.

(2) Diseases causing muscular spasticity in the presence of intact sensation, such as cerebral palsy and multiple sclerosis. Here the spasm and inco-ordination of the muscles of locomotion may make travelling to and from the lavatory, and transferring on to and off the toilet-seat, impossible without aid. Furthermore, spasm of the perineal muscle, buttocks, and external sphincter may predispose towards the development of constipation by obstructing rectal evacuation.

(3) Diseases causing flaccid muscular weakness or paralysis, with intact sensation, for example, muscular dystrophy.

In all these conditions, the weakness or paralysis of the muscles of the limbs, makes swift transfers difficult or impossible, and also weakness or paralysis of the lower muscles of the abdomen, the anciliary muscles of defaecation, make it difficult to assist by voluntary movement in the performance of this act.

In the context of the particular disability affecting any one patient, the following measures should be adopted and adapted for the prevention of constipation.

Diet

A high roughage, high protein, low carbohydrate diet is generally the most suitable for a disabled patient, both to encourage regular bowel action, and to prevent the development of obesity with its many deleterious effects. This type of diet will need appropriate modification for the many disabled patients who develop gastric and duodenal ulcers, or hiatus hernias (*see* page 135).

Fluid intake

This should be as high as a patient can tolerate without being incommoded by the increased frequency of micturition which results (*see* page 144).

Aperients

Aperients should be avoided whenever possible. Daily administration of I-so-gel mucilaginous granules, the inclusion in the diet of certain foods of known laxative values such as prunes and figs, and the daily use of glycerine suppositories are preferable. If, however, a regular bowel routine is not attainable by the method described, then the aperient chosen should be used in the smallest possible amount, as a daily stimulus, and employed for as short a time as possible. The administration of the aperient should be considered as a training mechanism to obtain a regular bowel action, and not as a permanent institution, and it is therefore important that it should be given at the same time each day, and that its dose should be gradually decreased once regularity has been established. Violent purgatives and the use of cascara and liquid paraffin in particular, are contra-indicated.

Defaecation

Since the transport of patient to lavatory or commode, or of bedpan to patient, is often a lengthy procedure, it is important that a time for defaecation is chosen which is mutually convenient to patient and helper, and that sufficient time is allowed for the rectum to be fully emptied.

The administration of hot drinks before defaecation, followed by abdominal massage and pressure, by the patient himself when possible, and by repeated contraction of the abdominal, buttock or adductor muscles of the thigh for those patients who can carry out these voluntary movements, are helpful in initiating a bowel movement. It is also helpful if the patient can defaecate while in the physiological position for the act, sitting upright, with the hips and knees flexed. Whenever possible, therefore, a patient should be sat on a toilet-seat or commode for the purpose, and not laid on a bedpan in bed.

When long sessions on the receptacle must be avoided, gentle massage of the anus with the finger-tip using a vaseline-lubricated, rubber finger-cot, will often induce rectal contraction.

Place of defaecation

Whether a patient is ambulant or chairbound, an architectural barrier to the toilet may be the critical factor which precipitates the onset of constipation. If the lavatory is upstairs and the patient lives downstairs, if it is outside, if it is reached through a narrow door from a narrow passage, or if it has a step, then reaching it becomes impossible without help. Unless that help is forthcoming when the need to defaecate is felt, defaecation is postponed and constipation soon develops.

When the architectural barriers are insurmountable, the provision of a 'sanichair' or commode may enable the patient to develop a regular routine independent of help, with the simultaneous instalment of a hoist when the disability demands it.

For some, the management of clothes and their perineal toilet are the prime factors mitigating against toilet independence. Appropriate alterations on the advice of a skilled occupational therapist can be prophyllactic measures against the development of constipation.

Review of drugs

Many disabled people are regularly taking a variety of drugs, whose efficacy should be regularly reviewed in relation to their side effects. Thus amputees and arthritic patients in particular, may need analgesics for persistent pain, the cause of which cannot be removed. Certain analgesics have a greater constipating effect than others, for example the codeine family, and should be avoided when possible in susceptible patients.

It should be remembered that almost all analgesic tablets tend to have some constipating action, and that their use should automatically point to the need for adjusting the diet by the inclusion of increased bulk to counteract this tendency. Conversely, mefanamic acid (Ponstam) often produces severe diarrhoea.

Similarly, many disabled people take nightly sedatives, most of which predispose to constipation by their depressant effect on the mobility of the gut. Certain groups carry an increased risk of producing this effect (particularly barbiturates) and should be avoided if their constipating effect outweighs their sedative value.

If constipation has become established, it is important to ensure that there is no underlying causative abdominal or pelvic pathology. Abdominal and rectal examinations will often reveal the presence of obstructing faecal matter, or may indicate narrowing or occlusion of the lumen of the gut by spasm, neoplastic or scar tissue.

In the presence of established constipation, as in the presence of true or apparent incontinence, it is essential to rid the lower bowel of accumulated faecal matter before beginning a programme of bowel retraining. Small daily enemas should be given or manual removals undertaken until both rectal and abdominal examination indicate that all hard lumps of faeces have been removed, and the bowel is again capable of unobstructed action.

FAECAL INCONTINENCE

A patient is said to be incontinent of faeces when he is unable to control his bowel action and defaecation occurs involuntarily. Full control of defaecation entails the synchronization of several reflexes, and these in turn need an intact sensory and motor supply to the involuntary muscles of the gut, and also to the voluntary ancillary muscles of defaecation of the abdomen and buttocks. Any interference with this balanced reaction, either by interruption of the nerve supply or by development of pathological change in the muscles concerned, may adversely affect the ability to achieve full control, which demands awareness of rectal distension and the synchronized muscular action necessary to relieve it.

Faecal incontinence may be real and permanent, or apparent and able to be corrected. It can be remedied when normal rectal and anal competence is present, and in the presence of an intact anal sphincter and of sufficient cerebration to enable the need for defaecation to be registered, inhibited until the lavatory is reached or the bedpan is available, and finally satisfied when defaecation is initiated by muscular action.

It is essential to establish whether or not incontinence is true or apparent, before any attempt is made to institute a new bowel regimen for a disabled patient diagnosed as faecally incontinent. A comprehensive history and clinical examination will usually yield the necessary information to do this. The history will reveal the amount of bowel training received, the appetite and eating habits of the patient, and the possibility of some pathological condition in the gut. Abdominal examination will demonstrate the presence of hard masses of faecal matter in the pelvis descending and even transverse colon, and the existence of a spastic colon. Rectal examination will reveal the absence of anal and rectal sensation, the presence of a flaccid or hypertonic anal sphincter, the existence of prostatic or cervical enlargement, polyps or neoplastic growth, and the presence of a faecal ball valve obstruction.

Apparent faecal incontinence may be found to occur either when adequate bowel training has never been given or when regular habits of defaecation have been allowed to lapse with the onset or progression of disability.

Adequate bowel training is often neglected by those who care for disabled children, either because in the presence of mental retardation or physical disability, they have considered that the introduction of further physical difficulty or stress into the children's lives is unjustifiable, or because they have not realized that faecal continence is attainable, or because they just have not bothered to make the effort needed.

Regular habits of defaecation may have been allowed to lapse for similar reasons. Chronic illness of one of its members entails the reorganization of an entire household. When faulty diet and lack of exercise make it no longer possible to defaecate at a given time, a patient must be content to wait until the commitments of his helpers permit him to be assisted to the lavatory, and irregularity of bowel action and constipation follow.

However it develops, the resulting constipation may produce such a degree of obstruction, that the distended gut may only evacuate involuntarily once every few days or else permit an intermittent trickle of liquid faeces to bypass the obstructing faecal mass, leading to the erroneous diagnosis of incontinence or diarrhoea.

Such apparent incontinence may be corrected in almost every patient by training, or retraining, provided that this training is extended to include the patient himself in addition to his bowels. But no method of training can be effective until the lower bowel is empty. Enemas are often ineffective, and regular manual removals of faeces from the rectum must be performed until no further faecal masses can be felt, and the faecal matter in the rectum is of normal consistency.

When true faecal incontinence is present as in paraplegic and tetraplegic patients, or children with spina bifida, the incontinence cannot be rectified but it can still be organized so that the patient has a fixed bowel routine and knows the time of day at which a reflex bowel evacuation will occur. Other daily activities can then be planned around this time, and can be undertaken with confidence that they will not be interrupted by unforseen bowel actions.

The keynote for the organization of such a bowel routine is the production of the requisite conditions under which an essentially rhythmically acting organ can function in a rhythm convenient to the individual patient.

Training

As in the production of a satisfactory bowel regimen in any disabled patient, the first concern must be with the diet. This should contain added bulk in addition to a plentiful supply of roughage and should be colourful and appetizing, with as wide a variety of food as possible.

Exercise is the next consideration. Patients should be encouraged to take whatever exercise is possible for them, even if this is limited to transferring themselves from bed to chair, standing up from the chair, or changing their position in bed.

The timing of defaecation is also important. Defaecation is the terminal event of a cyclical activity, and if a patient has a regular daily timetable for other activities and meals, it should be equally possible to establish a regular routine in which a definite time is set aside for the reflex evacuation of the bowels. This routine must be a matter of choice for each patient, depending on the nature of his disability and the demands of his situation, that is, whether he goes out to work, or whether he is dependent on helpers who have other commitments. The patient may defaecate daily, every other day, or twice weekly, and rarely only once a week; but his final decision should be related when possible to the rhythm of his bowel action prior to the onset of disability.

Laxatives should be used with caution. Of the 3 main types of laxatives, bulk producers, lubricants and softeners and stimulants, only the former 2 should be used as regular aids; recourse to stimulants being reserved for infrequent administration when bowel routine has become upset or during the training programme to establish a bowel routine.

If aperients of the stimulant class are used, then they should be administered in the smallest effective dose. As far as possible, they should be avoided in favour of more natural and accessory physical stimuli, used to supplement the combination of the gastrocolic reflex and abdominal straining. Thus rectal stimulation with the finger, anal massage, or the insertion of 1–2 glycerine suppositories on the morning on which bowel action is desired, may all be effective in initiating a rectal evacuation.

The mucilaginous seeds of I-so-gel combine the attributes of bulk producers and softeners, and in all incontinent patients the daily administration of I-so-gel or other bulk-producing mucilage is recommended. This produces a soft, formed, bulky faecal mass, increasing reflex peristalsis and preventing the formation of hard faecal lumps. It is best given night and morning, in doses varying from 5–10 ml.

A good routine which is adequate to ensure a complete rectal evacuation for most patients is a hot drink before breakfast when the mucilaginous bulk preparation is given; breakfast itself (consisting of a cooked breakfast, fresh fruit and hot coffee) and then the insertion of one or more suppositories. If these are inserted while the patient is still in bed, he can then be hoisted or transferred onto the toilet, and the evacuation allowed to occur, before washing and dressing.

If it is not possible to get a routine of regular spontaneous evacuation established, a daily manual evacuation may be substituted, preceded if necessary by the insertion of a glycerine suppository. When I-so-gel is being taken regularly, the rectum is full of soft faeces and are easily removed by the gloved finger, the whole procedure being completed in about 15 minutes.

The faecal retention which can ensue when a regular bowel routine is neglected can lead to a variety of symptoms, such as increased spasm, headache, and diminished concentration, appetite and muscular power, and later to symptoms of intestinal obstruction, such as abdominal pain, nausea and vomiting.

As with the management of micturition, bowel training can lead to considerable improvement in the patient's level of independence and may be the key factor in determining complete independence or social acceptability for employment or training.

The management of the bowels is closely related to the management of micturition. Patients who are continent of urine should have a daily bowel-action routine, for constipation can precipitate urinary incontinence. If, however, it is not possible to establish a satisfactory controlled regimen of micturition, then the bowel action can be less frequent (say 2–3 times a week).

ORAL HYGIENE

Severe physical disability imposes many additional stresses upon an individual, and any activity is accomplished by a greater effort than is required of the non-disabled. Impairment of upper-limb function is frequently most restricting in activities involving lifting the hands up to face level, particularly feeding and grooming. Whereas most patients will naturally make an effort to feed themselves, and women in particular will take great trouble to care for their appearance, care of the mouth and teeth is an activity which is frequently neglected. Severe physical disability is often associated with factors which specifically militate against the maintenance of oral hygiene. Muscular dystrophy, for example, is often associated with macroglossia and protrusion of the teeth; patients with rheumatoid arthritis often are unable to open their mouths fully because of involvement of the temperomandibular joint: hemiplegics have a facial paralysis with inability to control cheek and tongue on one side. Sjorgen's syndrome in a mild form is present in many patients with severe rheumatoid arthritis and leads to dry mouth and difficulties in mastication, aggravating the general problem of oral hygiene.

Many drugs used in the treatment of physical disability may affect the salivary glands: thus phenylbutazone may cause a soft generalized swelling and diminished salivation, while propantheline bromide (Propanthine) has an atropine-like effect and causes dry mouth which increases the difficulty of maintaining mouth cleanliness.

Angular stomatitis, associated with dribbling due to incoordination, paralysis or excessive use of the mouth to supplement deficient upper limb function, is common. Barrier creams are a helpful prophylactic, and creams containing lanolin at night are the simplest form of successful therapy. But as the cause cannot be eliminated, the condition may be a persistent nuisance, and prophyllaxis and treatment must be on a long-term basis.

Gingivitis, aphthous ulcers and thrush are relatively common among the severely disabled. Mouth-washes and dental care are the most important prophyllactic measures and, for those unable to cope adequately, oral hygiene should be supervised by an assistant. Hydrogen peroxide mouth-washes after meals are simple and effective. Sodium perborate buffered mouth-wash is theoretically more effective and can be regarded as at least a partial substitute for teeth cleaning, but it is very expensive and the taste is unacceptable to most patients.

Many of the severely disabled are on long-term antibiotic therapy or intermittent courses of antibiotics, particularly for urinary infections. This increases their liability to fungal infections which may present as ulcers in the mouth or as thrush, as well as the more common enteritis, or as vaginitis in women.

Nystatin lozenges and mouth-washes will usually control mild cases of thrush, but resistant cases can be treated with local applications of gentian violet 1 per cent in aqueous solution. Dequalinium chloride lozenges or paint is useful for all mouth and gum ulceration. Aphthous ulcers usually respond symptomatically to hydrocortisone pellets, but if they persist, may be cauterized by careful application of phenol direct to the ulcers.

Dental care presents a major problem for severely disabled patients retaining their teeth. Not only is adequate tooth cleansing difficult, but many disabled are physically unable to attend the dentist, either because they cannot get out, or because there is no local dentist with an accessible surgery. The wheelchair-bound and severely arthritic need to attend surgeries without steps, which are either on the ground floor or else accessible by lift. The local authority or local dental executive council will usually provide information on accessibility of dental surgeries. However, many of the more severely physically disabled will need to have their regular dental supervision arranged at hospital both for reasons of accessibility and for safety, as they often present greater anaesthetic risks. They may have restricted mouth opening, limited cervical mobility, poor respiratory function and an inadequate airway. This situation is further complicated in rheumatoid arthritis where cervical instability is often present.

The recent introduction of the electric toothbrush should do much to improve the dental hygiene of the severely disabled, making it easier both for the patient or assistant to achieve adequate tooth cleansing.

Too many severely disabled children and young adults present with carious teeth and generalized gingivitis. Simple routine measures can prevent much discomfort, an early recourse to dentures and an unnecessarily unpleasant appearance.

OBESITY IN THE PHYSICALLY DISABLED

Too often there is not enough money, time or thought spared for the care of a patient whose mobility and usefulness is drastically reduced by physical disability. Food is often chosen for its cheapness and for its easiness to prepare, convey to the mouth and chew. Fish, lean meat and green vegetables do not come into this category, and the diet of the physically disabled is often rich in carbohydrate and lacking in protein, roughage and variety. Many severely disabled patients are overweight and will admit to an increase in several stones since onset of disability.

When obesity is due to fat deposition from overeating, then in the absence of any medical contra-indication, it is invariably beneficial to put the patient on a low-starch diet together with a non-amphetamine appetite depressant. The severely disabled find dieting even more difficult than the non-disabled, and the administration of an appetite depressant (such as diethylpropion hydrochloride) is often the only way to obtain the necessary co-operation from patient and family. It is often unnecessary to continue appetite depressants for longer than one month, because by then the patient is used to the diet and is able to continue with diet alone, but sometimes the depressants may be continued until the desired weight loss has been brought about.

The physically disabled benefit from loss of excessive weight in various ways. Transfers become easier both for patients and helpers, and a greater degree of independence can be achieved in consequence. Frequently, respiration is improved. Patients relying on diaphragmatic breathing due to cervical-cord injury, or anterior poliomyelitis with involvement of the intercostal and abdominal muscles, need as little resistance to the excursion of the diaphragm as possible, and intra-abdominal and intra-thoracic fat deposition can provide a very formidable resistance to this. Circulation improves when obese limbs are thinner and more easily mobile, and digestion and constipation improve on a more balanced diet. Control of micturition in females is helped by reducing obesity. Perineal tone improves, and prolapse, cystocoele and rectocoele become less likely complications of disablement.

Thus, for many reasons, the physically disabled should be strongly encouraged to control their weight, and those who are overweight should be actively assisted to reduce their weight to standard proportions.

MENSTRUATION IN DISABLED WOMEN

It is often difficult for an able woman to remain personally and socially acceptable throughout the duration of her menstrual flow. For a disabled woman it may be impossible. Not only may the mechanical effort of performing her perineal toilet be beyond her capabilities, an efficient perineal toilet demands a considerable number of synchronized movements, but the menstrual flow itself may be heavier than normal, and preceded by severe premenstrual tension. The heaviness of the flow is possibly secondary to pelvic congestion from prolonged sitting, and premenstrual tension may be exacerbated by the enforced inactivity of a chairbound woman.

Furthermore, insertion of internally worn tampons is usually impossible for seriously disabled women, who are therefore compelled to use external padding. This causes considerable discomfort to patients confined to bed and chair, particularly when they need, but hesitate to request, frequent changes. The inability to cope with the perineal toilet, and the need to ask the assistance of a relative or nurse, may not only embarrass but greatly distress a patient, and may be the single factor which prevents her from achieving complete personal independence.

It therefore seems desirable to attempt to relieve disabled women of the monthly exacerbation of the discomforts which their disability entails. This may be done in several ways, provided simple general measures have first been tried. In the first place, the heavy flow and abdominal pain may be reduced to a certain extent by ensuring efficient bowel-emptying, at least during and immediately preceding the menstrual flow. Simple modifications of diet, such as increasing bulk and roughage content of the food consumed, may be sufficient to produce this. Aperients are not indicated, because in disabled patients, the administration of aperients may well lead to apparent incontinence if the patient is unable to transfer to the toilet as quickly as the aperient necessitates. For the same reason, the prescription of diuretics premenstrually is also contra-indicated, although it is effective in reducing premenstrual tension and the volume of the menstrual flow.

If the flow is heavy and dysmenorrhoea of first-day type occurs, the resulting pain may be eased by appropriate analgesics or antispasmodics. Rest in or on the bed, with a hot water-bottle or hot pad on the lower abdomen, is always comforting and frequently effective.

When these measures have been tried, and the menstrual periods still constitute times of distress, in the absence of anaemia or of pelvic pathology the treatment of which might be expected to bring further relief, it seems justifiable to suppress the monthly menstrual flow.

The volume of the loss may be decreased by the interrupted administration of one of the many brands of contraceptive tablets. By this means a small, regular, oestrogen withdrawal bleed is substituted for a large and possibly irregular menstrual flow. Pain, volume of blood-loss and premenstrual tension are all diminished, but the need for an effective perineal toilet remains.

In certain cases there may be valid reasons for considering complete suppression of menstruation. There are 3 methods available: (1) radium or irradiation menopause; (2) hysterectomy; (3) hormonal therapy.

The best way of preventing vaginal bleeding is to perform a simple hysterectomy. Either the vaginal approach is employed, if the patient is multiparous, or the abdominal approach, through a low transverse incision, if she is nulliparous. In either case the ovaries are spared, and post-operative symptoms of oestrogen deficiency are avoided. Conversely, such symptoms are very likely to follow high-energy irradiation of the ovaries, or a radium menopause, particularly in younger women, while their correction by means of oestrogen implants is contra-indicated, lest vaginal bleeding recommence through the reactivation of the endometrium.

But many patients do not wish to discard the idea of a possible pregnancy, however undesirable or unlikely this may actually be. Others consider regular menstruation as a single link with physiological normality. And for others again, a hysterectomy entails surgery of a major type, which they are not physically able to stand. For such patients, the suppression of the periods for long intervals by continuous administration of hormones offers a welcome alternative.

Long-term suppression of periods has often been attempted for women suffering from endometriosis, using either a progestogen tablet, or else one containing both oestrogen and progestogen. During the last two years, both types of tablet have been used separately in our Disabled Living Unit to suppress the periods in a limited number of seriously disabled women, with varying degrees of success.

Regimens

It is possible to suppress menstrual periods completely by prescribing a tablet containing 2 mg of ethynodiol diacetate and 0·1 mg mestranol. Owing to the inhibition of the normal, rhythmically fluctuating secretion of follicle-stimulating and luteinizing hormones by the pituitary, induced by this hormone therapy, ovulation is prevented, the uterine endometrium regresses, and menstruation does not occur. One tablet is given daily for 9 months without remission, the dose is increased only if vaginal spotting occurs. The dose is then held at a level sufficient to ensure the complete suppression of vaginal bleeding. After each 9-month interval, the tablets are withheld until 1 withdrawal bleed and 1 normal menstrual period have occurred; their administration is resumed on the third day of the next cycle. Such a regimen of recurring 9-month intervals of amenorrhoea is acceptable to most women and to their medical advisers as the natural one of pregnancy.

Contra-indications

Contra-indications to this treatment are hepatic or renal damage, and a history of jaundice in the first 3 months of a pregnancy. For this reason, liver and kidney function tests are necessary for all patients who wish to start on this programme, and should be repeated at regular 9-monthly intervals. Where possible, it seems advisable to take regular cervical smears from patients involved.

Advantages

On such a regimen, most severely disabled women experience considerable general improvement and many report a positive sense of well-being. Low haemoglobin levels rise, bedsores tend to heal, patients are less depressed and many are glad to be relieved of the physical problems of perineal toilet.

Disadvantages

The disadvantages of the method are considerable, and have caused many women to stop taking the hormone tablets spontaneously. The side effects of headaches, nausea, vomiting, weight increase, angina and bronchial spasm, ankle oedema, breast tension and an increased incidence of muscular spasms have variously been reported, and there is a risk of deep-vein thrombosis.

Most of these side-effects appear to be attributable to the oestrogen component of the tablet, and may be relieved by simple measures. Thus, the administration of perphenazine (4 mg) with the hormone tablet each day is effective in preventing nausea and vomiting. Some of this weight-gain may be offset by adjustment of the diet, but the component attributable to fluid retention is difficult to offset. Few severely disabled patients may safely be urged to limit their fluid intake, or conveniently be given a diuretic.

More serious is the rise in the serum glutamic pyruvic transaminase (SGPT) which occurred in a patient, who, having had 2 complete 9-month intervals of suppression, was anxious to begin a third. This appears to indicate that the higher doses of oestrogen which are used continuously in this method, relative to those in current combined oestrogen/progestogen contraceptive tablets, used intermittently, are causing liver damage. This method of period suppression should probably be abandoned.

Daily progestogen administration can be used to suppress

menstruation, but it is usually accompanied by unacceptable side-effects, such as acne and severe depression.

The beneficial effects of period suppression have nevertheless given a strong indication that some sort of period regulation should be attempted for those disabled women who experience distress at this time. Hormonal suppression may indicate to a patient the advantage of a hysterectomy or radium menopause, or if she cannot tolerate complete suppression, at least the hormonal therapy will considerably reduce her menstrual flow and pre-menstrual tension.

M.M.L. No. 655 born 1944 female

Diagnosis: Rheumatoid arthritis (Still's disease)

This patient contracted polyarthritis at the age of 7 years and had recurrent acute attacks until the age of 11 years, after which she had no further evidence of acute arthritis. The attacks were severe and generalized and she was eventually left with ankylosis of the majority of her limb joints, with sparing of the metacarpophalangeal joints of the hands and the interphalangeal joints of most of the toes.

After many manipulations, she had been given arthrodesis of both knees in extension; and arthroplastics of the right elbow and left hip. She was able to walk about 100 yards using gutter crutches, and had a Ministry of Health pushchair in which she was taken out. She had been assessed for a Ministry of Health electrically-powered tricycle (E.P.T. Model 64) with modifications to the controls, and was awaiting the supply of the necessary shed when she was first referred to the Disabled Living Unit. She was able to transfer from bed, chair and toilet independently at heights of 20–22 in (51–56 cm) and with the use of various long-handled aids, she was virtually independent for dressing. Some minor problems still existed in daily living activities and these were overcome with additional long-handled aids (such as toilet stick) or adaptations to clothing (for example, Velcro instead of buttons). She was able to wash herself as far as face and trunk were concerned. In addition, her mother gave her bed-baths and at intervals a bath.

One major recurring problem was that of menstruation. She had heavy irregular periods and she was physically incapable of coping with her perineal toilet. Furthermore, she had marked premenstrual depression and irritation. This was a major factor in preventing her from accepting training in a residential institution.

Her education, naturally, had suffered but she had had correspondence courses and obtained English language and mathematics G.C.E. 'O'-levels over a period of 18 months.

At the time of this first admission, she was caught up in a vicious cycle. She wanted to work, but was considered unsuitable for residential accommodation because she needed attention for bathing and sometimes help with toilet. She was unable to get a job, since she had no qualifications (apart from the 2 G.C.E. 'O'-levels) and she had no means of getting from home to place of employment. She was not accepted onto the Disabled Persons Register as it was considered unlikely that she would achieve employment. Many modifications to her home, such as grab-rails and pulleys had been promised but not executed. At this time, she was very depressed.

On reviewing the wheelchair situation, it was found that she was capable of propelling a semi-reclining wheelchair and, when cushioned to the correct height, she could get in and out of it herself. The only adaptation necessary was the fitting of a small wooden support to maintain the legs in a comfortable, slightly everted position. On the first admission this chair was ordered.

The other line of attack was towards the one severe area of dependence and associated depression and irritation, her menstrual periods. After full discussion, check of kidney and liver function tests, she was started on hormone suppression therapy.

When she was admitted to take delivery of her new wheelchair, 3 months later, she felt very much better. She had lost much of the depression, noticed complete relief from premenstrual tension and her morale was much helped by not having to ask for increased help each month to cope with her perineal toilet. She still did not have the outdoor vehicle, but already felt that she was on the way to increased independence.

Eleven months after her first admission, she was readmitted to review the hormonal suppression of menstruation and check liver-function tests. As planned, she had had a withdrawal bleed, followed by a normal period a month later, and then had re-started the hormone tablets. Liver-function tests and kidney-function tests were normal. She had had a slight initial rise in weight but this had been controlled by dieting and eventually she had managed to reduce her weight by several pounds. She was originally 8 st 4½ lb (52 kg) and now was only 7 st 10 lb (49 kg).

She reported that her outdoor transport had just arrived and had been modified so that she could get in and out of it.

On examination it was noted that she had gained movement of the hip which had had an arthroplasty to such an extent that the backrest of the self-propelling wheelchair needed considerable adjustment. This was an expression of her increased mobility over the preceding months.

Nearly a year later she was reviewed again (November 1968). She was holding a full-time job as a clerk and switchboard operator in a local welfare department. She had been at the job for 8 months except when she had a suspected fracture of the elbow after a fall on a wet slippery floor. She was working a full 5-day week (8.30 a.m.–5.20 p.m.) travelling from home to work (about half a mile) in her tricycle. All the planned modifications to her home had been carried out and she was clearly very happy.

Finally, after discussing with her the possible complications of continued hormone suppression of menstruation, she decided not to continue the tablets. She planned to work 3 months and see whether she noticed a return of premenstrual tension and irritability, whether she could now cope more adequately physically, and whether this degree of dependence affected her new, more active way of life. Should she wish, she could restart the hormones or ask for a hysterectomy.

Comment

Although this young woman had been well-treated and many plans were in hand, she was depressed and frustrated and indeed aggressive when first seen at the Disabled Living Unit. A reappraisal of her capability at self-propelling in a wheelchair gave her some increased independence, but it was the suppression of menstruation which had a most dramatic effect.

Her general sense of well-being enable her to make the most of the additional independence. This general improvement in outlook enabled her to accept the necessary delays, and as the plans previously set in motion came to fruition, she was able to take full advantage and organize herself into full-time employment in spite of considerable adversities.

RESPIRATORY INSUFFICIENCY OF LATE ONSET

In severely disabled patients with rapidly progressing muscular weakness, little may be gained by attempting to improve respiratory function when general deterioration is having an even greater impact. In patients with a stable disability, however, it is vitally important that respiratory function should be maintained at its maximal efficiency, since the onset of respiratory insufficiency can prejudice the synchronized action of all the systems of the body. Such maintenance demands constant watchfulness and prophyllactic care, and the rapid institution of therapeutic care when necessary.

Some deterioration of respiratory efficiency is an inevitable consequence of severe disability. The degree of deterioration may be minimized by counteracting wherever possible the direct and indirect adverse effects which severe disability has upon the respiratory system.

These adverse effects are direct when the respiratory apparatus is structurally affected by the disabling condition. They are indirect when the function of a potentially normal respiratory system is jeopardized by the dysfunction of other systems affected by the disability.

Direct involvement of the respiratory apparatus may be caused by:

(1) Weakness or paralysis of the main muscles of respiration, the diaphragm, intercostals and abdominals, as in anterior poliomyelitis, muscular dystrophy, tetraplegia, syringomyelia.

(2) Deformity of the thoracic cage from scoliosis, following bony abnormality or muscle inbalance, as in muscular dystrophy, anterior poliomyelitis, cerebral palsy and idiopathic scoliosis.

(3) Rigidity of the thoracic cage, as in ankylosing spondylitis.

(4) Weakness or paralysis of the laryngeal muscles and the accessory muscles of respiration, as in anterior poliomyelitis, syringomyelia, muscular dystrophy.

Indirect involvement of the respiratory system will follow the development of any severe disability, irrespective of its cause. It is partly due to the immobility which severe disablement confers on the patient, and partly to the sequelae of this immobility.

Therefore, disabled people with drastically reduced mobility need a reduced respiratory excursion and a correspondingly decreased expansion of the lungs to satisfy their oxygen needs. They tend to take fewer deep breaths during the day than an able-bodied patient who has several periods of increased activity in his usual daily routine.

Furthermore, in the presence of upper-limb paralysis, the brachiocostal accessory muscles of respiration cannot assist respiratory excursion. Also the confinement of many disabled patients to wheelchairs mitigates against deep respiration; if unbraced, patients with weak trunk muscles may slump in their chairs, so that the abdominal contents impede diaphragmatic movement; if braced, patients have to breath against the increased resistance offered by the brace, and this may offset the advantage of improved posture.

The dysfunction of the gastrointestinal system, often associated with severe disability, has several adverse effects upon the respiratory system. Constipation is an almost constant sequel of severe disability, and the loaded bowel which it produces may seriously impede diaphragmatic action. Wind is another unpleasant symptom which occurs frequently in patients with weak or paralysed abdominal muscles. The distended bowel may cause respiratory embarrassment to a disabled patient with diaphragmatic weakness, by pressing upwards against the unresisting cupolae. Disabled people frequently become obese by indulging in diets which are unwise in quantity and quality. The raised intra-abdominal resistance which large deposits of perivisceral and omental fat can produce may further impede diaphragmatic action.

Respiratory function

The degree of respiratory insufficiency present in a disabled patient is not always directly proportional to the degree of dysfunction of the respiratory system. Insufficiency indicates an inability to meet a need and is therefore dependent both on demand and supply. If the diminished air supply of a disabled respiratory system is adequate for the demands of the disabled body which it serves, then no respiratory insufficiency results. If, on the other hand, the primary disabling condition has affected the respiratory system so greatly that it can no longer satisfy the demands of the rest of the body, a state of respiratory insufficiency develops.

It is, therefore, important that examination of a disabled patient should include an assessment of respiratory function so that appropriate advice may be given on the maintenance and possible improvement of respiratory efficiency.

Estimation of respiratory function

Respiratory function is a complex physiological process, and the usual investigations to estimate its efficiency tend to be either rather inaccurate and unhelpful, or else complex and time-consuming. Simple measurements such as that of vital capacity and forced exspiratory volume do give some indication of function, but are relatively inaccurate when used as comparative measurements. Blood-gas estimations are often difficult to arrange and are preferably carried out in a laboratory equipped for the purpose. Perhaps the simplest over-all test, which is remarkably reproducible, and the repetition of which gives a reasonable guide to a patient's progress, is the timing of his ability to hold his breath. This activity involves many of the various aspects of respiration and requires little skill and co-operation. Records of the breath-holding time can give a useful indication of changes in respiratory function.

A preliminary but often effective estimate of the sufficiency or insufficiency of the respiratory system in any particular patient, and therefore of the need for further investigation, may be made by observing the patient during the course of his daily activities. If he can perform all these without becoming breathless, then his respiratory function is adequate for his needs under normal conditions.

Management of respiratory system in severely disabled people

The management of the respiratory system of a disabled patient has 4 main parts.

(1) The employment of active measures to maintain maximal respiratory efficiency.

(2) The provision of supplementary mechanical aids when simple measures do not enable a patient to attain respiratory sufficiency.

(3) The introduction of intensive treatment for respiratory infection when this supervenes.

(4) The recognition and treatment of respiratory insufficiency of late onset.

The maintenance of maximal respiratory efficiency

In the presence of weakness or paralysis of any of the main muscles of respiration, a patient should be given breathing exercises to encourage the use of any ancillary respiratory muscles which are still functional. Whenever possible, he should also be taught glossopharyngeal breathing as it is one of the simplest methods of supplementing respiration.

Glossopharyngeal breathing (or frog breathing)

Patients with adequate glossopharyngeal musculature can usually learn this technique from a skilful frog-breather, and can increase the vital capacity by 1,000–1,250 ml. To frog breathe, the patient gulps in a mouthful of air, closes the lips and nasopharynx, and then pumps the air down the trachea by forcibly depressing the tongue which acts as a piston. This action of gulping and swallowing air is continued as long as the chest can be expanded. The mouth is opened and nasopharynx relaxed to allow expiration. Once acquired, this skill is a most useful adjunct to respiration; but it has the disadvantage that it is tiring to use for long periods, particularly towards the end of the day.

Case history No. 250 illustrates its effectiveness.

M.M.L. No. 250 born 1933 female

Diagnosis: Anterior poliomyelitis

This patient had a severe attack of acute anterior poliomyelitis at the age of 23 years. She was treated in a tank respirator for $2\frac{1}{2}$ months and then was weaned on to a rocking bed and a cuirasse. Finally, she was weaned off both of these; she was left with complete paralysis of both lower limbs and severe weakness of shoulder girdle and some weakness of the rest of her arms. The trunk and respiratory muscles were also severely affected.

She is looked after by her mother but works at home as a translator.

When admitted for review in 1968 (12 years after her attack of poliomyelitis) her vital capacity was only 400 ml, but the arterial partial pressures of oxygen and carbon dioxide were within normal limits. Normality of blood gases was maintained by glossopharyngeal breathing and by this technique she could increase her vital capacity by 1,250 ml.

General measures

Whether or not the primary disability involves the thoracic cage, various other general measures should be urged to maintain respiratory efficiency.

Patients should be encouraged to sit in as upright a position as comfort will allow, and their chairs padded, if necessary, to assist them to do so. They should be urged to take whatever exercise is possible for them within the limits of their disabilities, and should be strongly advised to avoid becoming constipated or overweight.

Regular deep breathing, with about 10 deep breaths each hour, is also beneficial, and should be included in the daily routine of every disabled patient. This expands the lungs and promotes the production of the surfactant substance responsible for alveolar patency. Without the adequate production of this substance, alveolar function is affected, gaseous exchange is diminished, and alveolar collapse may occur.

Smoking should either be stopped or reduced to a minimum. Apart from its carcinogenic properties and deleterious effect on the cardiovascular, gastrointestinal and possibly urogenital systems, it reduces the air taken into the lungs, and decreases the oxygen-carrying capacity of the blood by the formation of carboxyhaemoglobin from the absorption of the carbon monoxide which it produces. In a system already so greatly and adversely affected by severe disability, such interference with the content and use of the inspired air is completely unjustifiable.

Mechanical aids

The second part of the management of the respiratory system involves the provision of mechanical aids to supplement natural respiration, if this cannot meet the needs of a patient. Provision of a rocking bed, Radcliffe positive-pressure respirator, cuirasse or tank respirator for use during the night may enable him to live a relatively active life during the day. A minority of patients with gross respiratory dysfunction will need to use a respirator constantly, and yet another group will need to use one only when they develop respiratory infections.

Respiratory tract infections

Prolonged disability tends eventually to reduce the standard of a patient's general health, and therefore the resistance to infection. The capacity of a patient to deal effectively with established respiratory infection is dependent both on the direct and indirect effects of disability on the respiratory apparatus.

Thus, when there is paralysis of the muscles of respiration or deformity or rigidity of the thoracic cage, coughing ability will be diminished and sputum will tend to accumulate in the lungs and upper bronchial tree. When the function of the respiratory apparatus is impeded in addition to its structure being pathologically changed, coughing ability is further diminished, and an upper respiratory infection may rapidly develop into a serious chest infection leading to pneumonia, respiratory obstruction or pulmonary collapse.

Any upper respiratory tract infection in a severely physically disabled patient must be regarded as dangerous. The prompt exhibition of antibiotics and the institution of adequate pulmonary drainage by suction, postural drainage and physiotherapy is essential. Patients prone to these problems should understand the need for prompt medication and those caring for them can be taught to institute simple measures, such as the administration of expectorants and antispasmodics, with bronchial antispasmodic inhalations and the use of postural drainage, and assisted coughing when this is possible. If the infection does not respond adequately to these measures, then admission to a unit equipped to deal with respiratory emergencies is necessary without delay.

Reassessment

The fourth part of the management of the respiratory system involves the regular reassessment of the clinical condition and respiratory function of seriously disabled patients, in particular those patients who suffered from paralytic anterior poliomyelitis in the past with accompanying respiratory involvement. Such reassessment is aimed at detecting respiratory insufficiency of late onset, and in providing adequate supplementary respiratory aid to halt the otherwise inexorable progress of the condition.

During the convalescent phase of anterior poliomyelitis, most patients with respiratory involvement are able to be weaned away from their respirators for longer and longer periods. A few seriously affected patients with intercostal diaphragmatic and abdominal muscles severely weakened or paralysed, have to remain permanently in respirators, such as a tank or cuirasse; but by far the greatest number leave hospital without mechanical assistance, or with mechanical assistance only at night.

Over the years the respiratory function of these patients gradually deteriorates. Joints and soft tissue lose their resiliency, intercurrent infections decrease muscular tone, daily physiotherapy is lacking and daily exercises neglected, and the demands made on the patients increase as the memory of their illness fades into the background. Slowly and insidiously they drift into a state of respiratory insufficiency. In this state of insufficiency not only the respiratory system, but every system of the body is affected.

Possibly due to the plethora of symptoms with which respiratory insufficiency may therefore present, the condition often goes unrecognized until its increasing severity makes the diagnosis obvious. Meanwhile, undiagnosed patients may be termed as fussy, neurotic or psychological.

The earliest signs of respiratory insufficiency of late onset appear in the central nervous system when patients who have coped adequately with their disability for years suddenly feel that they can no longer do so. They complain of decreasing alertness and intellectual capacity, progressing to depression and even confusion, and of intense, easily-induced fatigue. In the respiratory system, breathlessness on effort, on talking and finally at rest appears with an increased susceptibility and diminished resistance to respiratory infections. There is usually difficulty in coughing and occasionally in blowing the nose.

In the gastrointestinal system, increasing constipation and decreasing appetite may occur, with increased frequency of micturition and stress urgency in the urinary system, and palpitations and angina in the cardiovascular system.

In the peripheral vascular system increasing oedema, cyanosis and coldness of the extremities appear with possible weight increase due to fluid retention, and proptosis in the more severely affected patients.

The finding of this syndrome by clinical examination and interrogation, should be followed whenever possible by a detailed respiratory function assessment, including a blood-gas analysis.

Symptoms of respiratory insufficiency may sometimes be relieved by applying general measures for the maintenance of the health of the respiratory system, combined with instruction in glossopharyngeal breathing, and the provision of a night respirator or rocking bed. When, however, the patient is highly motivated and wants to make use of the maximal degrees of mobility of which he is capable, the provision of a small, portable positive-pressure respirator (PPPR) may give him mechanical assistance during the day, without tethering him to a large unwieldy respirator.

Such a respirator can be made by a relatively simple process of converting a small commercial vacuum-cleaner, weighing only a few pounds and measuring a foot in length. A flexible outlet-tube is attached by a plastic cup to the exit aperture of the vacuum-cleaner with a filter chamber incorporated in the distal part of the cup. Over the entrance tube a further filter is fitted.

Such a respirator may be powered by a 12-V battery or the 240-V mains electricity supply. It sucks in air by a fan and delivers it in a jet, the strength of which may be initially controlled by incorporating a resistor in the circuit.

To use the respirator, the end of the plastic outlet-tube is placed in the mouth and the stream of air inhaled during a single, moderately deep inspiration. The tube is then either removed from the mouth, or closed by the tongue, or by biting with the teeth, or else is directed onto the roof of the mouth during expiration. This procedure is repeated for periods of increasing length, until the patient is inhaling air under such conditions for about 5 minutes 4–6 times a day. Once a patient has been trained, he is able to regulate his use of such an apparatus and work out the optimum time and duration of his periods of assisted respiration, to fit in with his meals and his work schedule.

The use of such a respirator rapidly produces an over-all improvement in the condition of the patients. Fatigue is less, work output greater. Depression is alleviated and concentration and memory improved, with less drowsiness during the day, appetite is keener, frequency of micturition lessens, palpitations occur less frequently and there is less ankle swelling. Weight may be lost due to decreased oedema, or gained when appetite improves. Coldness no longer is a constant complaint. Patients use their accessory muscles of respiration less and are able to talk, eat and move with less breathlessness. Clinical examination often shows a marked decreased in peripheral oedema and cyanosis.

While it is apparent that the question of treatment of disabled patients with pulmonary insufficiency of late onset is not completely answered by the use of such respirators, it is nevertheless felt that they have a definite contribution to the total plan. Although these techniques are mainly applicable to patients suffering from residual paralysis after anterior poliomyelitis, there is some evidence that other static disabilities inducing respiratory insufficiency could be similarly managed.

Case history No. 769 illustrates the value of this form of management.

M.M.L. No. 769 born 1921 female

Diagnosis: Poliomyelitis

This patient had a severe generalized attack of anterior poliomyelitis at the age of 28 years. She was in a tank respirator for 3 weeks and then gradually weaned out of it over the period of about a year. After discharge from hospital, she continued slowly to improve and was able to run her home and help in a village shop which she and her husband owned. She was able to walk short distances using long leg calipers, but spent most of the day in a wheelchair. After about 15 years, she began to notice increasing fatigue, her ability of work in the house and shop diminished considerably and she suffered from increasingly frequent and severe attacks of sleepiness. She was diagnosed as having narcolepsy and treated unsuccessfully with amphetamine. At night, she had increasingly frequent attacks of twitching of her limbs and shouting, nocturnal frequency of micturition, and often woke breathless, cyanosed and having palpitations.

In 1967, she had dyspnoea on effort, she was cyanosed and had brawny oedema of both legs and thickening of both arms. Her face was thickened and she had a marked proptosis. She was referred to the Disabled Living Unit for advice on daily living activities.

On the assumption that many of her symptoms were due to hypoxia and not narcolepsy, she was admitted to a Respiratory Unit, where a diagnosis of hypoxia was confirmed (arterial P_{O_2} 57·8 mm Hg, P_{CO_2} 67·2 mm Hg). She was then supplied with a rocking bed and returned home. Reassessment 2 months later showed a general clinical improvement. However, 6 months after, she was readmitted in respiratory failure with a return and exacerbation of her original symptoms and signs. After an initial period in a tank respirator she was supplied with a PPPR and then discharged home once again, using a rocking bed at night and the PPPR at intervals throughout the day.

Six months after this admission, she had continued to improve. The gross oedema had dispersed; she had lost 2 st (12·7 kg) in weight. The cyanosis and proptosis had considerably diminished. She had had no episode of chest infection. She no longer had periods of sleepiness, nor were her nights disturbed by muscular twitching. Her urinary infection had cleared and her pilonidal sinus had healed for the first time in 10 years.

What was more significant was that her mental alertness and competence had returned and once again she was able to undertake considerable activity in the shop and home. By now, her arterial P_{O_2} was 70·1 mm Hg. and arterial P_{CO_2} was 46·5 mm Hg.

5—*Functional Problems*

INTRODUCTION

Functional assessment forms a large part of the work of occupational therapists, and also of physiotherapists concerned with the care of the more severely disabled. Although the assessment of a patient is a continuous process and involves integration of disciplines and activities, it is convenient to separate some of the major problems for the purposes of description. The 3 activities of major importance which are performed daily by able and disabled alike are sleeping, eating and using the toilet. For the customary performance of each activity in a separate room, a certain degree of mobility is essential.

TOILET

For the severely disabled, using the toilet is frequently the most difficult of these 3 activities to achieve, and yet is frequently the most critical activity for attainment of personal independence or acceptance into a community, either domestic or institutional. Incontinence has been referred to as a clinical problem (*see* Chapter 3) and is often easier to manage than intermittent incontinence or urgency or stress incontinence in the physically disabled.

The problems of toilet usage for the disabled are mainly problems of access; problems of transfer on and off the toilet; and problems of toiletry in a wheelchair.

In general, the disabled require more space for manoeuvring than normal people and since, as has been previously mentioned, the lavatory is usually the smallest room in the house in the most inaccessible corner, the majority of the problems are architectural (Chapter 8). The problems are different for individual patients and houses. Thus the Functional Assessment Unit requires facilities for practical tests with the patient and access to accurate plans of the home situation. It is even better, when possible, to carry out the preliminary assessment in the patient's own home, but the provision of solutions to the problems involved usually needs a variety of aids and appliances and is easier in a Functional Assessment Unit.

Access to the lavatory is the first problem which presents. Narrow corridors, awkward corners, narrow doorways, stairs and steps are common hazards or barriers to easy access. Outside lavatories are common in both country and town. Non-slip floors, gentle ramps or shallow steps with handrails and good lighting are the essential requirements for the approach to a lavatory. Access can sometimes be improved by simple rearrangement of furniture and fittings, reversing the hang of the door or fitting a sliding door in place of a hinged one. Outside toilets can be made accessible by ramping the back doorstep and providing a covered way. However, as the disabled are usually slower than normal, adequate heating is an additional need in outside toilets.

In order to save extra exertion, it is best to have a wash-basin in the lavatory when it is separate from the bathroom. Due to the extra effort which seriously disabled people have to make to perform each action, perineal and anal cleansing are often inadequate. This makes it particularly important for disabled people to be able to wash their hands after using the toilet, and if necessary, the perineum as well.

In general terms, a lavatory compartment for the ambulant disabled needs to be 2 ft 9 in by 5 ft 9 in (84 cm × 180 cm) with grab-rails along each side wall. For the wheelchair-bound disabled, the size of the lavatory should be 5 ft × 5 ft 9 in (160 cm × 180 cm) with grab-rails both behind the pedestal and to one side of it (*see* Chapter 8).

Reconstruction to improve accessibility will usually involve integrating bathroom and lavatory, thereby merging two accessibility problems in one. In the final analysis, there will be some patients with insuperable accessibility problems, and the installation of a commode may be the only practical solution to their difficulties.

Within the lavatory, the siting of the pedestal may be critical. For the wheelchair users, sideways transfers are facilitated if the pedestal is set further out into the room than usual; while many ambulant disabled have difficulty in manoeuvring onto the seat and require more 'elbow room' than is customarily available. A pedestal set out 12 in (30·5 cm) from both the rear wall and the side wall usually allows adequate room for these requirements. The majority of the disabled prefer a seat which is higher than normal and 21 in (53 cm) is the height most often preferred.

The type of seat provided can make a considerable difference to the convenience and comfort of its users. Horse-shoe shaped (open at the front) makes perineal cleansing easier for some, but may be too unstable for others. The old-fashioned wooden bench-type seat is often the best, as it is very stable and virtually acts as its own sliding board for transfers. For those with stiff hips, an inclining seat can be installed.

The size and position of grab-rails are often a matter of personal preference, but in general, horizontal and vertical bars are better for stability than inclining bars. Bars with a matt finish are easier to grip than polished chromium plate; and bars which are $1\frac{1}{2}$–2 in (3·75–5 cm) in diameter are easier to grip than the slimmer varieties. A few practical tests will usually reveal a patient's individual requirement.

The next problem is that of transferring. If a wheelchair patient can be trained to stand up, take two paces, turn round and sit down, then many of the problems of toilet independence are solved. This ability is well worthwhile striving for throughout a rehabilitation programme. However, for the permanent wheelchair user, transfer techniques will have to be adapted both to the patient, and if necessary, to the available lavatory. Sliding-boards and bench-type lavatory seats are common solutions to transfer difficulties, but some patients will need to transfer through the back of the wheelchair or to transfer forwards and sit on the pedestal back to front.

Transferring through the back of the wheelchair requires a zip in the back canvas and this invariably causes trouble. Zips are not designed to take the strains imposed on the back-canvas of a wheelchair and they are subject to frequent failure. Furthermore, many patients with disabilities of the upper limb will have considerable difficulty either in undoing the zip, or in doing it up. But for some paraplegics, or for patients who have a particular architectural problem and can transfer to a special chair for toilet purposes, this solution is applicable. Some patients may be able to use a sanitary chair, wheeling themselves (or being wheeled) over the toilet, and then transferring to another chair after dressing.

Dressing, undressing, cleansing and washing must all be assessed in conjunction with the use of the toilet. These activities have to be accomplished within the small confines of the lavatory, or other techniques and activity programmes must be devised. Adaptations to the clothing, particularly underclothes, can make the various manoeuvres easier. For some, simple aids such as a toilet stick, are helpful. The use of a bidet, or a lavatory pedestal which will dispense warm water followed by hot air may solve the problem of perineal cleansing, but these are expensive installations.

Night access may have to be considered as a separate problem. If the lavatory which is accessible by day is outside, then its use at night is likely to be unfeasible, and an alternative method must be available if micturition or defaecation are needed during the night. Patients with urgency of micturition, or patients using appliances, such as artificial limbs or calipers, cannot put these on at night just to use the toilet. In these circumstances, a night commode is likely to be the easiest solution to the problem. A further important consideration is that the partner, or relative, looking after a disabled person is often heavily committed by day and needs an unbroken night's sleep. If it is possible to organize the nights so that they are not disturbed, it may mean that they can continue looking after the disabled member of the household for much longer than otherwise might be the case (*see* Appendix O).

EATING AND DRINKING

The practical problems which eating and drinking present to the severely physically disabled are a part of the over-all problem of personal independence and can only be solved in the context of the individual circumstances. Patients living at home within a family are unlikely to have more than one meal a day on their own, thus, it is probably easier and quicker to plan for a simple snack which can be left available, rather than organize a complicated and possibly hazardous arrangement for the preparation of a more elaborate meal, necessitating considerable effort by the patient himself. A disabled person living on his own can usually have several main meals a week provided by 'meals-on-wheels' service or prepared by a home help, and this arrangement may be safer and easier than trying to organize complete independence in the purchase of food and its preparation. It is the young and middle-aged severely disabled patients wanting to be independent and to become integrated in society who face the greatest difficulties in achieving and maintaining independence in this respect, together with the disabled housewives continuing to strive to cater for their families and to retain the normal family inter-relationships.

For such patients, the installation of a telephone facilitates catering by enabling food to be ordered, rather than purchased on tiring shopping expeditions. The erection of a strong shelf at a convenient height outside the back door makes it easier to collect the delivered articles, and when delivery-men realize the circumstances of their clients, many of them are willing to bring their boxes into the kitchen and lift them onto the table.

The types, levels, modifications and arrangement of kitchen furniture and equipment are of the utmost importance to the preparation of meals by the disabled, and are dealt with elsewhere (Chapter 8).

The actual programme of action associated with mealtimes and the consumption of the meals themselves also needs careful assessment and often meticulous planning, if independence is to be achieved.

Social confidence may depend upon the patient's ability to eat and drink with dexterity in company, and an ability to accept help gracefully when needed is an important attribute for a disabled person. Dexterity is often the key. There are many people with congenital absence of the upper limbs who are so skilful with their feet that they can use these in public for many everyday activities without attracting attention. Should they use artificial arms, when relative awkwardness of movement draws attention to the disability?

When a patient's ability to be independent during mealtimes is being considered, the accessibility of the dining area and dining-table must be estimated. Approaching a table and adopting the most convenient position for eating may be complicated for both the ambulant and wheelchair disabled. The heights of tables and chairs are often critical, and extra space around them is usually needed for manoeuvring.

Modern dining-tables are frequently flimsy in construction and often do not provide adequate clearance for wheelchairs. Similarly, patients with stiff hips and knees need higher dining-chairs and tables than those usually manufactured. The size and position of the table needs careful assessing. Heavy tables against a wall or in a corner can provide adequate support for patients with inco-ordination or spasm, whereas a patient using a powered indoor wheelchair may find a lightweight cantilever table or a special tray on his chair more useful.

For those likely to spill food, such as disabled children or patients with severe upper-limb disability, plastic surfaces and a rim to the table or tray may save much time and trouble. Tables which adjust in height, or tilt are also available. For patients with ataxia, a special table with fittings to hold plates or bowls can be constructed.

Aids and appliances for feeding include overhead slings, mobile arm-supports (*see* Chapter 7) and specially designed crockery and cutlery. Mobile arm-supports were originally introduced as a feeding device for patients with severe upper-limb paralyses, and are still referred to as 'ball-race feeders' by some departments. Fitted to a wheelchair, or in special circumstances to a dining chair, they provide a balance movement of the forearm, together, if necessary, with pronation and supination. Correctly fitted, they assist the movement of the hand from table to mouth (*Figure 5.1*).

For a few patients with coarse, slow tremor or ataxia, ball-race feeders can be fitted with their movement dampened down by inducing friction in all the mechanical linkages, but success in the use of these adapted feeders is very limited. Head tremor is also difficult to overcome, and although winged headrests can be helpful in mild conditions, severe head tremor is virtually unsurmountable and

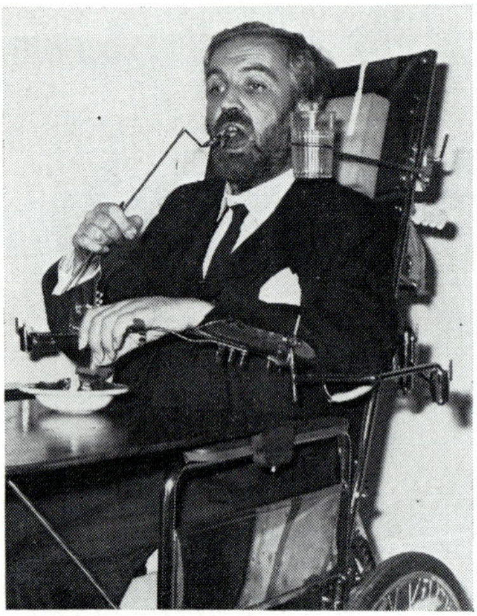

Figure 5.1. Mobile arm supports, an extended swivel spork and pusher

makes independent feeding an unrealistic goal for those who suffer from it.

Patients whose primary difficulty in feeding arises from weakness of the hands and forearms may usually be successfully assisted to independence by stabilization of the wrist by a splint, coupled with the use of adapted cutlery. There is a wide variety of such adaptations available. Some may be simply and cheaply carried out in most occupational therapy departments, and recently specially designed cutlery and crockery for the disabled is commercially available (Manoy ware). Such adaptations may be to the handle ends or to the effector ends of the cutlery or to both. Thus enlargement of the handles makes them easier to grip, while angling them facilitates access to the mouth, and extending them or fitting them with swivels compensates for a diminished range of elbow and wrist movement. Combination of the structural characteristics of two implements in the effecter end of one, will also combine their functions. Thus a spoon with its bowl divided into wide prongs combines the function of spoon and fork (spork), while a serrated knife with a curved, pronged tip combines those of knife and fork (cheeseknife).

The problems posed by independent drinking are somewhat different, but their solution is usually readily provided by a trained occupational therapist. Straws or polythene tubes clipped to the cup or glass, or containers on stands are simple to construct. The bottle carriers as used by long-distance cyclists can be attached to wheelchair or bed and fitted with a long straw or tube. Children's training beakers are non-spillable and insulated plastic camping mugs prevent undesirable cooling of their contents for those patients who are very slow in eating and drinking.

Some of the problems can be avoided by correlating the content, preparation and presentation of the diet with the disability of the patient. As limited mouth-opening (for example, rheumatoid arthritics), and poor dental hygiene may further increase the feeding difficulties of patients with upper-limb disabilities, meat should be served minced or cut up into small pieces rather than in slices requiring cutting, biting and strong mastication. Conventional salads are difficult for the disabled, but well prepared shredded salads which have been mixed to an even consistency with salad cream or oil (for example, Russian salad) can be handled with a spoon or spork. Rich soups and broths are more easily drunk from cups or through a straw than from a soup-plate. Many of the foods prepared for babies and available in tins provide a rich source of easily digested nourishment.

A patient with epidermophytosis bullosa who presented difficulties in feeding because of upper-limb disability and restricted mouth-opening (case history No. 1060) also had severe iron deficiency anaemia associated with bleeding from ulcers on her skin and in her gastrointestinal tract. Change to a diet of food of appropriate consistency and of high nutrient content, and the use of supplements (for example, Complan) improved her general health and her anaemia in a matter of months. Previously, she had persisted in attempting to cope with the same diet as the rest of the family.

M.M.L. No. 1060 born 1952 female

Diagnosis: Epidermophytosis bullosa

This girl suffers from epidermophytosis bullosa of the severe kind. Her arms and legs in particular, blistered and ulcerated from any form of minor trauma. During early childhood, the digits of the hands and feet became encased in blisters which later epithelialized, thus rendering her extremities equivalent to friable amputation stumps as far as function was concerned. The digits retained some

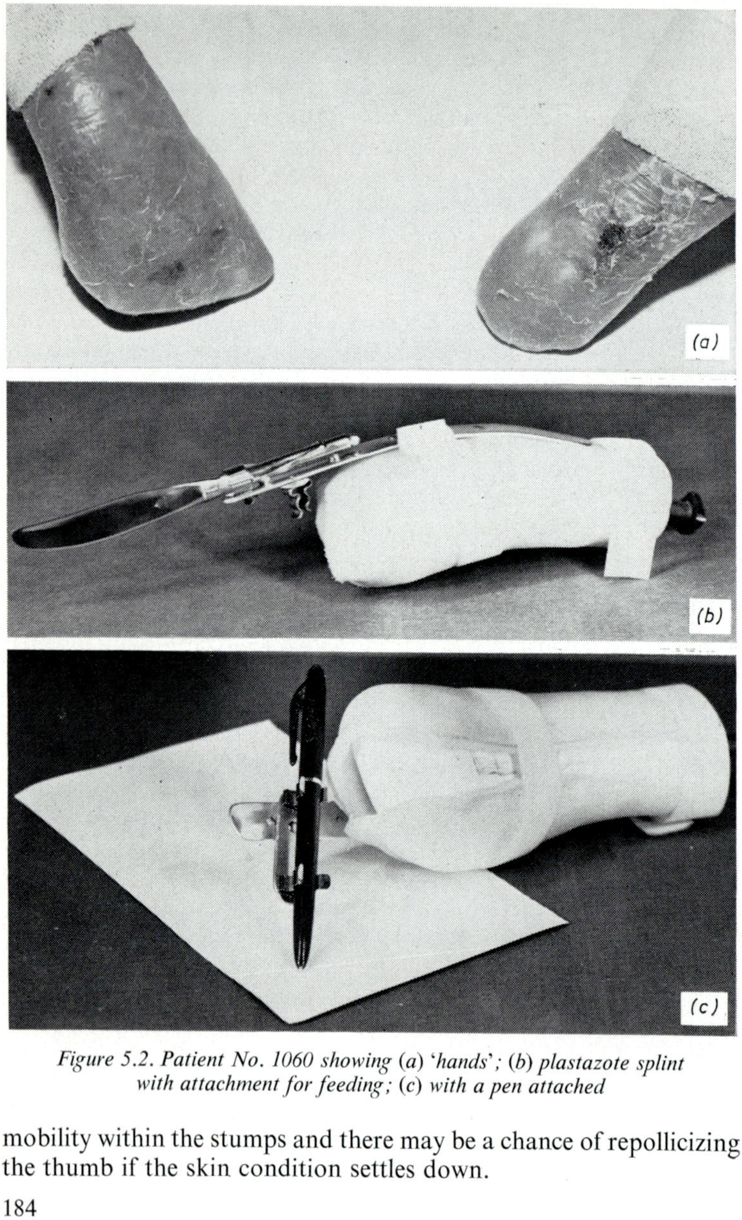

Figure 5.2. Patient No. 1060 showing (a) 'hands'; (b) plastazote splint with attachment for feeding; (c) with a pen attached

mobility within the stumps and there may be a chance of repollicizing the thumb if the skin condition settles down.

She was referred to the Disabled Living Unit on leaving school in order to reassess the likelihood of increasing her independence. She was of average intelligence but sexually immature as a result of prolonged steroid therapy (now discontinued). Her mouth was small,

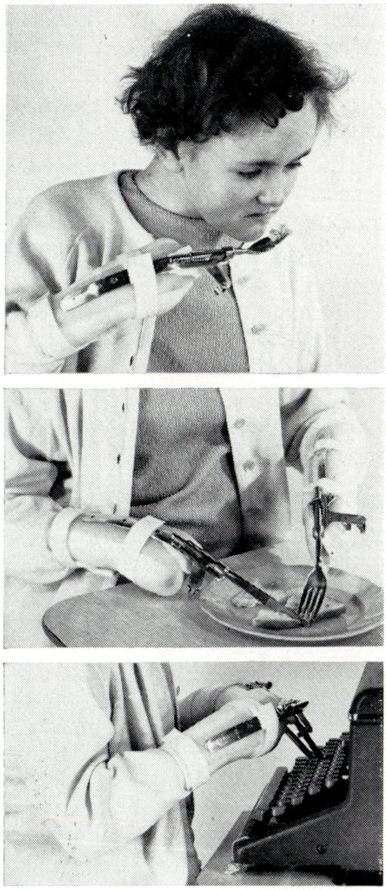

(*d*) (*e*) (*f*)

Figure 5.2 continued—Patient No. 1060 showing plastazote splint with (*d*) *spoon attached;* (*e*) *knife and fork attached;* (*f*) *typing attachment*

with limited aperture, friable mucosa and poor teeth. As a result of her poor diet and frequent bleeding from ulcerating blisters, her haemoglobin was only 41 per cent. The hands were enclosed in bags of skin and allowed her no useful grip.

She was able to feed herself somewhat laboriously using a two-fisted grip, but needed help in cutting-up and preparing her food, and she required help also with dressing and undressing.

She had no training for employment but felt she would like to try to be a telephonist or to do some simple clerical job. Thus, the main reason for her referral was to investigate the possibility of appliances which would help achieve this degree of independence.

The main difficulty in fitting this patient with any suitable prostheses was the pathological sensitivity of her skin, particularly to irritation, friction or localized pressure. These characteristics precluded the provision of any of the conventional prostheses, which were too heavy, and produced pressure sores. However, some simple stump appliances, similar to those used for congenital upper-limb amputees, were made from Plastazote (aerated polyvinyl) with fittings to accept cutlery or a typing stick. These were applied over her usual dressings, or if the skin was clear, over cotton stump-socks. Non-adhesive silk dressings were found to be preferable, being less likely to cause bleeding from ulcerated areas.

The splints proved successful, they were light and distributed pressure evenly. She began using them for only very short periods. Over an interval of 5 weeks she worked up to a total daily use of $3\frac{1}{2}$ hours without any ill effect. She was using the splints for eating, writing and typing on readmission, and was happier and less frustrated in consequence (*Figure 5.2*).

Other lines of management included the successful treatment of the anaemia by dietary improvement (advising her on how to obtain the most nutritious and high protein food in the soft form which she could manage), and with iron preparations by mouth. Alterations to her clothing and simple adaptations to eliminate buttons and zips enabled her to become more independent at dressing.

WASHING AND GROOMING

A disabled patient planning his daily washing routine needs access to hot water, but not necessarily access to a bath or wash-basin. Unless a wash-basin of the correct height is available to him, in a suitable situation within an accessible room, it is preferable to bring the hot water to him, rather than bring him to the hot water. And in planning this operation, the composition of the bowl used to contain the water, its height, support and position must be considered, in addition to the technique necessary to fill it with water of the correct temperature.

Correct assessment of these features of the chosen washing equipment are particularly important to a chairbound patient for whom special trays or lap-boards may be necessary to support lightweight plastic bowls. Hoses or thermos flasks are possible sources of supply of hot water which eliminate the fatigue of carrying heavy jugs; but any plan entailing the use of hot water needs careful practical trials before final adoption, for hot water is a considerable hazard to those with physical disability.

It is unrealistic to expect a patient with severe limb disability to be able to wash himself all over without help. Even if he can overcome the physical difficulty of achieving the considerable number of movement complexes which a thorough wash demands, he is likely to be exhausted by the effort entailed in doing so, and to be so slow that the prolonged privacy which he needs will constitute a nuisance to others. In addition, a slow, prolonged over-all wash is a chilling procedure, and it seems preferable to accept some help and lose a little independence, rather than retain it and suffer the accompanying fatigue, chill and inconvenience. If no help is available, a daily over-all wash should be avoided, and a timetable should be worked out by which different parts of the body get a thorough wash on certain days in a warm comfortable room.

Those who cannot reach all parts, or who cannot exert enough pressure or control to cleanse thoroughly, must also accept the use of aids (for example, long-handled sponges or brushes, hand-showers) or accept the need for regular help with washing. There are various aids for holding the soap, which either enclose it in a mitten or fix it to a container. Tricks for washing can be devised; for example, one foot can be used to soap the other or the forearms can be used instead of hands.

Drying presents the problems of gripping and controlling the towel, reaching the extremities and applying adequate pressure. A length of roller towel with the ends turned back to make 'mitts' will enable some patients to dry their back and legs. For others, a hot, wrap-over bathtowel or towelling cloak large enough to cover most parts, will act as an effective drying agent when the patient wriggles his body beneath it.

Thick-towelling mittens can be used for patients with severely impaired grip. But a warm room, and a method of warming the towels before use are probably the most useful requirements.

Teeth-cleaning can present problems for patients with upper-limb deformities whether it is concerned with dentures or natural teeth. For many patients with weak grip and reduced mobility, an electric toothbrush is most helpful in combining effective brushing with independence. Similarly, shaving is relatively easily organized with an electric razor which can be fixed at a suitable height on a suitable bracket, or fitted into a leather socket with elastic hand-loops and used in conjunction with mobile arm supports.

Grooming is primarily a matter of looking after the hair, the nails and, for women, making up the face. It is particularly important to encourage the severely disabled to take a pride in their appearance. Without this, the very necessary social contacts are more difficult to establish or maintain. For disabled girls, lessons in make-up can be the first stage of integration and acceptance in a community. Too frequently, they have missed the opportunities for learning the art of make-up, because of their disability. A mirror at the correct height in a good light is the first requirement. Special holders with long handles can be devised for all the necessary apparatus and accoutrements (powder-puff, lipstick, eyeliner) for those with restricted movements.

A woman's hair is so important to her appearance, that it is well worthwhile spending considerable time in helping her to achieve a suitable manageable style. Regular washing and the use of appropriate shampoos should be recommended to reduce seborrhoea and dandruff, which is more likely to appear in those who are unable to brush and groom their hair as frequently as the ordinary person. This also means that short simple styles are most appropriate. Unless the patient can afford regular hairdressing with permanent-waving and setting, styles involving waved hair are best avoided, as such styles need dexterity of fingers to maintain and their management after washing can be difficult.

Sometimes finger-nails can be managed with files appropriately adapted, or with nail clippers fixed to a board and with an extended lever, but this is hazardous for patients with diminished sensation or inco-ordinated movements. Few severely disabled can manage toe-nails, nor should they be encouraged to do so. If this cannot be attended to by the family, relatives or friends, it is important that the patient arranges for the regular attendance of a chiropodist.

BATHING

Taking a bath is a difficult and strenuous activity for the elderly and slightly disabled. For the severely disabled it is often very dangerous. Bathing is usually performed in a small room, difficult to reach and with awkward fitments and corners. The surfaces involved become wet and slippery. The atmosphere is hot and steamy and conducive to fainting, and considerable agility, including the ability to stand on one leg, is necessary to get in the out of a standard bath successfully.

When assessing a severely disabled patient for bathing and washing, it should be done under the following headings:

(1) Access to the bath

(2) Transfer in and out of the bath
(3) Taps and fittings
(4) Washing and drying
(5) Assistance needed and assistance available

Showers and baths

For many patients an appropriately designed shower provides a much more suitable method of washing than taking a bath, easier to manage, easier to manipulate and more economical. But the British in general have a strong antipathy towards the shower, probably in part engendered by the coldness of the average British bathroom. Whereas a hot bath is warming, a shower demands a warm bathroom for comfort.

For those with stiff joints a shower with a shower seat is much safer than struggling in and out of the bath. A shower fitted over the bath can be a useful compromise, so that the patient can sit on a bath-seat with his feet in warm water and can use a hand-shower to complete the washing process. Such a shower is economical in its hot-water usage, and demands less in effort from the user. Furthermore, it is easier to use to clean the bath rather than by scrubbing in the usual manner.

A fixed shower with shower-seat is a rare finding in the average British house, and even when such a fitment has been installed, the rose of the shower is usually overhead. This is unsuitable for the disabled patient who is likely to be sitting down on the shower-seat, and who does not want his hair wet during every routine shower. Thus the shower rose should preferably be situated at chest height, and should also be removeable so that it can be used as a hand-shower and facilitate showering all over from the sitting position.

Special showers have been designed to fit over a lavatory pedestal so that the patients can shower themselves down and cleanse their perineum after defaecation. This manoeuvre saves changing position and may be particularly suitable in certain circumstances; but once again, it is necessary to assess the capabilities and the needs of each individual in terms of safety, conservation of effort for patient and helper and efficiency of the operation as a whole.

Access

Although not so ill-designed for disabled living as the average lavatory, bathroom are notoriously difficult of access and are usually lacking in space for manoeuvring.

Whereas when planning a new house for a disabled person it is possible to allow space for wheelchair access to both rooms, it is often very difficult to convert the conventional bathroom for use by a chair-bound patient. Sometimes it is possible to remove a dividing wall between the bathroom and lavatory and thus improve access to both and make manoeuvring for necessary activities easier. Doorways are often awkwardly placed, and frequently the journey from bedroom to bathroom is through a narrow hallway or passage which precludes easy turning in a wheelchair.

Thus the assessment of the ability of a disabled patient to use the bathroom must be preceded by an assessment of his ability to reach it. If this shows that access is impossible without structural alteration to the approaches, it is then necessary to ensure that the use of the bathroom will be safe and successful before reconstruction is recommended (*see also* Chapter 8).

When planning the arrangements and activities within the bathroom, safety must be one of the prime considerations. Non-slip floor coverings and well-sited grab rails help considerably in the achievement of this. Hot towel rails must be covered up or dispensed with as so many disabled patients either have some defect of sensation, or else of muscle tone with consequent inability to relax their grip, that they may be badly burned if they use heated towel rails as grab rails in an emergency.

Old-fashioned baths, standing free and without the sides boarded in are often far more suitable for disabled people than are their modern counterparts. Their higher legs leave room for the feet of a helper and make assisted washing easier; they leave room for the footplates of a wheelchair and so facilitate transfers; they can readily be mounted even higher to give the 9–10 in (23–25 cm) clearance necessary for the feet of a portable hoist. Their rims are rounded and provide better grips for transferring patients who use them for support.

Grab rails fitted to the wall over the bath are often found to be of considerable help in transferring. These are best if fitted horizontally and vertically rather than diagonally. A tubular grip rail about $1\frac{1}{2}$–2 in (3·75–5 cm) is most widely acceptable, and it needs to be set 3–4 in (7·5–10 cm) above the rim of the bath, to be about 2–3 ft (60–100 cm) long, with a vertical rail of similar dimensions at each end, extending up from the horizontal bar. This combination of rails enables most patients to pull up, to pull forward, to push up, or to hold on to when getting in and out of the bath. The usual grab rails are finished with chromium plate, and this is very slippery when the hands are wet. It is preferable for them to have a non-slip surface or else to be covered with plastic-tape material to give a stable grip when wet.

Most showers have a basin or pan under them with a rim some 6–9 in (15–23 cm) high. This may be difficult to negotiate for a disabled person, and once again the provision of grab rails at the sides of the shower and shower-seat are necessary. It may be possible to install a shower without a rim to the pan if the shower is downstairs and a suitable sloping base with a floor drain can be fitted instead, but it is rarely possible to install this type of fitting upstairs.

Transfers

Transfers between wheelchairs and bath depend on the height, type and size of the bath. The height of the bath is critical for many wheelchair transfers. The rim of the bath should be at the same height as the wheelchair seat or slightly below, particularly if independent transfers are aimed at and a sliding-board is used. If the transfer is to be accomplished with the aid of a helper, then the height of the bath should be related to the needs of the helper, and should be higher than usual to facilitate lifting and prevent backache. If, however, the transfer entails the use of a hoist, then the height of the bath should be related to the needs of the smaller members of the household, and unless the hoist is a portable one, needing clearance for its feet, the bath may be of a conventional low level.

Transfers from the wheelchair to the bath must be planned after trial of different techniques and practice in their use, starting with the conventional bath, or the one that is present in the patient's home. If it is not possible for the patient to transfer under existing conditions then the decision lies between accepting a different means of transfer (using a hoist or being lifted) changing the bath, or reconstructing the bathroom. The function of the Disabled Living Unit is to establish the various possibilities and to relate these to the existing conditions, to assess the patient's capabilities in the context of his present home, or his likely future accommodation. *Figure 5.3* illustrates the vertical and adjustable horizontal bar over the bath, the feet of the hoist under the bath and the all-in-one sling.

The transfer may be directly over the side of the bath, forwards, sideways, over the end of the bath or via a bath seat. In all cases, a bath which is shorter than usual, is safer, as in such a bath there is less likelihood of the patient slipping under the water, whether he is bathing unattended or attended by a helper. It is perhaps a wise precaution that a disabled person should never lock the bathroom door, and should only have a bath when assistance is to hand.

Transfer to a shower should usually be via a shower seat. The shower pan will inevitably be wet, and thus there is considerable danger of slipping. The other possible transfer technique when there is no rim to the shower pan is to use a chair of some kind and shower while seated in that chair. A wheeled chair may be used for access, and an old kitchen chair or plastic garden chair with rubber ferrules on the legs, can be left under the shower.

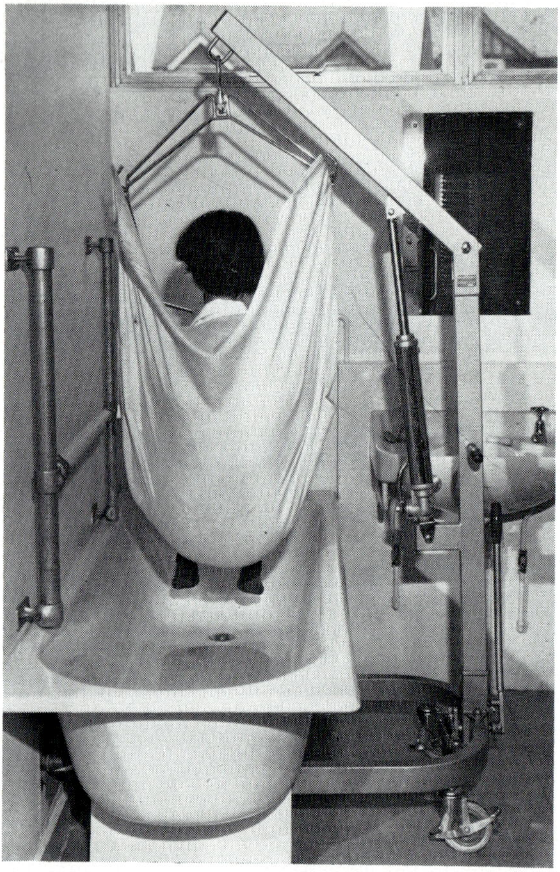

Figure 5.3. Patient being transferred to bath with a hoist

Taps and fittings

Taps are often used by the disabled as additional grab rails. This is a practice to be deplored, as their stability may be suspect, and a slip may not allow the patient to fall, but may also turn on the water and thus risk either a scald or drowning the patient. Taps fitted centrally at the side of the bath are easier to manipulate but rarely available. Lever attachments or lever-handled taps may enable the patient to operate them himself. Soaps, brushes and all other necessary appurtenances can be made accessible by standard bathroom shelves or bath fitments. A shower for a disabled person should have a thermostat control incorporated to prevent accidental scalding.

Assistance

Once a severely disabled patient is being catered for at home, or is striving to be independent, it is probably in the bathroom that assistance is most likely to be needed. Even though the situation seems to be satisfactory, regular visits from the appropriate welfare officer, or health visitor or district nurse are a wise precaution. In many areas, a bath service is available to avoid inessential demands upon the skilled services of the district nurses; but in any event, occasional visits to check on the patient's general state of health, cleanliness and freedom from pressure-sores or other skin damage may help to maintain the domestic situation and prevent further admission to hospital.

For further details and suggestions regarding bathing *see* Appen dixP.

DRESSING

Introduction

The necessary skills to dress and undress are taken for granted by the able-bodied, yet dressing is a process calling for balance, coordination, reach, strength and dexterity. It also requires insight into the task to be performed and a fair degree of spatial awareness, for example, hemiplegics with severe sensory loss associated with loss of spatial orientation or a distorted body image have more difficulty with their dressing, than those with only motor loss.

Rehabilitation of the severely disabled should be aimed towards independence in dressing as in other activities of personal care, but only in the context of each patient's circumstances. Maximum independence may be possible but unrealistic, and a patient who would be exhausted by the effort of dressing independently would do better to accept help and save his limited energy for more important and more enjoyable activities. For example, a man with traumatic tetraplegia (case history No. 257, Chapter 9, page 362) can almost dress himself but he takes a very long time and needs a great deal of effort to do so. It is quicker and more efficient for his wife to help him into his trousers, put on his shoes and socks and then transfer him to his wheelchair. He can then wash, shave and finish dressing while his wife organizes the breakfast and gets the children to school and is then ready for her to take him to work.

Assessment

An early and realistic assessment of the likely level of independence which a patient might achieve will establish in which activities need for training and practice exists. Given time and incentive, it is often possible to achieve more than originally estimated; but it is frustrating and discouraging for the patient if he fails to reach a therapist's over-optimistic goal. It is best to start with undressing, because in general, it is easier than dressing; and is normally done at a time less committed to the family routine. Starting with taking off the upper garments only, adding to this task that of undressing the lower half of the body, and eventually removing socks and shoes as well as speed and competence increase, many disabled patients will be able to achieve independence in this activity. A warm room, privacy and time to practice are essential requisites, and often an immediate assessment of the feasibility of independent undressing is not possible, because manipulative skill and trick movements may not be quickly acquired.

After undressing, dressing should be attempted. Once again, time must be allowed for this, perhaps waking up a few minutes earlier each day for the purpose. Breakfast and defaecation should rapidly be made to occupy fixed times in the rhythm of a disabled person's day and should not be altered, while waking time is more flexible in its adjustment. In dressing, as in undressing, a little at a time must be attempted, the upper half of the body being more easily dressed than the lower by most patients, and therefore being the better half to start on. Putting on the clothes of the lower half, pants, skirts and trousers, socks and stockings, girdles and corsets and finally shoes, often demands strength as well as mobility and may present difficulties which disabled patients cannot surmount.

When the assessing therapist has observed, advised and assisted, it is she who must help each patient to decide at what stage of dressing, his pain, slowness, weakness or stiffness should dictate the need to accept help. Such help may prove to be temporary only, particularly when the clothing has been suitably adapted, and the most efficient method of laying it out and putting it on has been devised.

Choice of style

As a general principle, clothes for the disabled should be chosen from those available on the market and in fashion. With the wide selection of garments currently available, it is almost always possible to choose something which is both fashionable and yet concealing, for example, slacks for women who have wasted legs or wear calipers. Specially made clothes, unless very skilfully designed and executed in contemporary colours and materials, will only serve to draw attention to infirmity or deformity.

Within the range of fashionable garments, it is often possible to select some of simple, loose fitting design with the minimum number of fastenings. Loose-fitting clothes with ample gussets and openings are not only easier to put on and take off, but are more comfortable to wear during long intervals of immobility, and last longer under the strain of assisted or unassisted transfers. They also have the ultimate advantage of looking smarter than tighter clothes which accentuate any deformity.

Shopping can be a difficult problem, and trying on clothes in a shop can be tiring and frustrating for the disabled. Some large department stores carry a wide range of clothes, will deliver on approval, or provide adequate fitting rooms, and are helpful in exchanging garments if the size or style proves to be unsuitable. Reputable mail-order firms now have an equally wide range of clothes that can be tried on in the privacy of one's own home, and for many this is the most practical solution.

For each patient there are many factors which determine the suitability of clothes. In assessing these factors, a therapist must always consider whether the requirements of the patient's particular disability modify what is generally found to be the most suitable form of any one garment.

From such considerations, various axiomatic statements arise:

If a disabled person dresses herself, it is easier for the clothes to have fastenings at the front; but if she is always dressed by a helper, it is easier to have fastenings down the back. A straight skirt is unsuitable for anyone wearing full-length calipers, it will restrict movement, ride up and get excessive wear and tear. Slippery materials that slide over one another make dressing easier, but when someone is liable to have extension spasm of the legs, the use of such materials will increase the tendency of the patient to slide forward in the chair.

A girl using a self-propelling wheelchair should choose a blouse with plenty of room across the shoulders, with raglan rather than inset sleeves, and with short or three-quarter length sleeves, as cuffs tend to get dirty on the wheels. On the other hand, a girl walking with axillary crutches will do better to choose a blouse with inset sleeves, as it will ride up less than one with raglan sleeves.

In general, the disabled are better wearing a size larger than expected. Wheelchair users, in particular, need slacks which are oversize in seat and crutch (it is easy to shorten the legs, if necessary). Belts and other tight fittings can be most uncomfortable for the disabled and elastic braces are advised in preference to these for men using crutches or sticks. They keep trousers well positioned and expand with extra shoulder movement. For women, flared skirts with an overblouse are often the most suitable form of clothing as these two-piece outfits are less likely to twist and ride up than most dresses.

As a general rule, pockets should be well forward, rather than at the side or hip. Adequate provision of pockets, suitably placed, adds to comfort and avoids the difficulty of carrying small objects, and leaves both hands free. The disabled often need to carry more with them, so as to prevent the need for extra journeys between various rooms to fetch each article as it is required.

It is necessary to analyse not only each patient's individual disability, but also his needs and circumstances when choosing clothes. It is also necessary to pay considerable attention to his comfort. A disabled patient may have to spend many hours in one position or one place, and have to wait a long time before someone can help him rearrange his clothing.

Comfort and choice of material

Whether the restricted mobility is secondary to weakness or diminished joint range, effort should be made not to further handicap the patient with heavy or constrictive clothing. The material chosen for the clothing of disabled people should be lightweight. It should also be warm, because the warmer the material, the fewer are the garments required. Thus dressing and undressing are considerably simplified and shortened if the daily wardrobe consists of only a few warm loose lightweight garments. A lined skirt, for example, may dispense with the need for an underslip, a brushed-nylon petticoat may serve as both vest and slip, and a quilted anorak is easier to put on and is more comfortable and warmer than a tweed jacket.

Stretch materials have many advantages when used for certain garments. Thus, when used in loose-fitting over-garments, of the same or of different material, stretch material is particularly suitable for collar and cuffs. It adds warmth, neatness and convenience to the loose garment, and in addition does away with the need for buttons and fasteners.

When used for undergarments, however, and in particular for underpants and socks, stretch material only makes further difficulties for disabled people. The openings of stretch socks and pants are small and difficult to locate and the garments tend to ruck up during use and to cling so that they are difficult to take off.

Underwear should be well-fitting and absorbent if there is any tendency to pressure-sores, and for this reason cotton materials are preferable to man-made fibres. Y-front underpants with elastic tops are probably the most comfortable for a man sitting in a wheelchair all day. For a woman in a wheelchair all day, it is helpful to move back suspenders round to the side. If a corset is not needed for support, a lightweight suspender belt is more comfortable than a girdle. If tights can be worn, they will dispense with the need for suspenders and are often more acceptable to patients who prefer to wear skirts.

The type of material can make a considerable difference to the difficulties involved with the long-term care of clothing. Clothes made of material that is easy to wash and quick to dry are the best choice. Garments which can only be dry-cleaned are not only an uneconomical buy, but the physical difficulties in getting them to and from the cleaners may present a further problem to the disabled patient.

Wool is relatively resilient, but will only stand up to frequent washing if great care is taken, and the same is true for wool jersey. Cotton is particularly useful when garments are likely to become soiled and stained frequently and may consequently require boiling and bleaching. Cotton underclothes, particularly women's pants, and cotton overblouses or shirts when food is likely to be spilled over them repeatedly, are ideal for this reason. Cotton jerseys, however, tend to lose shape. Rayon, though attractive in its surface appearance, is generally a most difficult material to care for. The recent widespread use of Crimplene for women's and men's overgarments has at last provided a material which washes well, dries quickly, needs no ironing, is elastic but not tight, is lightweight, but can be very warm, keeps its shape, and is available in a wide range of different weaves of varying weight, warmth and texture. Crimplene is also crease resistant, and as wheelchair-bound disabled patients tend to get their clothes twisted and folded Crimplene, in common with other crease-resistant materials, is therefore particularly suitable. Men's suits with terylene content will also be crease resistant, lightweight and warm, and in some cases, washable.

Easy maintenance is the advantage of most of the man-made fibres, though care in selection must always be exercised, since some man-made fibres must be dry-cleaned only, and shrink to an alarming degree if even lightly washed. Cotton terylene mixtures, nylon jersey, nylon, Terylene and Crimplene are all easy to maintain. With frequent washing by hand in water of the correct temperature containing detergent or soap to the right concentration, they will last well. Some garments in these materials need no ironing, some only minimum ironing. Machine washing tends to destroy the shape of many, and to loosen the seams of them all.

One disadvantage of some man-made fibres is their tendency to build up static electricity. This is especially noticeable in wheelchair users wearing too many nylon garments and may cause unpleasant shocks to the wearers.

Small-patterned materials show wear and spotting least. Dark plain colours such as navy, brown or black are difficult to keep free of fluff and so on.

Fastenings

Fastenings should be reduced to a minimum and where they are essential the type of fastening used should be that which can be managed by the individual. Velcro, zips or large buttons are some of the simplest types of fastening, and are manageable by the majority of disabled patients, whereas tied bows, hooks or buckles are to be avoided. Press-studs may be possible, if they are sited over a bony prominance (the iliac crests, for example). As a general rule, all fastening should be in front, near the mid-line and near the middle of the trunk, since the majority of the severely disabled have difficulty manipulating fasteners below the hips and above the shoulders.

Girdles, corset and brassieres present considerable problems, but even these garments can sometimes be managed if they have front fastenings of the appropriate type.

Tucking in clothes is also often difficult and skirts and blouses suitable for wearing outside the waistband of trousers and skirts should be chosen. Loose fitting clothes are usually more comfortable than tight ones, particularly with stretch edging, as described above.

Techniques of dressing and undressing

When the activities of dressing and undressing are planned for a disabled patient, the need for aids, equipment and special garments should be reduced to a minimum by the employment of a suitable technique. This will vary for each individual according to his personal characteristics and the nature of the dysfunction. There are, however, some general principles which can be applied to facilitate these activities for anyone.

Firstly, dressing and undressing should always be done in the same part of the same room, so that clothing need not be carried about and aids are to hand. Undressing should be something more than just taking the clothes off, it should also be a preparation for dressing. To save time and trouble in the morning, clothes should be prevented from falling to the floor and from turning inside out, and should be put ready for use the right way round and in the right order. The sequence of manoeuvres to be used during dressing must be carefully planned, for example, calipers and shoes first, before being able to stand, or pants and trousers first before a sideways transfer to a wheelchair. If help is needed for part of the process, it is necessary to decide whether this help is needed first, before independent dressing can proceed (for example, putting on a spinal brace) or whether it can be left till last (for example, putting on shoes).

Secondly, the timing of the disabled person's routine must fit in with the habits of the rest of the family, and must coincide with the most convenient time for his helper, if help is needed. Furthermore, the time when a patient is at his best may vary. Patients with rheumatoid arthritis experience stiffness and pain first thing in the morning, and many of them are more able to undertake the major effort of grooming in the evening. Conversely, some hemiplegics tend to become confused when tired, and are better advised to plan their major effort for the morning. The time actually taken to dress must be realistically assessed in the context of the patient's life; if he is going out to work, it must be possible to dress and groom reasonably quickly, and to organize their morning activities around toilet and dressing time tables. Continuous practice until new methods become automatic will gradually reduce the time necessary; but initially a calm, unhurried atmosphere is necessary for the disabled person to establish confidence and competence.

Thirdly, it is necessary to consider safety and this is usually related to place and position. Patients with impairment of balance or of spatial sense, such as a hemiplegic can start dressing on the bed, and should sit for most of the process, preferably with support on the affected side. It may then be quite safe for him to stand for a few minutes leaning against a wall or solid piece of furniture, while using his one good hand to continue dressing. Patients with areas of sensory loss must be trained to take special care to avoid skin damage on zips or fastenings. When balance is more severely affected or there is gross ataxia, dressing may be done wholly on the bed, possibly using a raised backrest.

Adaptations to clothes

When difficulties are experienced with normal clothes, then simple adaptations should be considered.

The most commonly used adaptations are as follows:

(1) Enlarging opening for ease of dressing.

(2) Extra openings, for example, zip in inside trouser seam for access to urinal.

(3) Moving fastenings within reach, for example, back suspender moved to side.

(4) Changing to more suitable fastenings: buttons instead of zip for one-handed, Velcro instead of buttons for weak hands, or zips for those with reach or co-ordination difficulties.

(5) Use of elastic to aid dressing and to keep clothes in position: elastic cuff-links or elastic in shoulder straps.

(6) Reinforcing clothes, for example, inside knee patches against excessive caliper wear.

If a patient's deformities or disabilities are such that even these adaptations are insufficient to enable him to dress independently or to be dressed easily, then major adaptations should be considered. By the application of dressmaking principles, it is possible to adapt standard home dressmaking patterns and achieve the reasonably smart appearance which is so important for a disabled woman.

Simple dressing aids

If techniques and simple adaptations to clothing are not enough to achieve some independence, then sometimes one or more dressing aid may be needed. These should be neatly made with no sharp edges to catch clothes or skin. They must be lightweight and portable and easily cleaned. Finally, they should either be durable, or cheap and readily available (*Figure 5.4*).

The most common useful dressing aids are as follows.

(1) Dressing stick, a simple reacher for pulling and pushing clothes, made from a length of wooden dowelling with a rubber thimble over one end, and a cleft or hook at the other end. Sometimes when necessary, a length of perspex or duralumin may be curved to individual needs.

(2) Long-handled shoe horn.

(3) Spring-steel button hook.

(4) Long-handled pick-up stick, for example, 'helping hand' or 'lazy tongs'.

(5) Stocking or sock aid, the simplest and most commonly used.

The severely disabled using equipment such as an electric bed or hoist can use this equipment to achieve some independence at dressing or to help an attendant to dress them.

A patient with muscular dystrophy and poor sitting balance may be able to dress independently on the bed if his back is supported and both hands are therefore left free. An electrically powered, self-operated bed will not only help such a patient to change his position in the night, but will also help him to be independent in dressing, by supporting him in a similar position.

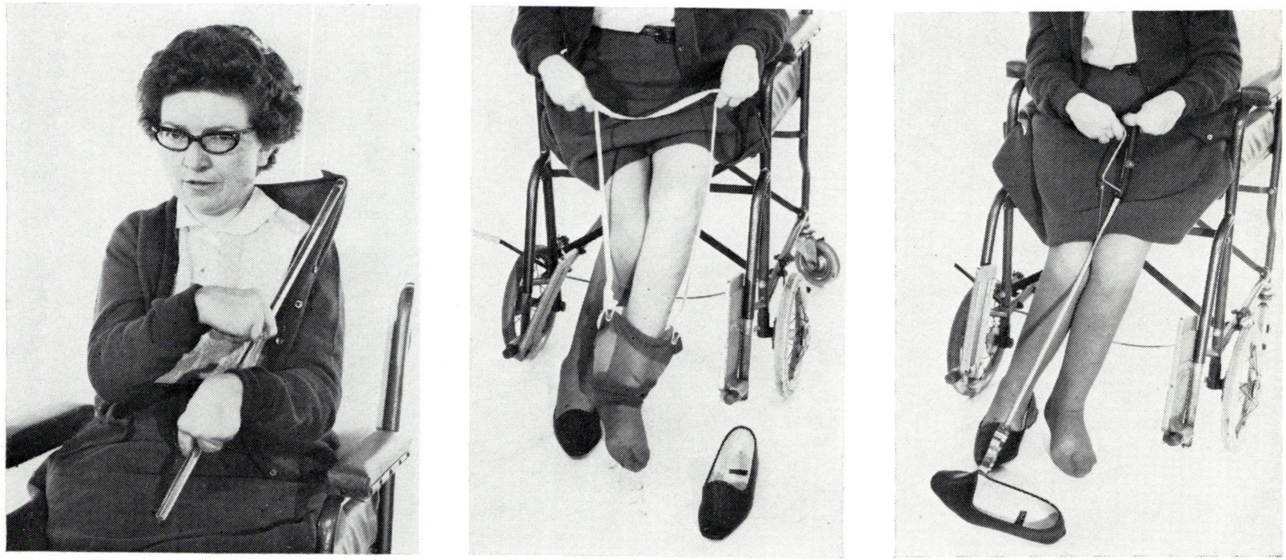

(*a*) (*b*) (*c*)

Figure 5.4. Patient with severe juvenile rheumatoid arthritis using (a) a perspex rod to assist dressing the top half; (b) a simple stocking aid; (c) a long handled pick-up stick to put on shoes

A simple monkey grip over the bed will enable a paraplegic to raise himself for transfers from bed to wheelchair, and will also enable him to pull his trousers up with his free hand.

A hoist over the bed will help a more severely disabled patient, or his attendant, to lift his body just clear of the bed and so enable clothes to be pulled down over the back of the shoulders.

COMMUNICATION

It is not usually realized that a high proportion of the physically disabled have some interference with their ability to communicate.

Those who have aphasia or dysphasia have an obvious difficulty in talking. Language is a function of the higher nervous centres, and its breakdown is common in brain damage, whether traumatic or circulatory in origin. When the dominant hemisphere of the brain is involved in the lesion, such breakdown is particularly likely to occur.

The breakdown may take the form of a receptive aphasia, when patients talk jargon or use the wrong words without appreciating that they are doing so. It may be an expressive aphasia in which they are unable to formulate words correctly. In the latter type of aphasia there is a failure to co-ordinate voice, tongue and lips. Nominal aphasia implies loss of memory of learnt words, and semantic aphasia implies loss of ability to construct sentences. Perseveration is a form of aphasia in which the same word or words are repeated meaninglessly. Verbal paraphasia (using wrong but similar words) dyslexia (inability to read), agraphia (inability to write) are all forms of aphasia.

Dysarthria is a neuromuscular disorder of speech not involving higher centres and more common in lesions of the cerebellum and bulbar nuclei. Speech disabilities are often amenable to improvement through speech therapy and their treatment must form an important part of rehabilitation.

Inability to communicate by means of the spoken word implies that in situations of danger or illness, help cannot be summoned and a means of summoning aid or of conveying a warning of imminent danger must be provided for such patients. Call bells and signal lights are the usual solution to these problems.

Inability to use the written word may be due to sensory dysfunction, loss of sight, mental dysfunction, agraphia or physical disability. The exact cause of the latter may be determined by a detailed physical assessment, and may be helped by the use of aids or appliances with suitable tables, writing aids, mobile arm-supports or prostheses. Typewriters with adapted keys, electric typewriters manually operated or controlled by sophisticated remote-control appliances are all available for the disabled through various charitable, educational and welfare organizations.

Providing the need for communication is understood and communication in all its aspects forms part of functional assessment, then many of the frustrations of the severely disabled will be avoided.

6—Problems of Mobility

TRANSFERS

Whether physically disabled or not, people require to sleep, eat and use the toilet every day, and unless they are completely bed-bound, this implies transferring from bed to chair and chair to toilet and back again as a minimum daily requirement. The techniques of transferring will depend on the patients' physical disabilities, the physical features of the appliances they use and the physical environment in which the transfers are to take place. The techniques depend also on the patients' will to undertake these activities, for many transfers entail considerable effort, and sometimes considerable discomfort.

Standing or ambulant transfer

The ability to stand and take one or two small steps reduces the problems of transference considerably. If the patient can get himself up off the bed, chair, or lavatory-seat, he may well become independent for many activities of daily living. The height of the bed, chair and toilet seat need to be the same, the bed and chair must be stable, and appropriate grab rails may be necessary.

Bed

For each patient there is an optimal height of bed. Some people find that this is the height which permits them to sit on the side of the bed, with their feet just resting on the floor during transfers. Many people are better suited by a hospital bed than by the usual domestic variety. Certainly, the conventional low divan style of bed is unsuitable for most physically disabled, particularly for those with stiff joints of the lower limbs, who transfer most easily when with buttocks resting against the edge of the bed, they are able to reach the floor with their heels.

A dimension which varies so greatly with the requirements of the individual may only be established by trial and error. There are, however, certain general characteristics which are common to all beds suitable for disabled people. The bed should be firm and stable, and preferably resting against a wall, so that a firm purchase can be obtained when the patient pushes up to achieve the standing position and to allow for the impact of the patient dropping back onto the bed again. Some patients employ the bounce of the bed to get up and therefore require a softer mattress than usual. In all cases, the mattress should be at least as wide as the frame of the bed and a narrow mattress should be avoided as it is liable to allow the skin of the buttocks to come into contact with the bedframe during transfers and thus cause skin damage. This is a common problem with the usual type of hospital bed, which should have a foam mattress with firm boards overlapping the frame as a precautionary measure.

Monkey bars, overhead chains, rope ladders, grab rails and other aids may be necessary to aid transfers in and out of bed. Sometimes, additional freedom can be obtained by using nylon sheets, which do not have the friction of ordinary sheets or sheepskins.

The bed should be placed in the room so that there is easy access, and its position can be easily changed, so that extra mobility may be obtained when necessary.

Lavatory

There is an optimal height for the lavatory pedestal, just as there is an optimal height of bed for each patient. The lavatory pedestal usually needs to be higher for the elderly and the physically disabled than for the able-bodied. Plastic or wooden clip-on raised seats are available, but they tend to feel unstable and most disabled patients do not like them. A firm seat can be built over the pedestal at the correct height and removed for other members of the household. Permanently raising the pedestal is a costly piece of plumbing and rarely warranted. However, it may be safer to arrange for the installation of a permanent, stable, high seat, providing appropriate footstools for other users, rather than to retain a conventional low pedestal with a cumbersome or unstable attachment for the disabled user. If the lavatory cannot be suitably adapted, then either a sanitary chair to wheel over the pedestal, or else a commode may provide an answer to the problem of the dissimilar family requirements.

Grab rails at the side and behind the pedestal are often necessary. These should be set horizontally and vertically so that the patient can both push up and pull up. The best position and height and shape can be found out by practical tests. The most useful dimensions and arrangements are indicated in the general recommendations of the Code of Practice (C.P. 96) issued by the British Standards Institution (*see also* Chapter 8).

Methods of wheelchair transfer

Wheelchair users who are unable to stand may be able to learn to transfer forwards, sideways, or backwards through the back of the chair. The technique used considerably depends upon the strength of their arms, and on whether they can use their legs as props or counterweights. Paraplegics who have full use of their arms develop powerful upper-limb and upper-trunk musculature, and can take their full bodyweight on their hands and arms, enabling them to transfer in different ways depending on circumstances. Those less physically strong, and patients with weakness or deformity of the upper limbs, will have greater difficulty in transferring, and will depend much more on having the chair, seat, bed and toilet at the same heights. For them, the position of the chair during transfers is critical, and needs careful adjustment. They may need such transfer aids as a sliding-board or monkey pole to help them.

Transferring sideways depends on the patient's ability to remove the armrests from an appropriate wheelchair. Such transfers are seriously impeded by particularly large (24 in, 60 cm) diameter rear propelling wheels, and by front propelling wheels; in both instances, the rim of the wheel is above the level of the side of the wheelchair seat.

Some patients, particularly double above-knee amputees, prefer to transfer directly forwards. Detachable footrests will enable the front of the wheelchair to be placed close to the bed or toilet. This particular manoeuvre is safer from wheelchairs with fixed armrests.

Many patients prefer a backwards transfer, having the back canvas of the wheelchair fitted with a zip fastener, for the purpose. The zip is best placed about 3 in (7.5 cm) to one side of the midline, on the easiest side to operate. A long leather thong or tag fixed to the zip will make manipulation easier. A zipped back is often difficult to do up, and the zip tends to become strained and break. It is easier to refasten if the zip opens upwards, but if the nib breaks, the zip will undo under the patient's weight. The strain can be taken off the zip by fitting an oversize canvas, and by inserting some system of overlapping straps to take the patient's weight. Laces or turnbuckles have been used for this purpose. This technique has many problems, but for some patients it is the only way in which they can obtain toilet independence.

It is possible to make a completely detachable back to a wheelchair out of a light metal or plastic material and to convert with cushioning. But such an adaptation must be individually made (*Figure 6.1*).

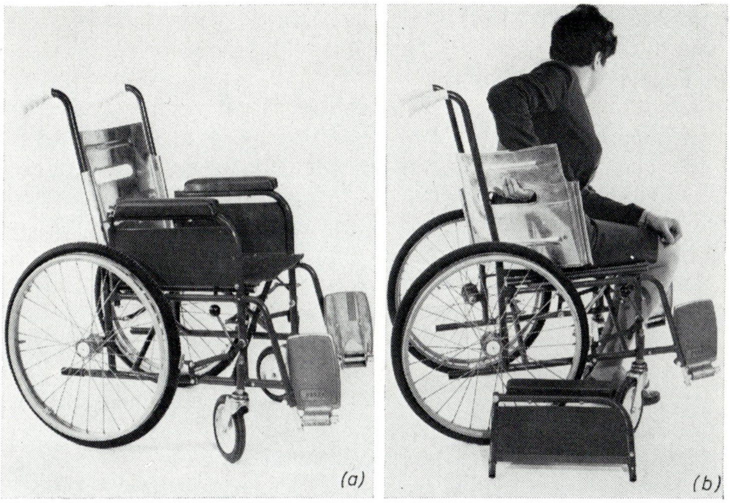

Figure 6.1. (a) the chair; (b) the back being detached (the armrest has been removed for the sake of clarity)

Aids

Sliding-boards are often used to bridge the gap between the seat of the wheelchair and the bed or toilet-seat. Such boards can be made of polished wood, or of wood covered with plastic or leather. The board is placed with one end on the bed and one end on the wheelchair. It is held in place by the patient's weight. The two ends must be level or the patient will have to go uphill in one direction. The width and length of the board depend on circumstances, but a useful general-purpose sliding-board is between 18 in (46 cm) and 28 in (71 cm) long and about 10 in (25 cm) wide.

In conjunction with a sliding-board, the best cushion is usually found to be one made of latex foam or similar material about 2 in (5 cm) thick, covered with smooth plastic or leather-cloth, and with a hard base (for example, plywood). The smooth, firm surface aids sliding and prevents damage to the skin of the buttocks and sacral area. Injudicious use of poor sliding techniques can produce unpleasant skin damage. Soft cushions are almost invariably an impediment to transfers for patients who do not have powerful arms.

Transfers on and off toilet

Toilet transfers may be perfected in the surroundings of a hospital or rehabilitation unit, but yet be impossible to reproduce in the domestic situation, where their success will depend on the architectural layout of the lavatory concerned. Unfortunately, most domestic lavatories are small and leave little room for manoeuvring by patients or wheelchairs.

Sideway transfers are only possible when there is adequate room to negotiate the wheelchair into position alongside the toilet pedestal. Where such room is lacking, the direct backwards transfer may sometimes be achieved, though not from electrically powered indoor chairs which have the batteries at the back and cannot be brought close enough for the purpose.

Some patients can manage a forward transfer and can thus use the toilet by sitting on it facing in the 'wrong' direction.

However, the patient who can stand and turn round, is much more likely to become independent for transferring on and off the toilet.

For all these manoeuvres, the modern low-flushing toilet suites are more awkward to negotiate than the old-fashioned ones, with a high cistern situated well out of the way. Grab rails and bars will be necessary in some cases and should be sited where the patient has a need for them.

Bath

Getting in and out of the bath is a complicated exercise, but with the use of bath seats at the right height for transfer from wheelchair and of steps down into the bath, many of the younger disabled can manage this manoeuvre independently. For the more severely disabled, and for the elderly, the use of mechanical devices such as hoists can aid the attendants, or even make the patient independent for these activities if he is capable of operating the hoist himself.

HOISTS

Many disabled patients, whether their arms are normal or mildly affected, can be trained to transfer from one seat to another. The common transfer problems exist in moving between bed and wheelchair and between wheelchair and toilet, but a further considerable problem may exist transferring in and out of the bath. When a patient is unable to achieve these transfers unaided, he becomes reliant upon relatives or other assistants, and is no longer capable of independent living.

In most institutions, whether hospitals or residential homes, the attendants usually prefer to lift the patients for these activities, finding that two attendants can often accomplish the transfer more quickly and with less discomfort to the patient than one attendant using mechanical aids. However, when the patients become very floppy or heavy, or if they have severe muscle spasm, manual lifting becomes more and more difficult. At home, there are often times when only one attendant is available, and lifting a severely disabled patient single-handed is difficult and dangerous, both to the patient and attendant. In these circumstances, hoists, particularly portable hoists, are of great value, but their efficient use demands experience and training. The correct technique can make all the manoeuvres easy and comfortable, whereas the wrong slings and inexperienced handing can not only hurt the patient, but make them fearful for future occasions.

Portable hoists

Several firms manufacture portable hoists; there are two main types. There is a stable and expensive type which lifts the patient in a lying or sitting position and which requires little in the way of slings. However, it is difficult for an attendant to manoeuvre the large model, and it is not really suitable for domestic use. It is relatively easy to use, requires little skill and is very safe.

The smaller, cheaper and more manoeuvrable hoists are much more complex to use because they involve the use of slings (*Figure 6.2*). However, if the attendant can master these complications, such hoists are very useful, even in small dwellings, as the patient can be swung through an arc of movement without moving the base of the hoist. Thus, the patients can be lifted off their wheelchairs and into bed, for example, without moving the hoist. This type of hoist can be pushed from room to room providing there is adequate door width and turning-space, and this can only be checked by trial. Pumping-up the hydraulic jack to lift the patient does not require much strength, but the attendant needs to be reasonably robust if the hoist is to be pushed from room to room, particularly if it is necessary to negotiate carpets.

When the hoist is used for bathing purposes, it is essential that there must be about 10 in (25 cm) clearance under the bath (and no side-panels (*Figure 5.3*) or else that the hoist can be manoeuvred into place and used from one end of the bath. The usual small bathrooms in conventional local-authority dwellings frequently present great problems.

Whether using a portable hoist or a fixed-track hoist, the physical proximity of bath and lavatory makes patient handling much easier,

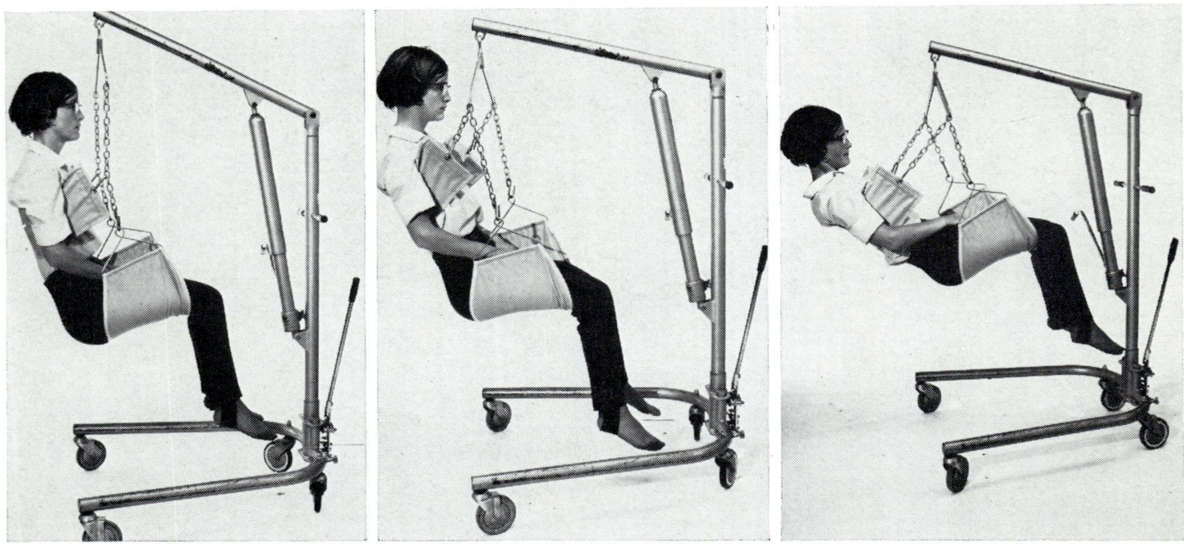

Figure 6.2. A portable hoist showing a patient being lifted in different positions, using two slings and adjusting the linkages of the suspension chain

and tracking direct from bed to bath or toilet can eliminate the number of necessary transfers for daily routines.

Portable hoists can be used for getting patients into motor-cars providing the car door is large enough, and the car has enough clearance to allow the feet of the hoist to go underneath (*Figure 6.3*).

Overhead hoists

A patient cannot operate a portable hoist on his own, but many patients can manage an overhead hoist. These can be fixed or tracked. Those that run on a track can be manually operated or fitted with an electric motor to drive them along the track (*Figure 6.4*). Either type of hoist can have a manually operated lifting device or an electrically operated lifting motor. The fitting of the overhead suspension or track will require professional installation as it is often necessary to undertake structural alterations to the house in order to strengthen the ceiling. If the track has an electric motor and is to run into a bathroom or toilet, then it is necessary to install an isolating transformer, and this installation is subject to the local by-laws and should be carried out or inspected by the local Electricity Board. A portable framework is now available and in certain circumstances may solve many of the installation problems and obviate structural alterations (*Figure 6.5*), but such an installation cannot track over long distances and the framework will occupy a considerable area of floor space.

Slings

There are many slings of different design, material and method of application. Materials used are usually nylon, canvas, or Covertex. Canvas and Covertex are firm and do not crease. Nylon is light. Nylon and Covertex are easily dried if it is necessary to wash them, and nylon mesh is particularly suitable for transferring patients in and out of the bath as it is porous and rapidly drip-dries. If the patient has to remain seated on the slings all day, or to lie on them at night, then one of the critical features of a sling is the extent which it tends to crease and fold.

There are two main slinging techniques. One employs 2 slings or 2 straps and the other one employs a hammock-type support.

The 2-strap technique

Although the simple 2-strap technique is simple to apply, it is limited in its application because it is poorly tolerated by patients with painful joints, especially of the spine, and by the elderly.

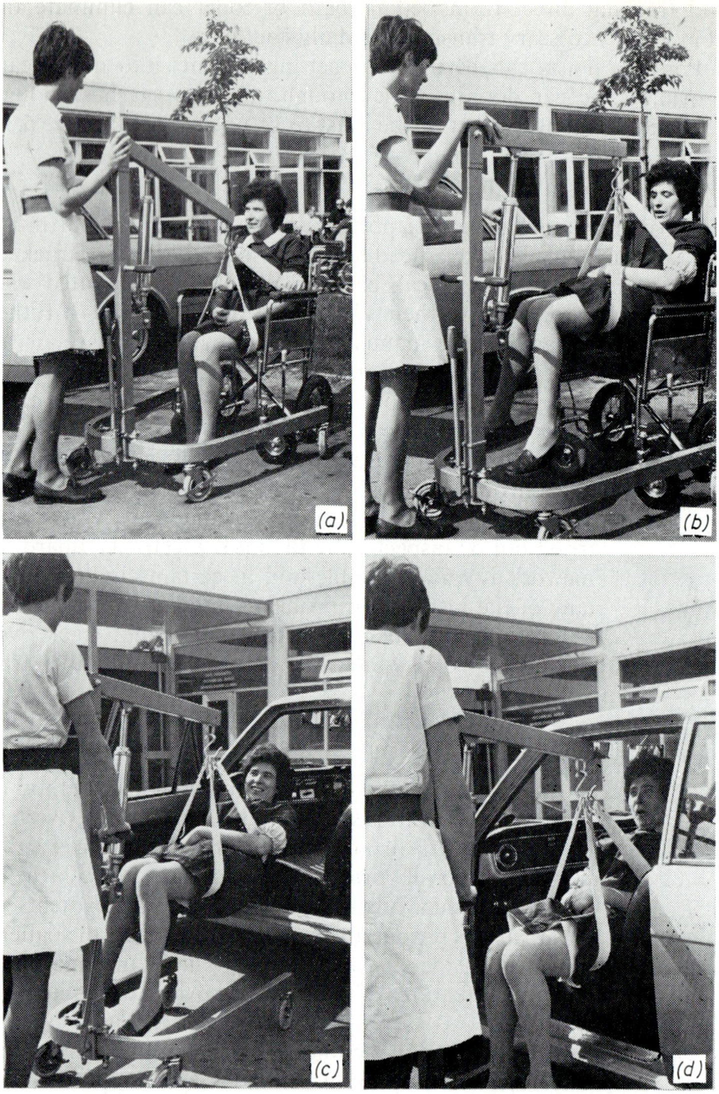

Figure 6.3. Lifting into a car using a portable hoist (a) slings in position; (b) lifting off the wheelchair; (c) negotiating the car door; (d) settling on to car seat

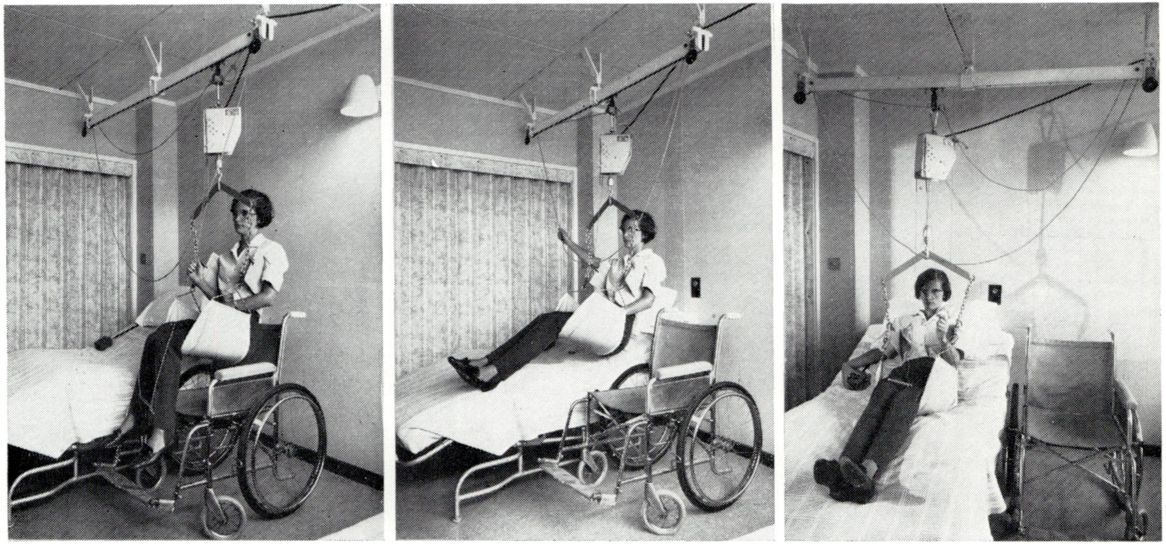

(*a*) (*b*) (*c*)

Figure 6.4. An electric hoist on a fixed overhead track being used to transfer from wheelchair to bed (*a*) *operating pull-switch of electric motor to lift off the wheelchair;* (*b*) *operating the cable to transfer from chair to bed;* (*c*) *controlling pull-switch with left hand and operating the controls of the bed with the right hand*

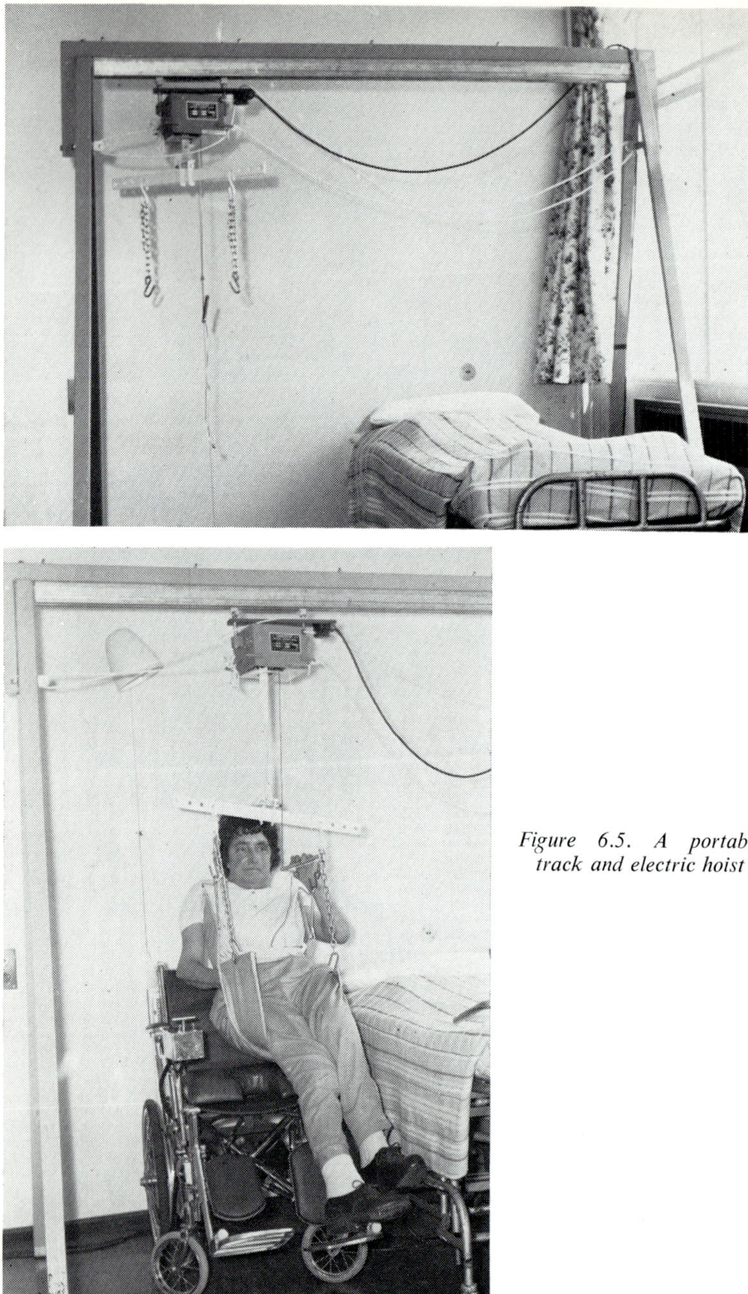

Figure 6.5. A portable track and electric hoist

The 2-sling technique

The 2-sling technique is similar to the 2-strap method, but wider slings are used which spread the load. This technique is somewhat less uncomfortable than the 2-strap, but severely disabled patients, particularly those with widespread weakness or paralysis tend to jack-knife and slip between the slings. The position and stability of the slings can be improved by judicious adjustment of the linkages which control them, enabling the patient to be transported in the sitting or reclining position.

Hammock sling technique

Patients unable to tolerate the 2-sling technique either because of pain, a tendency to slip between the slings or a tendency to go into spasm, are better using a hammock-type sling.

Various designs are available. Some provide head support, some have a toilet aperature, some have a split at one end to provide individual leg slings, giving separate support for each leg, and others are made like a full hammock.

In those with the split at one end, known as split-leg slings, the leg slings are easily slipped under each thigh and attached to a suspender. This type of slinging is convenient for toilet purposes as it allows the thighs to be abducted, and the leg slings are easily removable by the patient and thus absolve him from the need to sit on them throughout the day.

The complete hammock-type of sling is very safe and very comfortable once the correct positioning of the attachments has been worked out by practical trial. The patient's position during hoisting should be that which is most comfortable and does not induce any sensation of insecurity.

The child's hammock-sling is of simple design, easy to use, and supports the child completely. To avoid any manual lifting, the child can roll himself onto the sling laid on the floor or bed. The chains are then attached to the spreader bars and the child hoisted into his chair, where he sits on the sling throughout the day.

Spreader bars

Spreader bars are coat-hanger-like metal bars which separate the chains attached to the slings. These chains are hooked into the spreader bar at the appropriate linkage to obtain the patient's optimum position for hoisting. There are several sizes of spreader bar, and it is important that the correct one is used, because its width determines whether the slings grip or chafe the body during hoisting. In general, the spreader bar chosen should be the smallest one which can be used without chafing the body, since it will ensure that the sling grips the body well with little likelihood of slipping.

Chains

The slings are attached to the spreader bars by chains. Trials allow the assessor to find which link in the chain should be attached to the spreader bar for a particular sling on a particular patient. For hoisting a patient into a car, it is essential to use the shortest possible amount of chain to allow for manoeuvring through the limited space of a car door. Suspenders are supplied with hammock slings, and are individually designed to suit the sling (*see Figure 6.2*).

Sometimes the slings provided by the manufacturers are of unsuitable specifications. If any part of a sling needs alteration, it is usually wiser to arrange for the manufacturers or suppliers to make the appropriate adjustments. This may take longer, but it may also avoid an accident, and if an accident does occur, the blame for it cannot be attributed to unauthorized alterations by the therapists concerned.

The need for practical assessment

Practical trials of slings and hoists fulfil a dual purpose. They establish the competence of patient and relative to handle such equipment, and they also help to convince the local authority that the recommendation for their provision is a valid one.

Even when competence has been established in a Disabled Living Unit, its acceptance by relatives and patient must be confirmed. Exact measurements of the rooms where the hoist will be used are needed to ensure that there is enough space to manoeuvre and store a portable hoist. If a fixed-track hoist seems preferable, it is essential to find out whether the structure of the house is sufficiently strong to support such a fitment, or whether it is necessary and possible to install suitable scaffolding to take such a track.

The co-operation of a domiciliary occupational therapist is of the utmost value in these investigations.

Finally, clinical examination will establish whether the prognosis indicates that the patient is likely to get reasonable use from the installation of such expensive equipment.

WHEELCHAIRS

The ability to move from place to place, even if it is within the confines of one room, may make all the difference between some degree of independence and complete dependence with the frustration which this entails. Wheelchairs are, therefore, as important to many disabled patients as artificial limbs are to amputees. The same care in selection and training in manipulation is necessary for both types of equipment.

There is a slight preponderance of women among wheelchair users, 60 per cent. Of the total wheelchair using population, the majority are between 15 and 65 years of age, but a significant proportion, about 15 per cent, are under 15, and about 10 per cent are over 65.

Currently, there are about 100,000 wheelchair users in the United Kingdom, 20,000 to 25,000 of whom are permanently wheelchair-bound.

About 30,000 new wheelchairs are issued by the Department of Health and Social Security each year, but experience indicates that at least one-third of these are returned, or not used, because they are unsuitable for the patient.

The commonest cause of disability leading to the use of a wheelchair is arthritis. Osteoarthritis and rheumatoid arthritis each accounts for about 15 per cent of wheelchair users, the majority of whom are naturally in the older age groups.

The next most common disability amongst wheelchair users is multiple sclerosis, which also accounts for about 15 per cent of all users. This disease presents many problems, but the combination of ataxia, muscle spasms and pathological lack of insight into the disability make the successful prescription of a wheelchair a difficult exercise.

Cerebrovascular lesions account for about 13 per cent of users, and lower-limb amputations for 9 per cent. Double amputees, luckily rare, present particular problems because of the alteration in their centre of gravity which makes them likely to overbalance backwards in a standard general-purpose chair.

About 8 per cent of wheelchair users are drawn from patients with cerebral palsy, and a further 8 per cent from those suffering from paraplegia (including paraplegia due to spina bifida). The remainder are drawn from patients with a variety of disabling diseases, including some of neuromuscular, respiratory and cardiac origin.

The present conditions governing the provisions of wheelchairs are largely responsible for the high percentage of these chairs which remain unused. Wheelchairs may be prescribed by any hospital consultant, regardless of his speciality. Yet for many patients a correct prescription can only be made after expert assessment and practical trials by trained therapists and technicians. Furthermore, the standard prescription form allows a very limited amount of space for information from the prescribing consultant, the chair is usually delivered direct to the patient's home, little attempt is made to adjust the fittings to the requirements of the patient (for example, footrests), minimal explanation is given to him about the variations which are available in the individual parts of the chair, and seldom is any training provided in its correct usage. Lastly, the consultant prescribing the chair rarely has the opportunity of seeing the patient in it, and thus loses the chance of observing and rectifying the mistakes which he or anyone else has made.

Ideally, patients should be seen in wheelchair clinics attended by therapists and technical officers sufficiently experienced in this field to enable them to make an adequate assessment of the patient's needs, to make appropriate adjustments or alterations to the wheelchair after its delivery, and to give the patient any necessary training in the correct use of the chair.

Types of wheelchairs

Wheelchairs may be self-propelled or attendant-propelled. Self-propelled chairs must have one pair of wheels large enough for a patient to reach them without effort when propelling himself. Attendant-propelled chairs have small wheels which need not be within reach of the patient. Such a chair may be small (car transit), for easy transport in a car, or large when it is only intended for use within pushing distance of the home. In the latter case, the chairs are like large, well-sprung push-chairs, and indeed the chassis and handle-bars are designed rather like those of a child's perambulator. Comfort and not compactness is the dictating factor in their design. The size ranges are child, junior, adult and outsize.

General purpose chair

Folding, self-propelled, general purpose, wheelchairs with the propelling wheels at the rear, and the castor wheels in front, are the chairs most commonly issued (The Ministry of Health Model 8) (*Figure 6.6*). Approximately 80 per cent of all the chairs issued are of this basic design, but vary in weight, construction and accessories.

An all-purpose chair, the Model 8 weighs about 57 lb (20 kg) but is robustly made. The armrests are detachable, but the footrests are usually fixed, recent versions have swinging detachable footrests. The backrest recline varies from 10–15 degrees and variations of the chair include solid or pneumatic tyres. It is also obtainable in a lightweight form (*see Figure 6.6* (*c*) and (*d*)) which weighs about 36 lb (16 kg) with detachable footrests and armrests. The backrest reclines to about 8 degrees and may be hinged. This chair is being increasingly supplied for elderly patients or those who have difficulty with propelling. All Model 8 chairs are fitted with tilting levers and hand handles to enable them to be pushed by an attendant and tilted to negotiate kerbs.

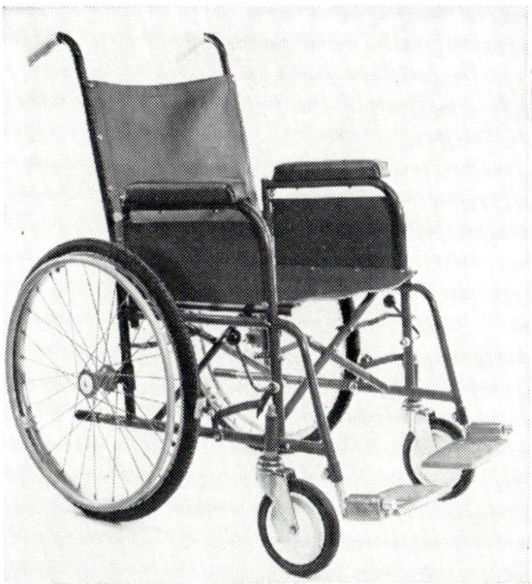

(*a*)

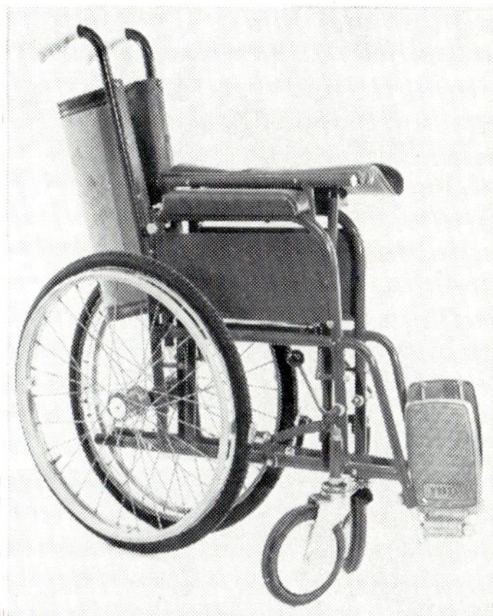

(*b*)

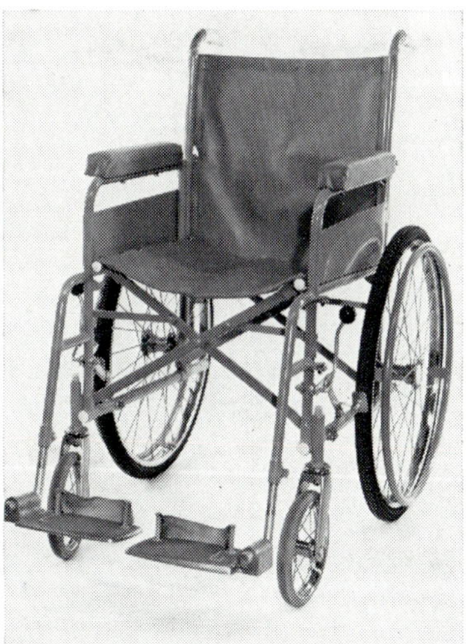

(*c*)

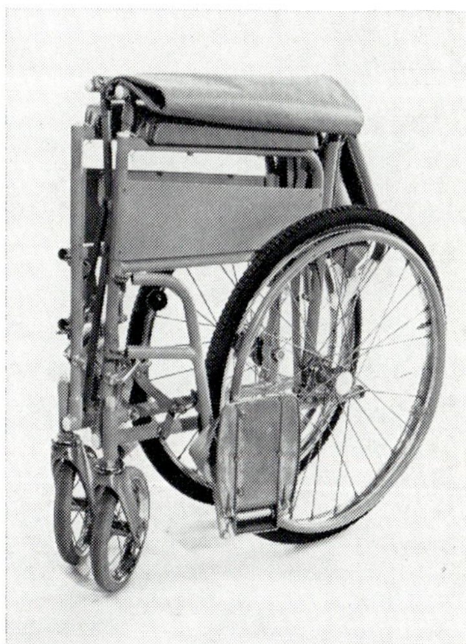

(*d*)

Figure 6.6. Model 8 standard general purpose chair (a) ready for use; (b) folded. Lightweight general purpose chair (c) ready for use; (d) folded

Indoor chairs

Indoor chairs usually have the large wheels in the front and the castor wheels at the back, making them easily manoeuvrable and enabling very disabled patients to move them around a room independently. The usually prescribed indoor chairs (Model 1) are made of wood and have comfortable upholstery (*Figure 6.7*), resembling an upright Victorian armchair on wheels.

Such chairs can be fitted with trays or commodes, and their

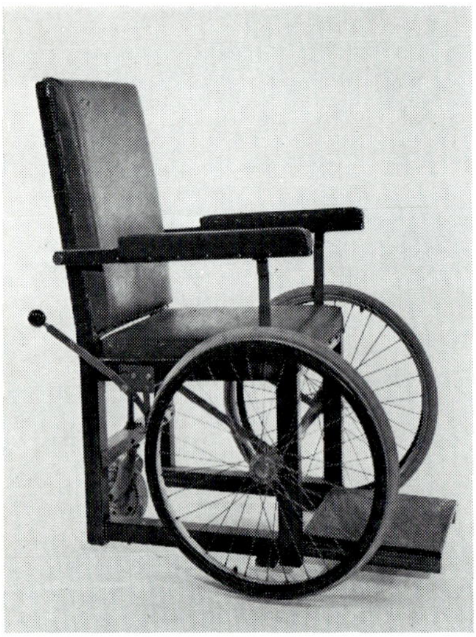

Figure 6.7. Model 1 wheelchair

cushioning is easily altered, but they have several disadvantages which limit their usefulness. They are dangerous when pushed by an attendant, as they are readily caused to tip by small obstructions such as a stone or step. They cannot be tilted backwards for an attendant to negotiate a kerb. Their large front wheels prevent patients from undertaking sideways transfers, and from coming sufficiently close to many working surfaces such as tables and sinks.

About 3–5 per cent of all chairs currently issued are in this group, and the majority of patients using them are elderly or severely disabled.

Outdoor chair

There are two main types of outdoor wheelchairs which are designed to be pushed by an attendant and do not have provision for the patient to propel himself. One type of chair is large and designed rather like a pram. It has comfortable upholstery, is well-sprung and is provided with a retractable footboard and an apron for inclement weather. Many elderly and arthritic patients are best served by this chair for their accompanied outings (Ministry of Health Model 13) (*Figure 6.8*), but it has several unfortunate disadvantages. Many of the attendants, who are often also elderly, complain about its

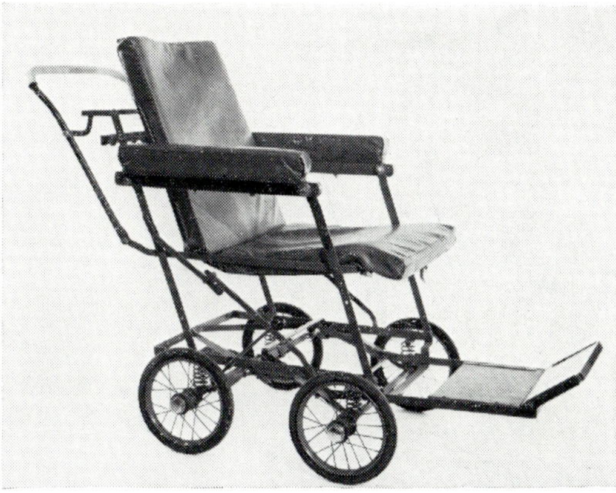

(*a*)

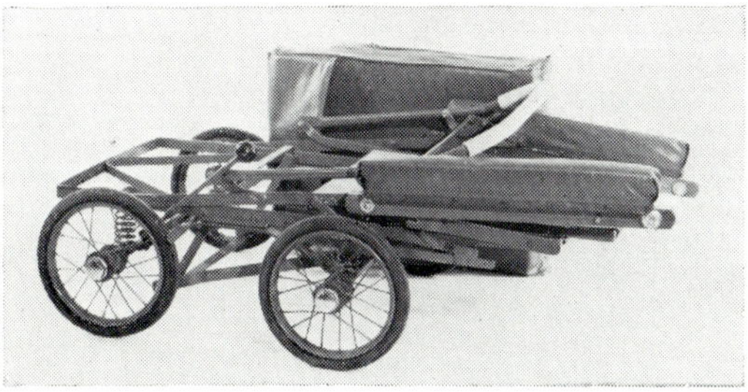

(*b*)

Figure 6.8. Model 13 standard push-chair
(*a*) *ready for use;* (*b*) *folded*

weight. In fact, it is the combined weight of the patient plus the chair which is relevant, and a chair some 20–30 lb (9–15 kg) lighter makes little difference to the total load. This push-chair is easier to push and can negotiate rough paths, kerbs and steps, but it is difficult to push round corners and to manoeuvre in a confined space because of the lack of castor wheels. The handle gives better purchase and leverage for tilting, the brakes, like pram-brakes, can easily be operated by the attendant's foot. It is undoubtedly much more comfortable for the patient. But the difficulty of getting the chair in and out of a house with old-fashioned narrow corridors and steps, the inability to transport it in the family car, the problem of storage in the usual small domestic hallway and the prejudice which exists against this model because it looks like an invalid chair often combine to outweigh its mechanical advantages.

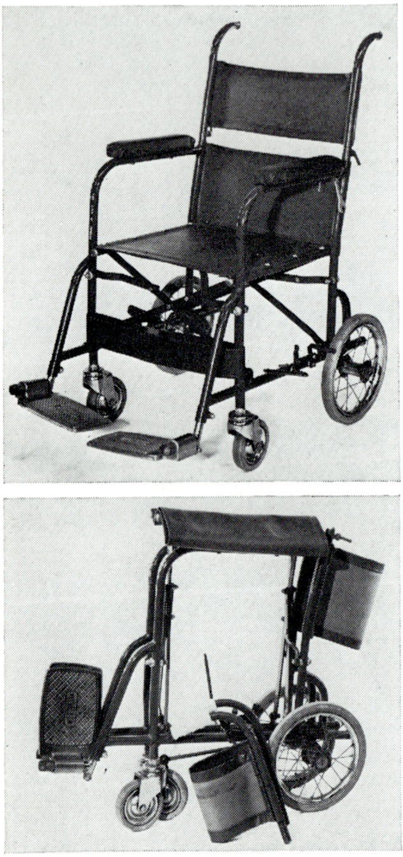

(*a*)

(*b*)

Figure 6.9. Standard car-transit wheelchair
(*a*) *ready for use;* (*b*) *folded*

The second type of outdoor, propelled chair is the car-transit chair, which is deliberately made small and compact so that it can be folded up and transported in a car boot. Such chairs have minimal comfort and are not suitable for pushing a patient for long distances. Whether a patient uses an indoor chair or an outdoor chair, if he requires to be taken out in a car for social or therapeutic purposes, then a car-transit chair provides a useful second wheelchair (*Figure 6.9*).

Prescribing wheelchairs

Selecting the best wheelchair for a particular patient is often an exercise in compromise. Most patients demand (1) comfort, which usually means roominess and cushioning; (2) minimal bulk so that the chair can be transported in the smallest car-boot; (3) a chair which is robust and reliable and yet very light; (4) a chair which is easy to self-propel and also easy for an attendant to push.

These features are practically irreconcilable, and as a compromise some variant of the general-purpose chair is chosen. Sometimes the patients may be best served by 2 (or more) wheelchairs. At present, about 1 in 5 wheelchair users has 2 chairs and 1 in 20 has more than 2 chairs.

Transfers to and from wheelchairs

When considering the appropriate wheelchair to prescribe, it is essential to establish the technique which a patient will use to get in and out of the chair, whether he will be independent, whether transfers will be standing, sliding, sideways or forwards and whether the transfers will need a hoist or merely help from an attendant (*see* Transfers, page 204). The technique to be used may determine the type of armrest (fixed or detachable), the type of footrest (fixed or swinging detachable), and the propelling wheels (front or rear).

Sides and armrests

The sides of a wheelchair may be fixed or detachable. Some patients need fixed sides to give them firm grip for manoeuvring in and out of the chair, or lifting the chair into cars. Other patients must have detachable sides to allow sideways transfers, and also to reduce the weight and size of the chair for folding it into a car boot, by removing the sides and lifting them in separately.

The height of the armrests may be critical for some patients, and the relative height depends on cushioning. A high cushion lifts the patient up and he may then find the armrests relatively low. This can be corrected by increasing the depth of the padding of the armrests. The detachable sides of some proprietary brands of wheelchair are supplied in different heights.

Sides can also have a shaped front which allows the wheelchair to approach closer to table or desk (desk armrests or domestic armrests), the front part of the side and armrest being cut away to fit under the table.

Some manufacturers make sides which are reversible. The patient may wish to have the domestic armrest shape to allow close approach to tables or desks for working, but may require to remove the sides and use the front part of the armrests at normal height to push on when transferring.

Wheels and tyres

The size of the wheels can be varied. The larger the wheels the greater the leverage, and the easier it is to propel the chair. However, large wheels present considerable difficulties for patients who are likely to transfer sideways out of the chair.

Rear wheels of 20 in (51 cm) diameter are usually completely below the level of the seat and present no hazard to sideways transfers. Wheels of 22 in (56 cm) may present slight hazards, but are usually negotiable, whereas 24 in (61 cm) rear wheels are a definite hazard to sideways transferring. Large front wheels of any size usually impede sideways transfers and they also prevent the fitting of footrests which can be swung sideways to make standing easier. Thus, front-wheel-drive chairs are normally restricted to patients unable to transfer themselves.

The tyres are important. Pneumatic tyres are better for outdoor use, as they have some element of springing and give a better grip on wet surfaces. But they are liable to puncture, and a puncture may render a severely disabled patient helpless. Also pneumatic tyres have a higher degree of friction with the floor than solid tyres, and thus make the wheelchair more difficult for the weak patient to manoeuvre, particularly on a carpet.

Therefore, solid tyres are easier to manage indoors and on a smooth (tiled or linoleum) surface and may allow a disabled patient to be independently mobile, whereas he might be unable to propel a chair with pneumatic tyres. Handrims and capstans can be fitted to aid grip. Although usually of metal, these can be varied, and the capstan knobs may be variously designed to enable patients to push with palm or knuckles.

Some severely disabled patients can manage a wheelchair on the flat but cannot manage to push it up a slope, tending to run back down the slope between forward pushes. There are two types of unidirectional brake available, one fitting on to the undercarriage of the chair, and one fitting on to the wheel. In each case, there is no impediment to forward movement, but the brake prevents the chair running backwards.

Single hand control (one-hand drive)

Wheelchairs are available with the propelling handrims for both wheels on the same side of the chair. This enables a patient to control his chair with one hand. Such chairs are very difficult to manoeuvre and although young patients with static lesions may become very adept at their control, elderly patients recovering from strokes are rarely able to learn to manage them successfully. *Figure 6.10* illustrates a wheelchair with the backrest partially reclined, 8 in pneumatic tyres at the front and 24 in pneumatic tyres at the rear. This chair has swinging detachable footrests and a double handrim on the left so that the chair can be propelled with the left hand alone.

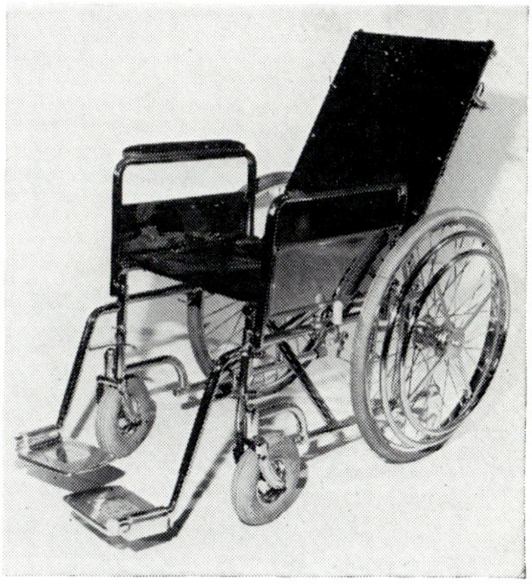

Figure 6.10. A one-hand drive wheelchair

A more easily acquired technique for these patients is the combined use of their good hand and foot. The hand propels the chair forwards (albeit tending to turn the chair towards the opposite side) and the foot is used to check the tendency to turn. Such patients can often manoeuvre the chair very accurately over short distance, either forwards or backwards.

Castor wheels are usually 7 in (18 cm) in diameter. If their diameter is any less, then it is difficult to negotiate even small obstructions such as a carpet edge or small stone or a step to an interior doorway. The combination of large (24 in, 61 cm) rear wheels and small (5 in, 12 cm) castors is particularly dangerous. Spokes are sometimes used for lightness, but they are liable to mechanical failure, and 7 in (18 cm) or 8 in (20 cm) solid castors are probably the best for general purposes. Castor wheels are subject to considerable trauma and need to turn freely for manoeuvring. Solid tyres are therefore preferable to pneumatic tyres, which are liable to puncture and also create more friction during turning.

Footrests

Fixed footrests constitute a hazard for patients with calipers and artificial legs, for patients with loss of sensation in the legs, and for patients who tend to get spasms. For such patients, footrests which are easily swung aside and detached are of considerable advantage. Some footrests can only be detached by attendants, or after the patient has vacated the chair. The most useful footrests are those with a simple swinging motion, which can either be swung aside or else easily detached and replaced by the patient while still seated in the chair. The footrests should be adjusted to such a length that a patient can place both feet on them, while he is sitting with thighs resting in the horizontal position on the chair seat. If the footrests are too high, the knees will be too high, and hips and knees will be uncomfortable. This position may also cause drainage problems for patients using incontinence appliances.

Elevating legrests are almost invariably the cause of difficulties. They are awkward for the patient to operate unless he can take the weight of his legs off the legrests before elevating and lowering them. They considerably increase the length of the wheelchair, making it difficult to manoeuvre in a confined space. Many patients find it uncomfortable to sit with their legs outstretched, and can only achieve comfort by sitting in a reclining position. But unless a wheelchair with a special reclining back is provided, comfort can only be obtained with considerable padding and cushioning. This will alter the patient's position in the chair and so necessitate alterations in the length of the footrests. Thus, elevating legrests often provoke more discomfort than that for which they were prescribed. It is often easier to advise the use of a simple footstool.

Backrests

As with ordinary chairs, the angle of the back which is most comfortable varies from patient to patient. Some patients like sitting upright and others prefer to recline. Too great a recline may make a patient slide down the chair. It may also make it more difficult for him to propel the wheelchair, or to sit comfortably for feeding or working. In the absence of specific reasons for providing a more reclining back, most patients are best suited by a chair with a near-upright back, reclining at about 5 degrees from the true vertical. The seat of this chair is angled at 90 degrees to the back, with the footrests raked at 5 degrees to follow the rake of the seat.

Although wheelchairs may be advertised as having a back inclination of 5–15 degrees, this may or may not take into account the rake of the seat. Thus a standard chair may be applied with back inclined to the vertical from 5–25 degrees. This is a further reason why practical trials are necessary before the prescription of wheelchairs. There are wheelchairs available with adjustable backs for patients who need more than 15 degrees recline, or else the facility to recline intermittently; but there are none with adjustable backs which can be easily operated by the patient. *Figure 6.11* shows a wheelchair fitted

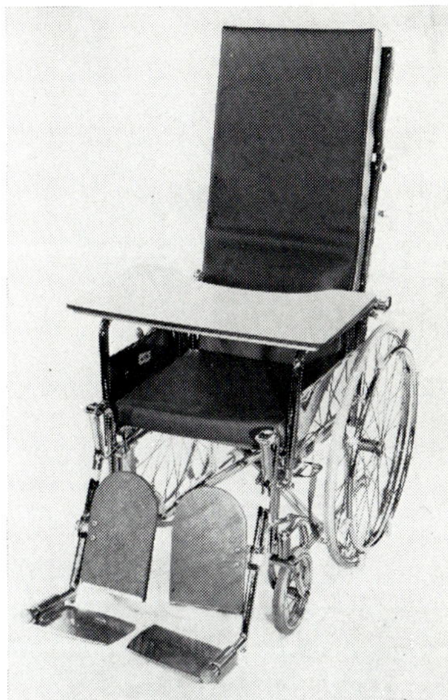

Figure 6.11. A wheelchair with an adjustable back

with a reclining back, a full-length cushion to include a headrest extension, capstans on the handrims, detachable swinging elevating legrests, 8 in solid-tyred spoked front wheel, 24 in solid-tyred rear wheels and detachable table.

Many wheelchair users sit in a hunched position, either because they tend to sprawl in the chair, or because they have a collapsing scoliosis. More efficient use of the chair can be obtained if the sitting posture is corrected. Lateral supports can be fitted within the wheelchairs as a form of cushioning. If the patient intends to use mobile arm-supports, it is particularly necessary to support the trunk. Without adequate trunk-support he may lean on the mobile arm-supports, and so cause them to support some of his body weight as well as his arm weight. In doing this, he will interfere with their mobility and efficiency. *Figure 6.12* illustrates a wheelchair adapted for a child with muscular dystrophy showing monodrive attachment, special footrests, side pads to control collapsing scoliosis, mobile arm-supports and the cushion to hold knees apart.

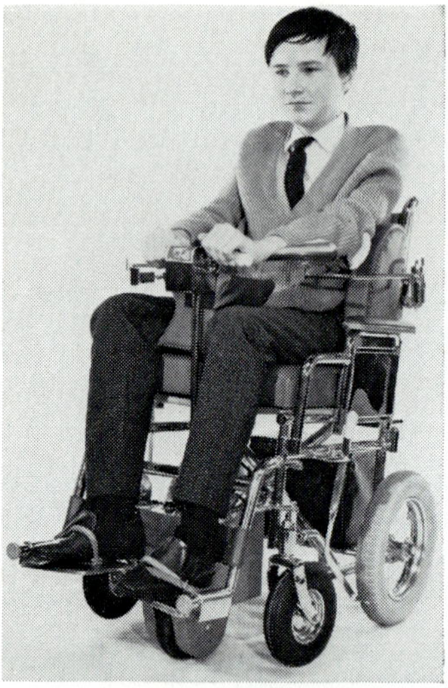

Figure 6.12. A wheelchair adapted for a child with muscular dystrophy

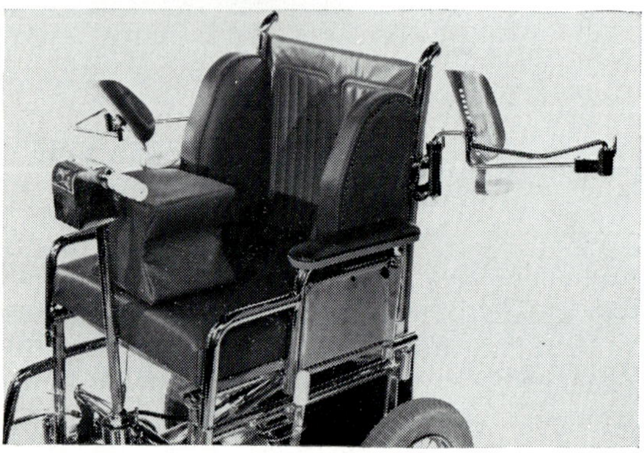

Seat and cushions

Cushions can make or mar the patient's comfort. Soft cushions, air-rings and similar emblems of comfort often cause discomfort and are sources of danger. Air-rings predispose to pressure-sores, and deep soft cushions successfully immobilize the severely disabled. As has been earlier mentioned, soft upholstery with a leathercloth cover on a firm plywood base provides the most suitable form of cushion, holding the patient up and allowing easy sliding transfers. These cushions have the further advantage that when used for wheelchairs of the folding type, they are easily removed before folding the chair, minimizing the space needed for chair storage in car boot or hall.

It cannot be stressed too often that the inter-relationship of the heights of wheelchair seat, toilet seat and bed are critical for transfers, and it is a matter of judgement to determine which is selected as the key against which the others must be adjusted.

Paraplegic patients are taught to ease the weight off their buttocks and to change their position frequently, but patients with weak or

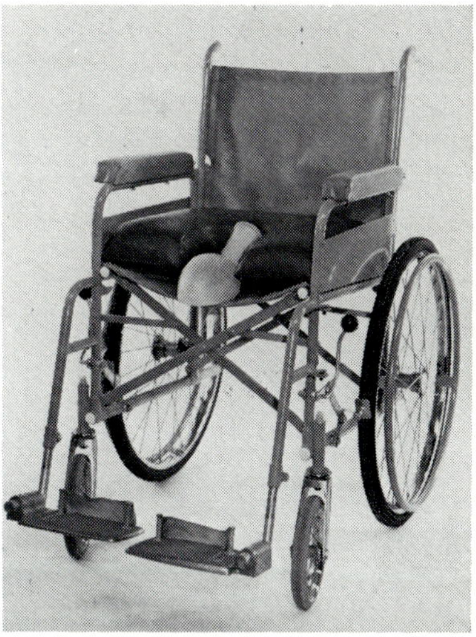

Figure 6.13. A lightweight chair with a paraplegic cushion with male urinal in position

deformed arms may need to rely on sheepskin covers for their seat cushions, or ripple (alternating pressure) cushions, or both.

Cushions with cut-out portions to accommodate urinals may assist with personal care (*Figure 6.13*) (*see* Problems of Micturition, Chapter 4).

Headrests often cause difficulties. Most wheelchairs can be fitted with a headrest extension, but this follows the line of the back of the chair and thus is often not in the best position to support the head. Simple neckrests and headrests can be made to attach to the wheelchair headrest extension, and they are best when custom-built. Attempts to support a very weak neck are most likely to succeed when the back of the chair is reclined at an angle of 30 to 40 degrees. It is particularly difficult to provide adequate support for the head of a patient with severe head tremor. A well padded winged headrest gives some support and exerts partial control of the tremor as well.

It is usual to find that the more complex the cushioning the less likely it is to be successful. Although it is often necessary to adjust the sitting-space to the patient, the cushioning provided for the purpose must be simple, repeatable, easily removeable and replaceable, and not restrict the patient. Otherwise it will be neither acceptable nor comfortable.

Spasms problems in a wheelchair

Muscle spasms are a frequent problem for wheelchair users. Flexor spasms of the legs tend to pull the feet off the footrests of wheelchairs into the track of the front castor wheels, thus making manoeuvring difficult. Usually the spasm, or the subsequent flexion deformities, can be partially controlled by the use of heel straps or leg straps behind the calves. Such straps have to be removed before the swinging detachable footrests can be removed, but modern straps are made with press studs and removal is not difficult for an attendant.

Extensor spasms are a greater problem. Severe spasms will cause the patient to extend the hips, and thus span the wheelchair, arching from the top of the back rest to the footrests or the floor. The patient will tend to slip off the chair or so alter his position that he is no longer reasonably comfortable, and may not be able to regain his usual sitting posture. Restraining a patient with these extensor spasms is difficult. The usual lap straps are inadequate, as the patient tends to slip under them when extended at the hips. A body-strap from the back of the seat of the chair over the lap, together with a pair of thigh-straps fixed to the side horizontals of the seat and through a loop between the thighs, together constitute a harness which exerts adequate control.

Shoulder and chest restraining straps may also be necessary for some patients.

The Amesbury Bantam Chair has been specially designed for children with cerebral palsy. It has a pommel to separate the thighs, and a special foot box which prevents the feet overlapping or slipping off the footrests (*Figure 6.14*).

Brakes

There are several designs of wheelchair brakes. Most depend on a mechanical linkage which enables a metal lever to bite into the tyre of two of the wheels. Solid tyres gradually wear away and the brakes become slowly less effective, whereas on wheels with pneumatic tyres the brakes exert a better grip. Efficient brakes are essential to prevent the chair from running away when the patient gets in and out of it, and as many patients push up from the chair and drop back into it

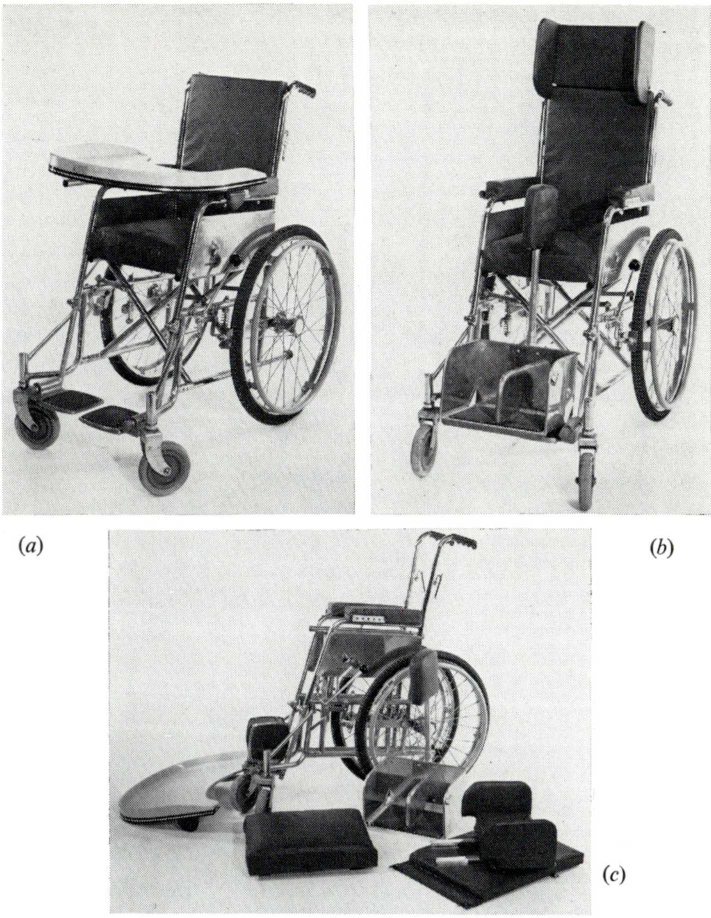

(*a*) (*b*) (*c*)

Figure 6.14. The Amesbury Bantam Chair showing (*a*) *tray;* (*b*) *thigh pommel, foot-restraining box and headrest;* (*c*) *folded chair with attachments removed*

when sitting, careful attention to brake maintenance is necessary for continued safety. For patients with only one effective hand, there are brakes operating from one side only with a cable connection to apply the brake on the opposite side. These brakes are unreliable, as the cable tends to stretch, so that one wheel is less efficiently braked than the other. Whenever possible the patient should be taught to use independent brakes. An extension to the brakes may make them easier to reach and easier to apply; but the extension lever may interfere with sideways transfers. Many standard chairs can be supplied with detachable brake-extension levers.

The majority of wheelchairs have brakes which are applied by pulling backwards on the brake lever, and this seems to be the natural action to stop a forward motion of the chair. Recently, some chairs had been supplied which had brakes operated by a forward push. This has confused some patients, and also has contributed to accidents, as patients propelling themselves have inadvertently caught the brake lever in their clothing, putting the brake on suddenly and thus ejecting themselves from the chair. The efficiency, stability, ease of operating, and avoidance of unintentional application are particularly important for the young disabled with unstable disabilities such as haemophilia and fragilitas ossium.

Wheelchairs for children

Children present particular problems. There is no standard chair available for the very small child and there is a serious gap in the sequence of sizes suitable for children during their growth between 9–13 years. The child's general-purpose chair (8C) has a standard seat width of 12 in (30 cm) and the next size (8J, Junior) has a seat size of 15 in (38 cm).

Now that more children with spina bifida survive and present as paraplegia or partial paraplegia, there is a growing need to provide suitable wheelchairs to enable a child to obtain mobility at the age when he would normally crawl. A small self-propelling chariot can be made quite cheaply (Chapter 3, *Figure 3.2* and *Figure 6.26*). As the child grows, he will graduate into standard child-size wheelchairs, but current models are heavy and difficult to fold. For a mother with a disabled child, lifting the child, folding the chair and getting both on to public transport is almost an impossibility.

For car travel, children are often better suited by proprietary seats designed to attach to the seat of the car. Sometimes these 'shells' are the most suitable form of seating for a child, particularly athetoids, and they can be attached to the framework of a Model 13C wheelchair. *Figure 6.15* shows how the footrest of the chair has been turned upside down to achieve the correct height between the seat and footrest.

Prone lying

Propelling a wheelchair from the prone position is occasionally necessary, as for example, to a child with spina bifida with completely flail lower limbs, who was draining from an ileal conduit. She also

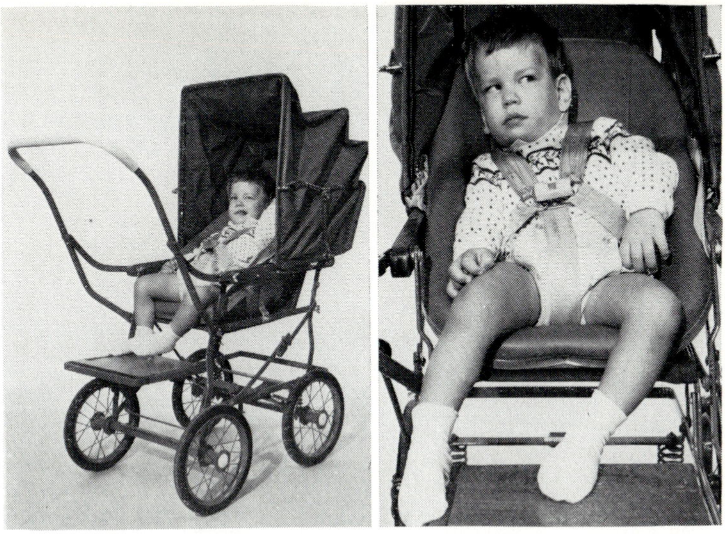

Figure 6.15. A commercially available child's car seat fitted into a standard Model 13C pushchair showing the inverted footrest and restraining straps

had a collapsing scoliosis and was unable to sit up, and for several years she had been pushed around in a converted pushchair. No suitable chair could be found which she would propel. A platform was built on the framework of a Model 1 wheelchair, with the wheelbase extended by resiting the castor wheels. This provided a stable base for her to lie upon (*Figure 6.16*). The platform was then built up with polyurethane foam and covered in plastic. The cushion was shaped to allow her to hold her head in a comfortable position in relation to her books, and a cavity was provided to accommodate the drainage bag for the ileal conduit. The child was now independently mobile within the confines of the residential school for physically handicapped children.

Toilet adaptations

The patient who is unable to achieve independence for toilet purposes, and who has to be left on his own for many hours, presents a considerable problem.

Although commode-chairs and sani-chairs designed to be wheeled over the toilet are available, their use involves transferring from one chair to another, and this is often a severe drawback for a very

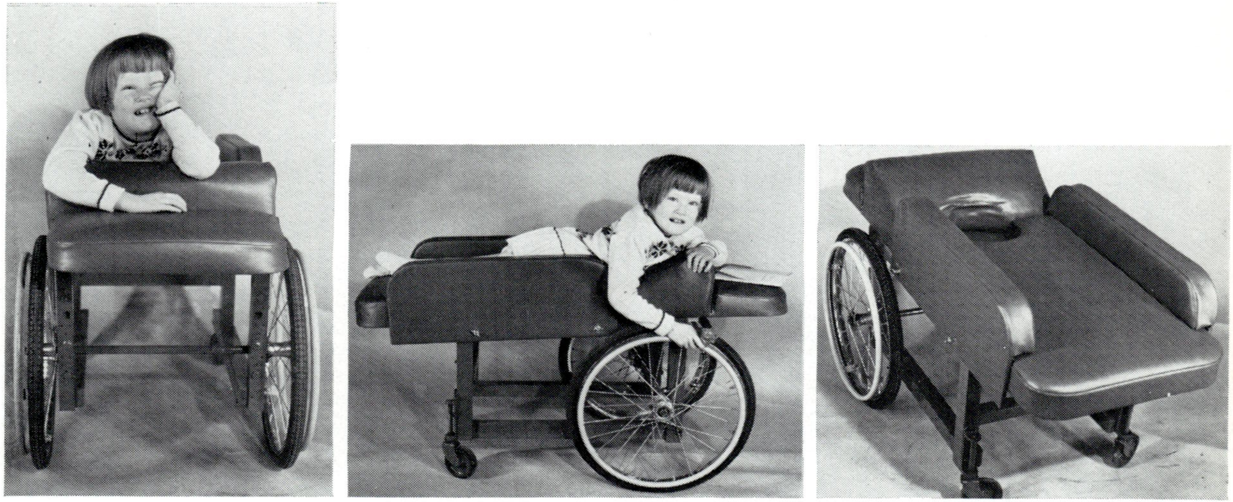

Figure 6.16. A prone-lying self-propelled wheelchair made from a platform built on the framework of a Model 1 wheelchair

disabled patient. However, a bedpan situated permanently beneath a chair is insanitary and a very unsatisfactory solution. Cushions which incorporate urinals or bedpans are also subject to many accidents and failures.

Foot propulsion

Wheelchairs need not necessarily be self-propelled by the hands or be pushed by an attendant, they can also be propelled by the feet. Some patients become exceedingly skilful at foot propulsion, either 'walking' the chair along or, if the large propelling wheels are at the front, by turning the propelling wheels with their toes. This form of propulsion is used by some children with cerebral palsy when their arms are so severely affected by athetosis that they are unable to use their hands.

Another group of patients who find this a useful method of progression are rheumatoid arthritics who normally require walking aids. Using walking frames or crutches or sticks precludes them from much active housework, as they are unable to carry anything around while they are walking with their walking aids. Some manage by walking with a tea trolley. Others can use a wheelchair by 'walking' the chair along, their hands remain free for carrying and for household activities such as cooking, whilst they are also obtaining active exercise for their legs, or 'punting' the chair with their sticks (*Figure 6.17*).

Many different types of wheelchairs can be propelled in this fashion: front-wheel self-propelling chairs, rear-wheel self-propelling chairs or car-transit chairs which have castor wheels. Here again, seat height is often critical.

There are also chairs available with 4 castor wheels which are even more manoeuvrable. Some patients even prefer to fit universal furniture castors on to the legs of a comfortable household chair and 'kick' that around. Practical trial will determine the most suitable chair for any individual patient.

Tables for use with a wheelchair

It is often difficult to manoeuvre a wheelchair into the most useful position at a table or working surface. This may be because of the style of wheelchair used or because of the height of the working surface or the plan of the accommodation. In these circumstances, it may be easier to bring the table or work surface to the wheelchair.

The height and shape of the wheelchair armrests, the height of the patient's knees and the wheelchair footrests are all features needing consideration.

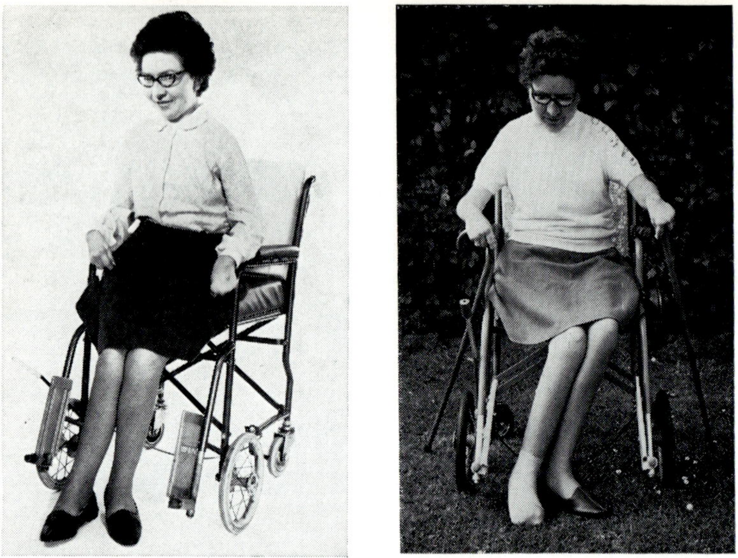

(*a*) (*b*)

Figure 6.17. (a) 'walking'; (b) punting. The chair is an obsolescent rear-castor car-transit model which is in this case the most suitable because of its manoeuvrability

Suitable tables for use with wheelchairs include:

(1) A tray to be fitted to the wheelchair is usually available as a standard extra, but may need adaptation. In some instances a special tray may have to be constructed (*see* case history No. 975, Chapter 9, page 331).

(2) Lap-tables can be made from plywood cut to fit within the wheelchair and shaped to come close to the patient's body. Commercial lap-tables are also available.

(3) Cantilever tables are also available commercially and can be adjusted for position and height. They tend to be slightly unstable for heavy use.

ELECTRICALLY-POWERED INDOOR CHAIRS

Introduction

Since July 1964, the Department of Health and Social Security has extended its provisions for the severely disabled to include electrically-powered indoor chairs. Such chairs may only be prescribed for

TABLE 6.1

Major Features of Wheelchairs Which can be Varied on Prescription

Type	*Frame*	*Seat back*	*Seat*	*Armrest*	*Footrest*	*Brakes*	*Wheels*
Folding	Single X Brace	5–25-degree tilt	Hard or soft (2–4 in)	Fixed	Fixed	Paired	Size 20 in, 22 in, 24 in
Rigid	Double X Brace	Semi-reclining	Soft on hard base	Detachable	Divided	Independent	Front propelling
Adult		Fully reclining	Paraplegic	Padded	Swinging Detachable	Extensions	Rear propelling
Junior		Zip		Desk Arms			
Child		Folding	Smooth cover	(Specific height)	Elevating		Single-hand propelling
Pushchair		Extension for headrest	Sheepskin cover		Heel loops, etc.		Hand rims
Self-propelling			Ripple cushion				Capstans
Transit							Solid tyres
Glideabout							Pneumatic tyres
Sanichair							Solid castors Spoked castors
Special							

patients who are not only unable to walk because of some disability affecting their legs, but who, because of weakness in their arms, are also unable to propel themselves in a wheelchair. There is one further proviso, powered chairs may be issued if, but only if, an electrically propelled indoor chair will help a patient to achieve some measure of independence in the home. By 1970, over 1,700 had been issued to patients.

The criteria of entitlement imply an assessment not only of the patient's physical disability, but also of his domestic environment. It is no use providing a powered indoor chair, if there is no suitable place to use it. Many small cottages or terraced houses are of such a design that a powered indoor chair would not confer any additional independence. In order to obtain one of these chairs, the patient is not only subjected to a rigorous medical examination, but technical officers have to make a practical assessment of the domestic situation. The two aspects must be carefully balanced, for even a limited degree of independent mobility can restore self-respect, and sometimes the provision of a powered indoor chair can be the beginning of a chain of events leading to a comprehensive revival of activity for a severely disabled patient.

It is sometimes difficult to assess the need and the effect of such a provision. Some patients do not strictly qualify because they are still able to propel themselves for short distances. But not infrequently a patient may be able to propel himself, yet in so doing may physically exhaust himself to such an extent that he is unable to achieve any useful activity other than propelling from one place to another. Furthermore, at centres, institutions, or schools for the disabled, or indeed at work, the distances or slopes involved are such that the patient cannot achieve the necessary mobility to traverse them. An electrically-powered indoor chair may be the means whereby the patient can achieve education or may continue at work. In such circumstances, a detailed assessment in the context of the home surroundings can lead to a correct solution of the problem.

Any vehicle which is powered and which is used outside the patient's private accommodation is subject to Road Traffic legislation, but the Chronically Sick and Disabled Persons Act 1970 substitutes a more flexible power to make special regulations relating to the characteristics of the vehicle. The regulations governing the patient's entitlement are geared to the requirements of the Road Traffic Acts, and the medical examination must establish competence to control a vehicle on the road. Consequently, the Ministry of Health appears reluctant to provide an all-purpose powered vehicle although they have certain mechanical advantages, and are the most suitable form of powered transport at, for example, special training centres for the severely disabled, or residential homes with extensive grounds.

Chairs available

Chairs have been made to operate by single levers, by toe, mouth, or finger, and indeed to climb upstairs, to sit the patient up, and to lay them down. Such special designs are expensive, and the need for them is relatively small. In the United Kingdom, 3 types of electrically-powered chairs are commonly available for indoor use, differing mainly in their control systems and in their seating arrangements.

For the severely disabled, both these features are critical, and the selection of the most suitable chair for any one patient revolves around the sort of problems already discussed (*see* Wheelchairs) as regards the seating, cushioning, legrests, sides, armrests and so forth, and also around the patient's capability to control the vehicle.

All the chairs currently available are powered by 12-V (or two 6-V) batteries, which are recharged by means of a portable recharging unit supplied with the chair. The amount of recharging necessary depends on the use to which the chair is put, and patients who use the chair for work or school, may need to recharge every night. The recharging problem imposes a need for appropriate electrical connections and assistance from attendants to arrange for the recharging.

Speeds vary from about $\frac{3}{4}$ mph to 3 mph, two types of chairs having several speeds. Although specifications are usually quoted for these chairs to climb gradients of 1 : 10, they rarely do, and a more realistic gradient is 1 : 12 or 1 : 15. When the battery is getting flat they have difficulty in coping with 1 : 15 slopes.

A.C. Epic

The standard electrically powered indoor chair Epic, provided by the Department of Health and Social Security, is very robust, reliable and compact. Early versions only had one speed, less than 1 mph. The seat, backrest and armrests are of one design only. The backrest is very low and there is no facility for significantly altering the angle of recline, cushioning or size nor can accessories such as mobile arm-supports be fitted. The arms, though hinged and able to swing outwards, on the non-control side, tend to interfere with transfers.

The steering and control are incorporated in one rotating handle. Close manoeuvring at tables or desks requires enough strength to overcome the friction and weight on the driving wheel. Normally, there is a 2:1 reduction gear on the steering, but a 4:1 reduction can be supplied. This requires less strength but more movement. Patients with ataxia and athetosis, however, can sometimes operate these controls when they are quite unable to manage more delicate or more precise mechanisms.

More recent versions of the Epic have powered steering, and the strength and range of movement necessary to steer the chair is very small. Control can also be achieved by means of microswitches or pneumatic switches for those severely disabled patients whose hands are too weak to manipulate the usual steering handle. The chair is very manoeuvrable and safe. Its built-in recharging unit saves time and trouble for the attendants, who have to recharge its battery frequently.

M.M.L. No. 1019 born 1923 male

Diagnosis: Cerebral palsy; spastic quadriplegia

This man with spastic quadriplegia had never walked, and only with considerable difficulty and discomfort had he managed to propel himself for short distances in a self-propelled wheelchair. He had a marked dysarthria.

During childhood, he had had various surgical procedures, including psoas and Achilles tendon tenotomies. He had been fitted with calipers, splints and spinal supports in great variety, but none had enabled him to achieve any increased function or independence. Furthermore, the amount of hospitalization which he had required had prevented him from achieving any schooling, although it may, to some extent, have limited the development of his limb and trunk deformities.

His movements were athetoid. He had severe flexion contractures of both arms and legs and marked limitation of movement of all joints. He had a severe scoliosis, with a convexity to the right in the thoracic region, and to the left in the lumbar region. This deformity made it very difficult to find a chair that was comfortable, and his combined deformities and athetosis prevented him from achieving a reasonable degree of wheelchair activity. As he spent much of his time inactive in the wheelchair, he had continuous complaints about its comfort and suitability. He was continually striving to improve his activities and felt thwarted by his inability to achieve the mobility which they demanded.

Since 12 years of age, he had lived in various institutions, hospitals, local authority and voluntary residential accommodation.

On admission to the Disabled Living Unit he was found to be able to sit in a standard electrically-powered indoor chair. This needed no alteration apart from the forward advancement of the chair seat by 2 in (5 cm) to support him adequately under the thighs, and the provision of extra padding on the right to control his tendency to slump to that side. To stop him from slipping off the seat, and to restrain his movements when they became inco-ordinated, a sheepskin was

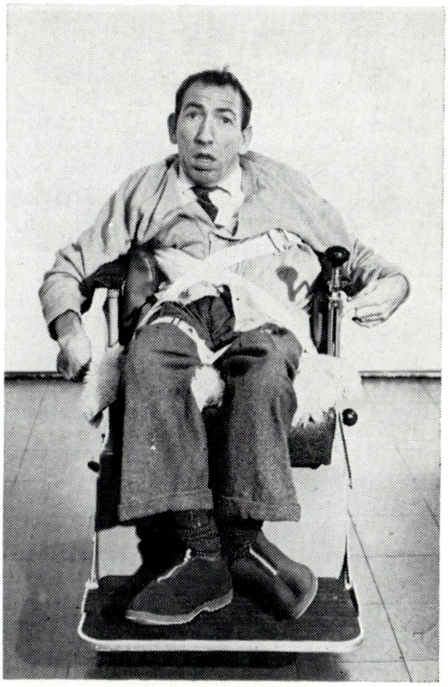

Figure 6.18. Patient No. 1019 with cerebral palsy in his Epic wheelchair with straps and sheepskin

laid on the seat of the wheelchair, and a harness was attached to the framework. This consisted of trunk and thigh straps, which were meticulously adjusted to retain him in a comfortable sitting position, without producing a feeling of undue restriction (*Figure 6.18*).

The achievement of independent mobility made him much more relaxed, reduced considerably his complaints about his chair, and enabled him to enter into the activities and spirit of the institution where he lived.

Monodrive unit

This Monodrive motor unit, with its detachable steering column, can be fitted to the front framework of Everest and Jennings Wheelchairs (*Figure 6.19*).

The patient can thus be provided with the appropriate chair and cushioning, and the power-unit added afterwards. The addition of the Monodrive produces a slight tilt in the chair (5–7 degrees), and may make it necessary to adjust the mobile arm-supports and cushions for some patients.

The chair is steered by a T-shaped handle-bar, and controlled by small levers below the handle-bars. There are fast and slow forward

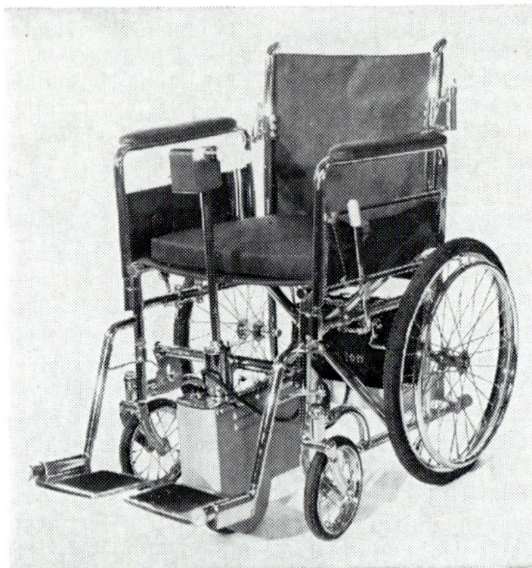

(*a*)

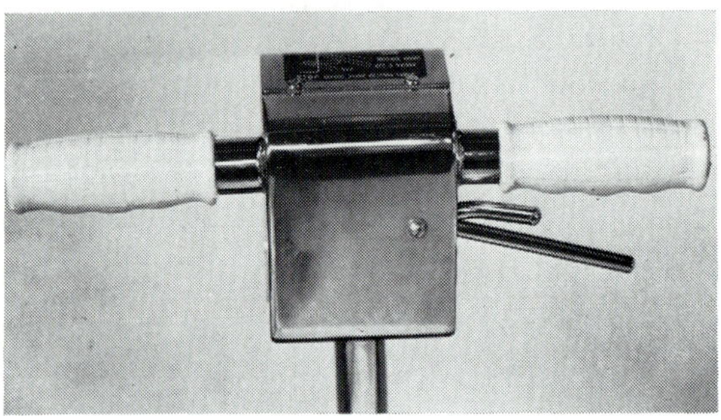

(*b*)

Figure 6.19. (*a*) *The Mondrive unit on a standard Everest and Jennings wheelchair;* (*b*) *hand-controls of Monodrive unit*

speeds, a free-wheel position and also a reverse gear. When the patient releases his grip the chair stops.

The provision and possible modification of an appropriate chair before the addition of the powered unit, gives this powered chair a great advantage over the Sleyride powered indoor chair. Both have the same motor and controls, but the structure of the latter chair is unadaptable and the position of its motor fixed. Monodrive units can also be fitted to reclining chairs, which can be supplied with the usual range of accessories. A further advantage of these units is that they may be fitted with an offset steering column, so that the position of the controls may be adjusted to the ability of the patient.

M.M.L. No. 168 born 1920 male

Diagnosis: Juvenile rheumatoid arthritis

Juvenile rheumatoid arthritis starting at the age of 4 years and remaining active until the age of 14 years, left this patient with complete ankylosis from head to foot, with the trunk and legs in a gentle curve convex to the left. The only movements available to him were those between scapula and thorax, and some minimal movements at the metacarpophalangeal joints. He had lived in hospitals or institutions for most of his life, and had no memory of ever being able to move himself or his chair. He had always remained in a pushchair.

By balancing a book or plate on his right shoulder, he was able to read and eat, and with a typewriter placed on his right he could use a typing stick in his left hand.

At the age of 41, he was provided with an electrically-powered indoor chair. Special cushioning had to be made to accommodate his rigid and curved body. The controls of a Monodrive unit were specially adapted and the steering column was altered to become a side tiller. The control box was situated at shoulder level and turned on its side. With these adaptations, he was independently mobile for the first time in over 35 years (*Figure 6.20*).

Powerdrives

The Powerdrive has 20 in (51 cm) diameter, pneumatic rear wheels, each of which is driven by a separate motor through a system of rubber belts and pulleys. The belt can be relaxed so that the chair can be pushed by an attendant in the conventional fashion. The control box is usually mounted on the outside of one armrest, but by appropriate brackets it can be placed elsewhere for the patient's convenience. Two toggle switches allow the user to select the speed. Steering control is by means of a joystick, operating switches to select forward and reverse motion for each motor. Steering is accomplished by pushing the joystick in the direction of choice. Only light pressure and slight range of movement (about $\frac{1}{4}$–$\frac{1}{2}$ in ($\frac{1}{2}$–1 cm) are necessary (*Figure 6.21*).

It is relatively easy to devise adaptations and extensions to the control levers and switches for hand, mouth or foot operation (*Figures 6.22, 6.23, 6.24*).

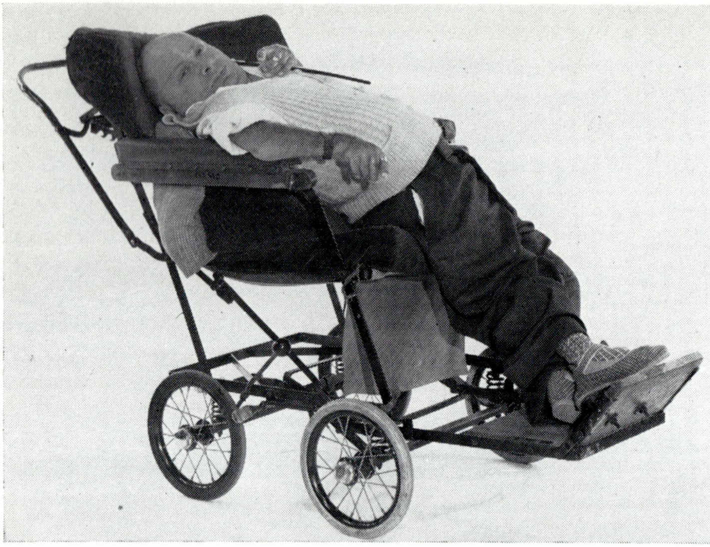

(*a*)

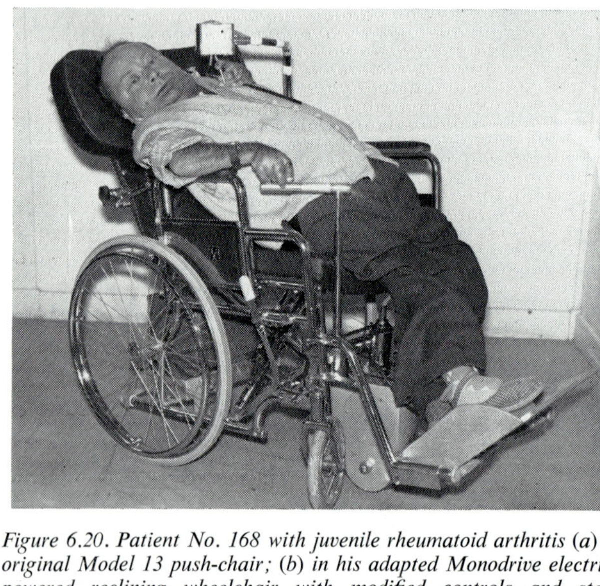

(*b*)

Figure 6.20. Patient No. 168 with juvenile rheumatoid arthritis (a) *in his original Model 13 push-chair;* (b) *in his adapted Monodrive electrically-powered reclining wheelchair with modified controls and steering.* (*Reproduced by kind permission of the Editor, 'Orthopaedics': Oxford*)

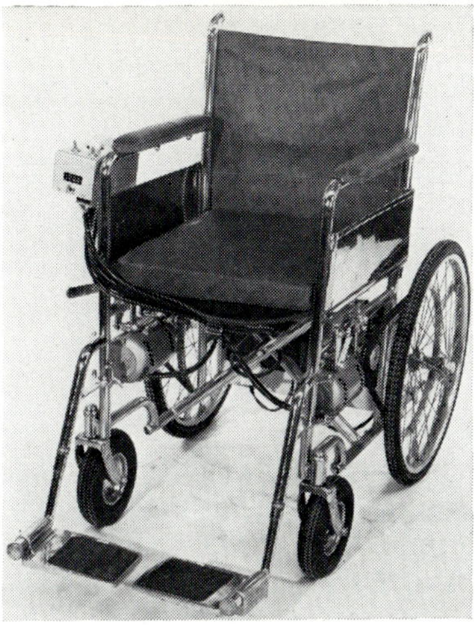

Figure 6.21. A standard Powerdrive electrically-propelled chair

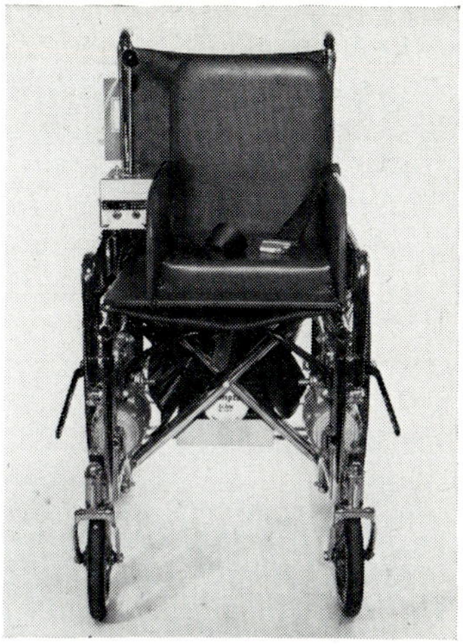

Figure 6.22. Powerdrive indoor chair adapted for a child with phocomelic arms

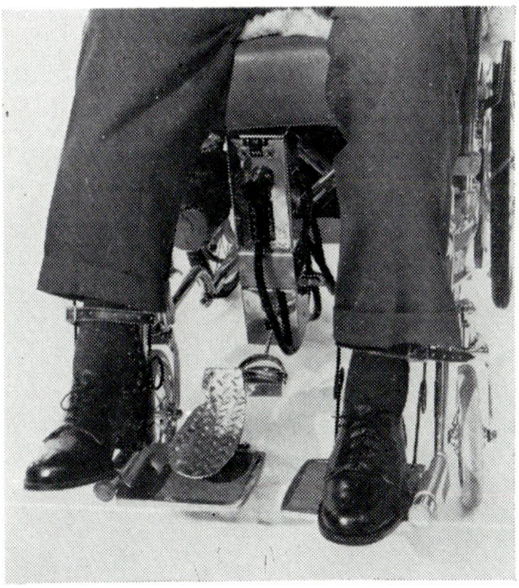

Figure 6.23. Patient's adaptation to Powerdrive chair enabling him to control it with one foot

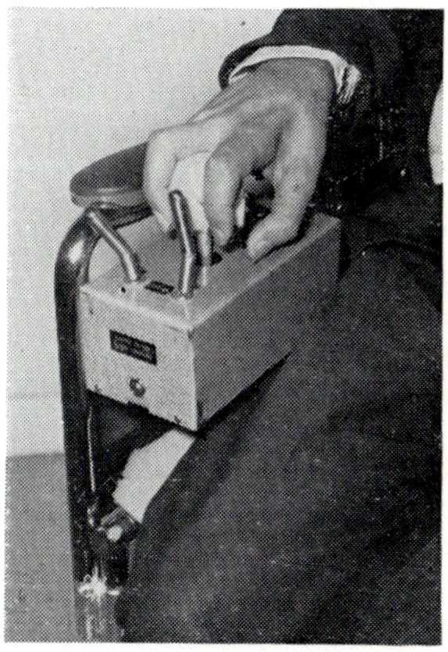

Figure 6.24. Control box of Powerdrive chair repositioned inside the armrest; padded T-bar attached to steering knob and extensions fitted to switches

The standard chair is fitted with 8 in castor wheels with pneumatic tyres, but these give rise to considerable friction when trying to turn sharply at slow speeds, and it is often advisable to exchange them for castor wheels with solid tyres. The standard chairs also have fixed armrests, but they can be alternatively supplied with detachable armrests and with reclining backrests and elevating legrests (*see* case history No. 288, Chapter 9, page 363). Some patients using mobile arm-supports have difficulty in controlling the Powerdrives, and they either have to abandon the arm-supports for driving, or else are better advised to use a Monodrive unit.

Comment

Other types of electrically-powered indoor chairs may become available, and the selection of the most suitable chair for a particular patient will be based on the assessment of his physical disability, the patient's chair requirement, his ability to operate the controls, and also the nature of the environment in which the chair is required to function.

The relevant questions are:

(1) Does the patient need a powered indoor chair?

(2) Will a powered indoor chair provide an additional functional facility?

(3) Can the patient sit comfortably in the standard model chosen, or can the chair be suitably adapted to accommodate the patient?

(4) Can he control the chair adequately with standard controls, or can the controls be suitably adapted?

(5) Will the chair cope with the architectural hazards, for example, ramps and corners?

(6) Can the patient negotiate the awkward corners which exist in his environment?

Like so many other appliances, there is often a need for compromise and the most satisfactory results can only be achieved by careful assessment of the patient and his environment.

M.M.L. No. 445 born 1964 male

Diagnosis: Werdnig Hoffman's disease

This little boy never walked, but as he grew he was able to support himself sitting up, although he could not get up from the lying point. When first seen at the Disabled Living Unit, he was 2 years of age. He was neither able to crawl nor pull himself along the ground (he spent his life in a small pram).

A simple self-propelled chair was made for him (*Figure 6.25*)

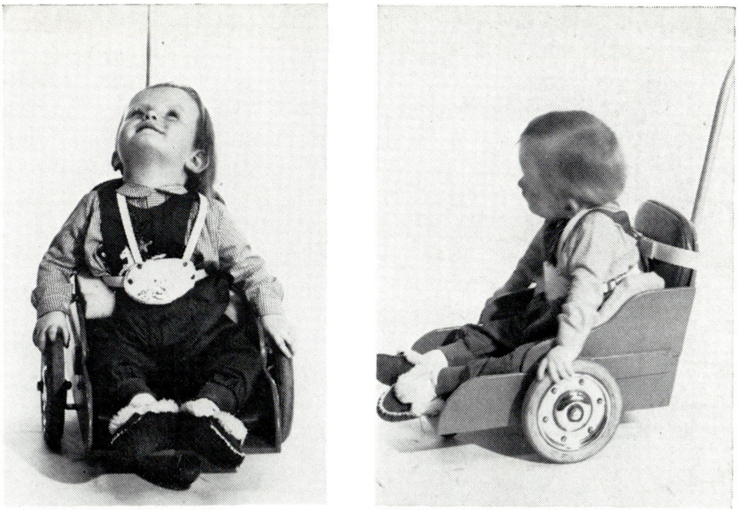

Figure 6.25. Patient No. 445 at 2 years of age with Werdnig Hoffman's disease in a simple self-propelled wooden wheelchair with detachable handle

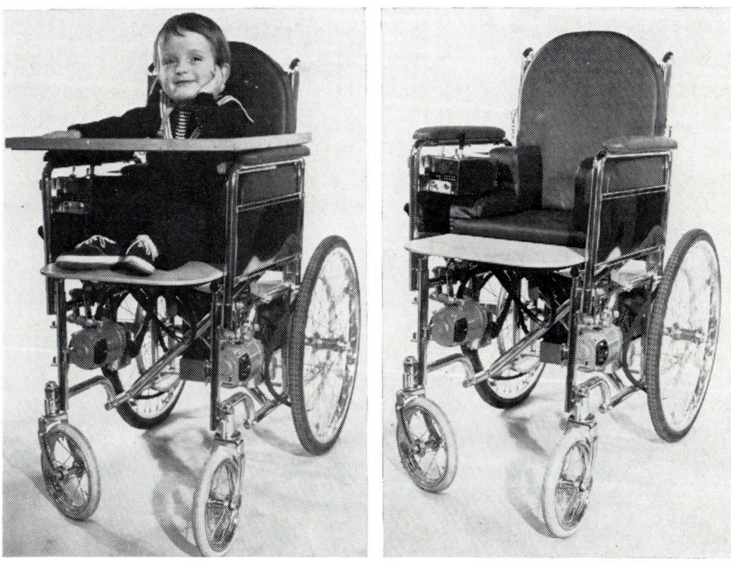

Figure 6.26. Patient No. 445 at 5 years of age using an adapted electrically-powered indoor chair

which he immediately found he could use for independent mobility. This gave the child obvious pleasure and also relieved his mother of the considerable strain of moving him wherever and whenever he wished. As he grew, he became more venturesome, and by the time he was 3 years of age he was too large for this home-made wheelchair, but he was still not strong enough to self-propel a small conventional wheelchair.

Thus, he was provided with a standard junior-size electrically-powered indoor wheelchair with simple controls. A seat insert was made as the chair was too large for him, and the control-box was repositioned inside one of the armrests (*Figure 6.26*).

This chair enabled him to retain his independent mobility and allowed him to start at a local primary school at the normal age. (A second chair for use at school was provided through the education authorities.)

POWERED OUTDOOR VEHICLES

Transportation to and from work, shops, or social activities, is often the greatest problem in resettling a severely physically disabled patient.

Powered outdoor vehicles for the disabled may be supplied on the recommendation of a hospital consultant, providing the patient is entitled to one because of his disability, and providing he is able to control the vehicle adequately. He must, in addition, pass a medical examination related to the legislative requirements, mainly associated with visual acuity and capability of controlling the vehicle in an emergency.

Once eligibility has been accepted, the patient may opt to have a cash grant towards the conversion of his own car for manual control, plus an annual grant for maintenance and tax relief.

Under current arrangements, a single-seater invalid tricycle may be provided for a disabled person who falls into one of the following categories.

(1) Patients who have one leg amputated above the knee and the other amputated either above or below the knee.

(2) Patients suffering from paraplegia or other defect of the locomotor system resulting in the total or almost total loss of use of both legs, so that to all intents and purposes they are unable to walk.

(3) Patients slightly less severely disabled who because of their disability, require a machine to get to and from work.

Persons whose walking ability is restricted by non-locomotor disability such as heart or lung disease may only be provided with a vehicle under the third provision, to help them get to and from work, although the respiratory or cardiac cripple may be more restricted than many suffering from locomotor disorders.

The alternative of a small 4-seater car is available to war pensioners and, since July 1964, has been available under the National Health Service to two members of the same family who are both separately entitled to an invalid tricycle, and to a husband and wife one of whom is eligible for a vehicle and the other is blind.

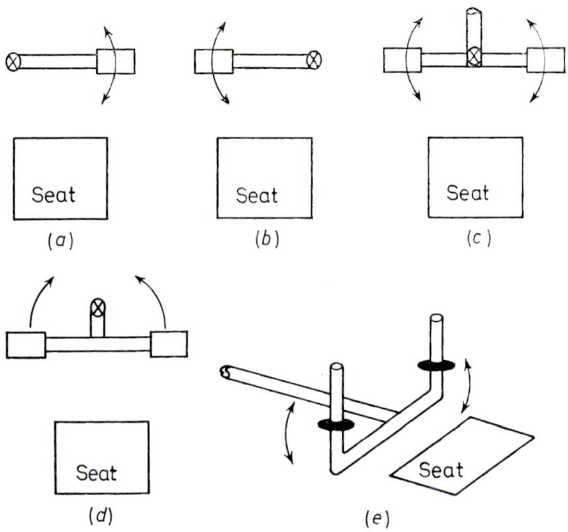

Figure 6.27. Alternative tiller controls (a) side tiller, right-hand control; (b) side tiller, left-hand control; (c) bicycle type (push-pull) control; (d) centre tiller (North-South) control; (e) aircraft type tiller

In February 1967, the Ministry of Health made cars available to the following further 3 groups.

(*a*) A disabled parent having the sole care of a child.

(*b*) Two relatives in the same household, not necessarily husband and wife, of whom one is eligible for a vehicle and the other is blind.

(*c*) Two relatives in the same household, both eligible for an invalid vehicle, one of whom is under 16 years of age.

Between 1,500 and 2,000 households will benefit from these additional provisions.

Criticisms are frequently made of the invalid 3-wheeler, they have a narrow wheel-base and are reputedly liable to overturn; the petrol-driven versions are noisy; although there are various alternative tiller controls (*Figure 6.27*), they are all difficult to control. The bumpy ride provided may well be the cause of discomfort for arthritic patients and cause repeated bleeding in elbows of haemophiliacs. Mechanically, they have a reputation for being unreliable, and because of their unique features, it is difficult to get urgent repairs carried out on the road.

Getting in and out of such a vehicle presents many disabled patients with problems, and lifting a wheel chair in and out is often very awkward too. Frequently, extensive and expensive alterations have to be carried out in order to enable a patient to achieve the ability to control it. In countries where large cars are common, and special invalid tricycles are not available, the motor-car industry has become expert at providing adaptations to standard cars which enable even the most severely disabled to drive independently, using hand-controls or foot-controls. The large size of the car increases stability and makes access easier for patient and wheelchair alike, while having sufficient room to enable the patient's family or friends to accompany him.

There is considerable evidence that the extension of provision of small cars or a financial contribution towards a car of the patient's choice might well be both more suitable and financially less demanding. However, the provision of motor-cars as a health service commitment is debatable and the inter-relationship between medical needs and social needs is blurred.

In England and Wales, there are over 6,000 invalid cars and 20,000 invalid tricycles on issue. In addition, over 3,000 car conversion grants have been issued and about 1,200 private-car maintenance allowances.

7—*Functional Upper-Limb Splints*

INTRODUCTION

Functional braces and splints for the upper limb are numerous and varied. The majority are designed for temporary use and their construction is cumbersome, complicated and lacking in cosmetic appeal. Permanent functional splints for the severely disabled must give an immediate and direct improvement in function. They must also be robust and reliable, yet light in weight, simple to apply and aesthetically acceptable. It is unlikely that any splint without these attributes will be accepted and used to maximum potential.

There are many classifications of upper-limb splints. Those used for the severely disabled can be divided into 3 main groups: (1) splints for wrists and hands; (2) splints for paralysed arms; and (3) supporting appliances for weak-shoulder girdles.

Within this grouping, splints can be further subdivided into those providing stability, positioning or immobilization, and those substituting absent or weak motor-power. Most functional splints incorporate both functions.

Splints may be static or dynamic. Dynamic splints are sometimes called 'lively' or 'functional'. Static splints may 'conform' to the limb and thus support it, or they may not conform and thus be 'corrective'. Functional splints may harness the patient's own movements, transmitting them directly or by cables, or they may supply additional (external) power through elastic bands, springs, pneumatic or electric motors. Many splints combine in one appliance the attributes and therefore the functions of static and dynamic splints. With these, they may also combine the effects of gravity, added external power and the actions of the patient himself.

Splints may be devised to fulfil a variety of purposes: to prevent deformity or correct deformities; to prevent increase in muscle imbalance; to assist weak muscle or to substitute for paralysed muscles;

to encourage function or to support a painful part by preventing movement; to transfer power from one point to another; or to assess the possible advantages to be gained by surgical reconstruction.

Although there are certain standard types of splints available for the severely disabled, prescription and manufacture of the individual splint will frequently be a very necessary individual process. Thus a Unit managing these patients requires some workshop facilities and technicians with experience in this work.

In order to prescribe a splint for an upper limb, the patient's functional requirements must be firmly established and the purpose of the splint clearly delineated. This purpose must be analysed and expressed in terms of support, correction and deformity, assistance provided for movement, method of control, means of attaching the device to the patient, and additional devices or appliances which may need to be attached to the splint itself.

The prescription of the splint will, therefore, usually be the outcome of collaboration between clinician, therapist, and technician, each contributing and understanding the difficulties and decisions taken by the others. A theoretical solution based on clinical appraisal may not be realistic in terms of functional requirements. Likewise, a requirement in functional terms may not be reasonable in terms of manufacture. Usually, splints are a compromise between the ideal and the realistic.

In all cases, adequate time should be allowed to a patient for training and adaptation to the splint. Minor mechanical alterations are often necessary, but the patient should not be parted from the splint for long intervals during the early training period, 'indoctrination period' is probably a more appropriate description. If the splint provides an immediate functional gain clearly noticeable during this indoctrination period, acceptance is usually good.

The appearance is important. A splint which looks unfinished and amateurish in construction does not inspire confidence. But a confident and skilful technician can carry a patient with him during the construction and fitting stages. By his attitude of guarded optimism, his insistence on accurate fitting and precision of action, and his final production of a well finished appliance, he can prepare the ground for the therapist's training and indoctrination.

FLEXOR-HINGE SPLINT

The flexor-hinge splint is based upon the principle of converting a flail hand into a three-jaw chuck, the index and middle fingers moving together to meet the thumb which is stabilized in a functional extended position. The rigid finger-pieces stabilizing the interphalangeal joints are hinged at the metacarpophalangeal joint on the radial aspect. Extension of the wrist closes the 'chuck' and flexion of the wrist opens the pinch (*Figure 7.1*). This action may be produced by the wrist extensors if they are powerful enough; M.R.C. Grade 3+ is necessary, or by a pneumatic McKibben artificial muscle (*see Figure 7.2*), or by a cable operated from the shoulder.

Whatever the source, the power available for dorsiflexing the wrist (extension) is available for closing the chuck and producing a pinch grip. Opening is performed by a spring. Although this may appear to be an unaccustomed movement, wrist extension to produce finger grip, it does not usually take long to learn, for in a normal grip the wrist extensors act powerfully to stabilize the wrist and a powerful grip is applied with the wrist in slight extension and the thumb in line with the radius.

The action of the splint mimics a surgical tenodesis of the finger flexors (so that the wrist extension produces passive finger flexion) coupled with arthrodesis of the thumb. The disadvantages of this surgical procedure is that the permanently extended thumb interferes with many activities, particularly transferring and wheelchair propelling.

The flexor-hinge splint is primarily intended to provide prehension and release and is particularly suitable for patients with cervical-cord lesions. The minimal requirements which must be fulfilled by any patient for whom such an appliance is contemplated are:

(1) Passive range of movements
- wrist: 40-degree flexion and extension; no radial or ulnar deviation during flexion/extension
- thumb: 50-degree abduction in a plane; perpendicular to the palm
- fingers: 0–90-degree flexion/extension of metacarpophalangeal joints of 1st and 2nd fingers
- forearm: full pronation from mid-position

(2) Muscle power (for muscle-driven flexor-hinge splint wrist): dorsiflexion of wrist of M.R.C. Grade 3+.

Slight wrist deviation may be acceptable, and wrist extension which is unable to activate a standard wrist-driven flexor-hinge splint may be able to do so if a hinge is inserted. This applies when extensor carpi radialis longus is the main surviving wrist extensor and tends to pull the hand radially during extension of the wrist (case history No. 776).

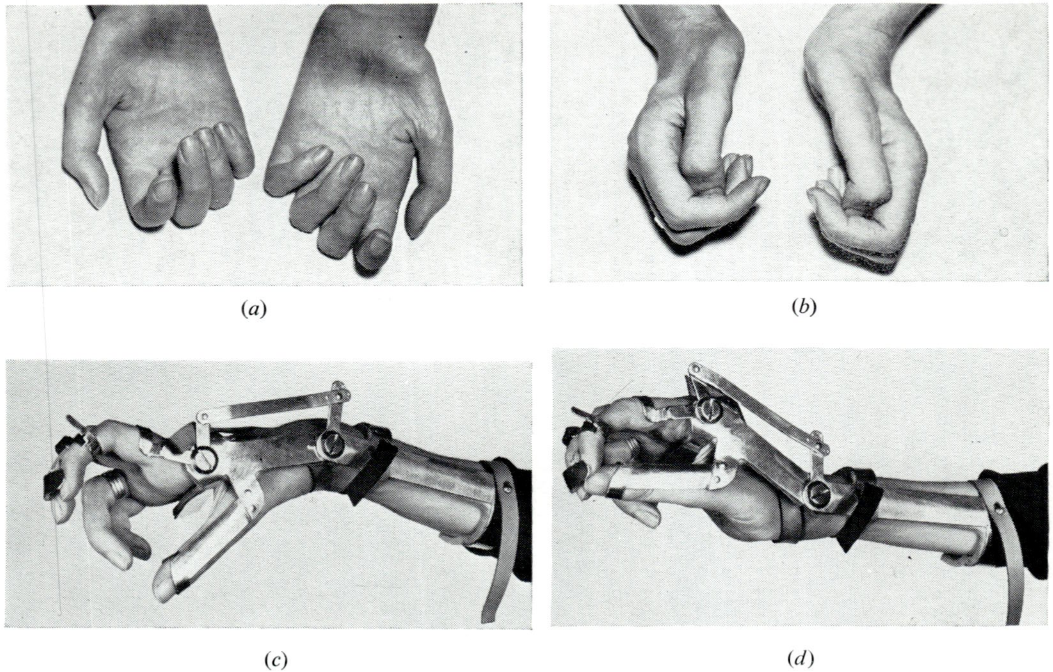

Figure 7.1. Patient No. 420 (a) with a C7 lesion; (b) active dorsiflexion of wrist; (c) flexor hinge splint in position with wrist flexed and grip open; (d) wrist extended and grip closed

M.M.L. No. 776 born 1922 male

Diagnosis: Ankylosing spondylitis; fracture dislocation C6/C7

As a young man aged 18 years, this patient was found to have ankylosing spondylitis which steadily progressed and involved the whole of his spine and both hips. At 43 years of age he fell from a ladder and sustained a fracture dislocation of C6/C7 with a resulting tetraplegia. He was hospitalized for about 18 months in a general hospital, then 3 months in a spinal injuries unit. After this, he was transferred to a rehabilitation unit.

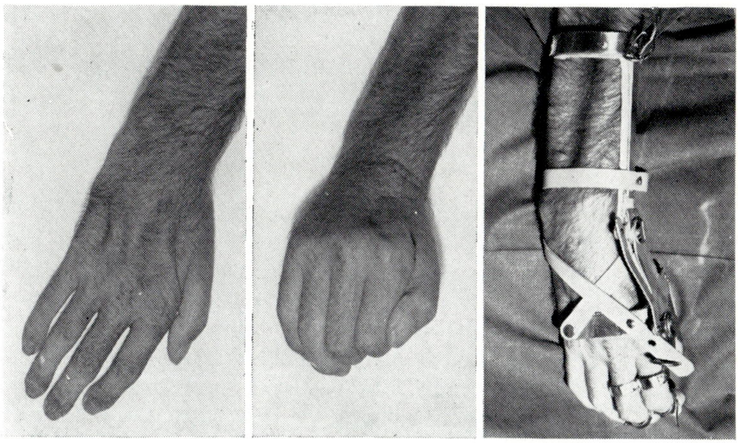

(*a*) (*b*) (*c*)

Figure 7.2. Patient No. 776 with right hand (*a*) *in neutral position and dorsiflexed showing radial deviation at wrist;* (*b*) *flexing on fingers due to flexion contracture;* (*c*) *with flexor-hinge splint—note polyethylene hinge and D-strings to assist self-application of straps*

At that time, in addition to the ankylosing spondylitis and tetraplegia, he had severe flexion contractures of the hips and knees. Physiotherapy improved the contractures and his eventual return home to a specially designed bungalow was planned. As he began to improve, he was admitted to the Disabled Living Unit to be assessed for a flexor-hinge splint.

His hands were by no means ideal for flexor-hinge splints. There were flexion contractures of all fingers and the web between index fingers and thumb was tight. Although he had active dorsiflexion of the wrist, this was weak (M.R.C. Grade 3) and it was accompanied by radial deviation (*Figure 7.2*). He was, however, very keen to try the splints as he wanted to attempt to return to some form of work.

Therefore, a splint was made for the right hand but he could not operate this, and it was thought that he would need a powered splint. As it appeared to be the radial deviation which was preventing him from operating the splint, a polyethylene hinge was inserted in the splint between the forearm cuff and the finger cage, and this allowed the wrist to extend and produce a finger grip (*see Figure 7.2c*). The grip was useful but small because of the tight thumb web.

He returned to the Rehabilitation Unit to continue his general rehabilitation programme and to continue practising the use of the right-hand splint. Three months later, he had become very adept at using the splint and was asking to have one for his left hand as well. This was provided. Like the right one, it also incorporated a polyethylene hinge to allow radial deviation to occur. Within a week or two he was able to undertake increasingly fine manoeuvres such as painting, writing and typing.

Comment

It is usually agreed that powerful wrist extension (M.R.C. Grade 3+ or 4) is necessary for successful operation of a flexor-hinge splint, and that wrist extension must not deviate. This patient showed that the introduction of a polyethylene hinge into the splint, to allow a few degrees of radial deviation enabled the splint to be operated by dorsiflexors which fulfilled neither of these criteria, since they were only graded M.R.C. Grade 3 in power, and produced a radial deviation of the wrist on contraction.

This same patient (case history No. 776) illustrated a further point.

One further advantage of the Disabled Living Unit is the independent flat for training the disabled patient. Although this particular patient has been in hospital for over two years, his wife had only been partially introduced to the problems involved in his daily care.

On his two admissions to the Disabled Living Unit, his wife was admitted with him and they shared the flat. She was, therefore, able to be trained in all aspects of his care, including his bowel and bladder routine and the daily stretching of the contractures of his hips and knees. After these two periods of 3–4 weeks, she was able to manage with great competence, which gave her confidence that she could cope when he was eventually discharged home.

Unfortunately, their house was very unsuitable for a wheelchair existence, yet about a year after the fitting of the splints and some 9 months after his discharge from hospital, the patient and his wife were still living there, with the patient confined to two rooms, unable to get out and somewhat depressed. Eventually, however, with the

Figure 7.3. A letter from Patient No. 776 one year after fitting flexor-hinge splints illustrating the quality of writing achieved

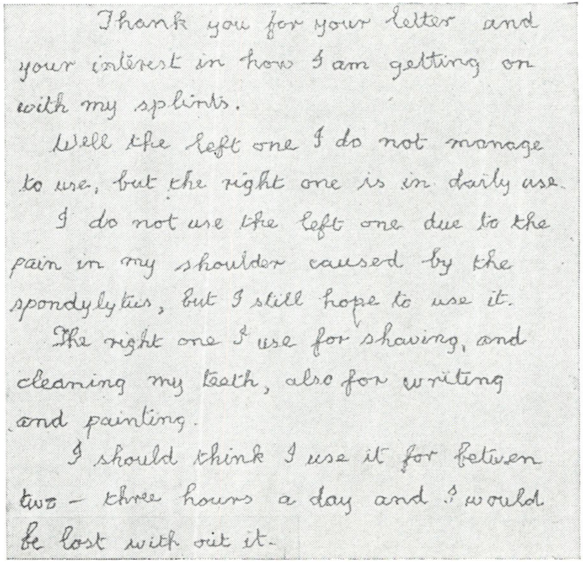

Thank you for your letter and your interest in how I am getting on with my splints.

Well the left one I do not manage to use, but the right one is in daily use.

I do not use the left one due to the pain in my shoulder caused by the spondylytis, but I still hope to use it.

The right one I use for shaving, and cleaning my teeth, also for writing and painting.

I should think I use it for between two – three hours a day and I would be lost with out it.

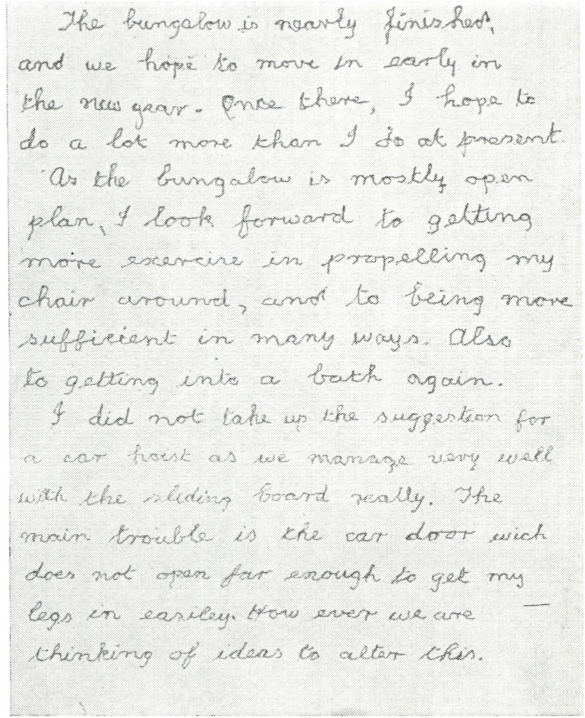

The bungalow is nearly finished, and we hope to move in early in the new year. Once there, I hope to do a lot more than I do at present.

As the bungalow is mostly open plan, I look forward to getting more excercise in propelling my chair around, and to being more sufficient in many ways. Also to getting into a bath again.

I did not take up the suggestion for a car hoist as we manage very well with the sliding board really. The main trouble is the car door wich does not open far enough to get my legs in easiley. How ever we are thinking of ideas to alter this.

aid of local social workers, they obtained permission to build a suitable bungalow in some land owned by the family, and so were finally more suitably rehoused. A letter from the patient at this time illustrates the standard of writing which can be achieved with this type of splint and also, from its content, indicates that with continual practice, and moral support, this severely disabled patient was continuing to progress in his own resettlement. (*Figure 7.3.*)

Powered flexor-hinge splints

When the wrist extensors are absent, or too weak to extend the wrist with the splint in place and against the power of the return spring, then external power can be used. The simplest powered flexor-hinge splint uses compressed carbon dioxide as its power source and a McKibben artificial muscle as its motivator (*Figures 7.4*, *7.5*). This is, in effect, a rubber balloon within a cover which, because of its helical weave, shortens in length when the baloon is blown up and increased in diameter. This type of splint can be used as a therapeutic adaptive splint as well as a permanent substitute, as is illustrated by case history No. 938.

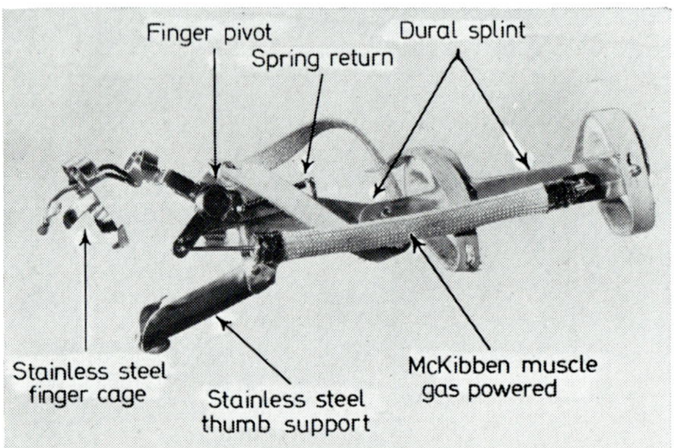

Figure 7.4. McKibbon muscle driven flexor-hinge splint

M.M.L. No. 938 born 1916 female

Diagnosis: Partial brachial plexus lesion

This lady fell downstairs and sustained a fracture of the neck of the left humerus, with considerable extravasation of blood into the surrounding soft tissue. At the time of the reduction of the fracture, she was found to have a partial brachial plexus lesion with weakness of the deltoid, triceps and paralysis of the triceps and all muscles of the forearm and hand.

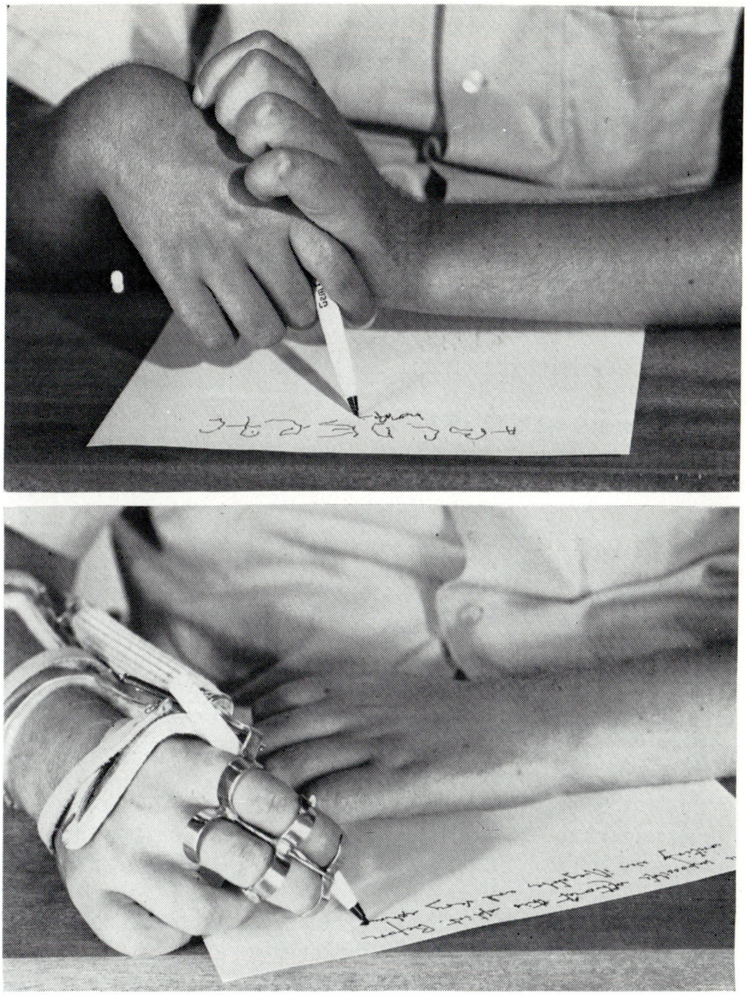

Figure 7.5. Patient No. 1002 with a C5/C6 lesion (a) usual two-handed writing technique; (b) using a McKibbon muscle-driven flexor-hinge splint

During the ensuing 12 months, she regained considerable power in the deltoid, triceps, biceps and spinatus longus, but there was no evidence of recovery in the muscles of the forearm and hand. She was referred to the Disabled Living Unit for the possible provision of a flexor-hinge splint operated from the shoulder. She was a difficult patient to fit, because the thumb web was very tight, and there was considerable stiffness of the fingers, particularly the metacarpophalangeal joints.

A cable-operated shoulder-driven splint was tried, but the shoulder girdle was still weak and she was unable to sustain the grip, so a McKibben artificial muscle was mounted on the splint and controlled by a valve operated from the shoulders. This splint was used for many everyday activities (*Figure 7.6*).

Gradually, the passive range of movement of the wrist and metacarpophalangeal joints improved. It had at first been suggested that she would need a capsulotomy of the metacarpophalangeal joints to obtain maximum use of the splint, but the splint gradually stretched them itself and the finger cages had to be altered to accommodate her increased opening span, and the decreasing swelling of the hand and fingers.

After a further 12–18 months, recovery was taking place in the hand and she was gradually able to discard the splint as active movement returned. This illustrates the value of a powered flexor-hinge splint as a therapeutic device to maintain and improve passive joint range and to maintain active wrist and hand function during the recovery period of the peripheral nerves concerned.

Training

The flexor-hinge splint is a sophisticated appliance requiring skilled manufacture and fitting, careful assessment and prolonged training. Its mode of operation can be varied, the action being controlled by wrist extension, or wrist flexion, or by cable controls from the shoulders. In some circumstances, it may be necessary to undertake surgical procedures to enable a suitable patient to use such a splint. Contracture of the thumb-web limiting the maximum opening of the pinch, fixed deformities of the fingers limiting movement available at the metacarpophalangeal joints, or contractures of the forearm muscles preventing pronation are all amenable to surgical correction if they do not respond to physiotherapy or prolonged practice with a splint.

Finally, it must be emphasized that it takes long practice to achieve skill and dexterity with these splints, and the number of patients with the necessary motivation and realistic ambitions for their use are few.

After intensive use of a flexor-hinge splint over a year or two, some patients can then discard the splint with little loss of function as they will be found to have developed muscle power and contractures, which are equivalent to an extensor tenodesis and although the thumb is not stabilized it is more in opposition than previously.

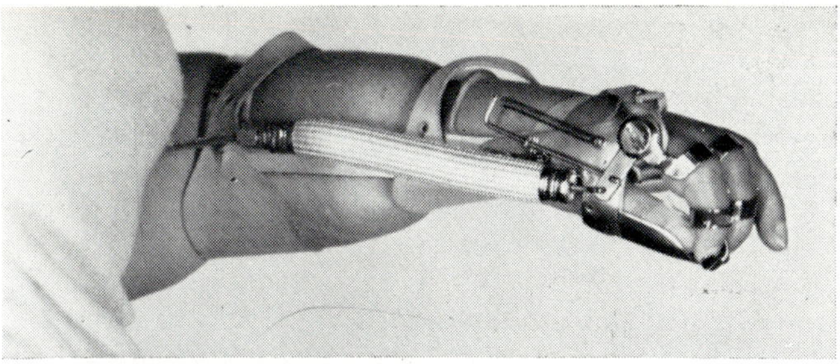

(*a*)

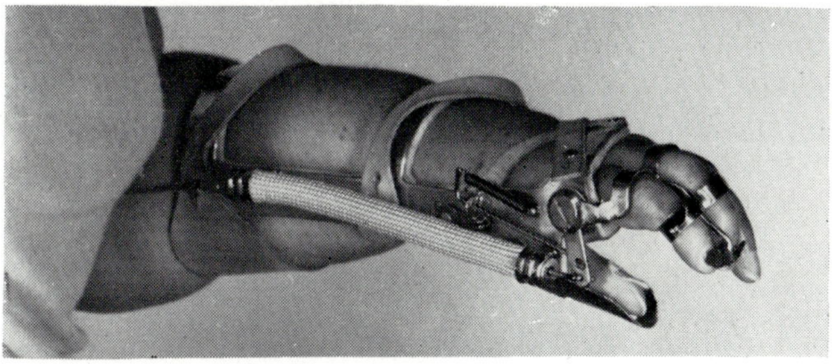

(*b*)

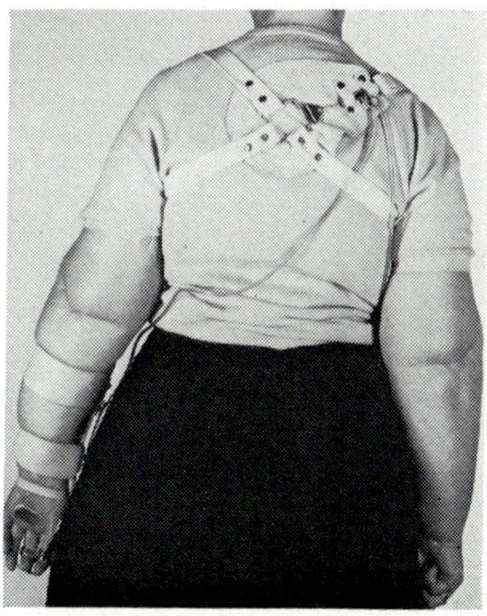

(*c*)

Figure 7.6. Patient No. 938 with partial brachial plexus lesion wearing a gas-powered flexor-hinge splint (a) splint open; (b) splint closed; (c) shoulder harness operating valve control

M.M.L. No. 1002 born 1942 male

Diagnosis: Incomplete tetraplegia following fracture C5 on C6

A fracture dislocation of C5 on C6 was followed by incomplete tetraplegia which was treated with traction followed by immobilization in a collar. He was in a spinal injuries unit for 10 months and then returned home. Initially he lived with his wife in his parents' house which had been adapted with a downstairs bedroom. His wife and his mother lifted him for all transfers even though his wife was small and his mother was liable to bouts of cardiac failure. They used no hoist, nor had they ever been able to try one. A male nurse attended daily to bath him.

Funds raised locally on his behalf enabled him to buy a house of his own and he had many visitors. However, he and his family gradually became tired of inactivity and eventually he started attending a local occupational therapy department. Later he expressed a desire to train for accountancy. Six years after the accident, he was referred to the Disabled Living Unit for general assessment regarding possible increased independence and further training.

Sensation was absent below the level of C6. Shoulder movements were present and of fair power, elbow flexion was present at Grade 3. Elbow extension was absent and wrist and hand movements absent apart from weak extension of the right wrist. There was severe clawing and contractures of all fingers and of the web of the thumb. He had no pressure-sores, but his urine was infected with pseudomonas pyocyaneus.

Psychological and educational assessment showed him to be of average intelligence and education, having left school at the age of 15 years. But he appeared to have little initiative for work. There were indications that he would not persevere with intensive training such as would be required for accountancy in which he expressed an interest. The general impression gained both by therapists and the psychologist was that with his insurance benefits and National Assistance, he was relatively independent financially, and to be worthwhile any employment would have to provide an income of more than £25 per week.

The bungalow was designed to give him maximum mobility and he and his wife had worked out their needs over the past few years with considerable skill and forethought. There were, however, many other ways in which he and his wife could be helped.

First, the provision of an electrically propelled indoor chair gave him a considerable increase in independent mobility. It was then decided that his family could be helped by the use of a hoist, either portable or electric since they were lifting him unaided for all transfers. A split-leg hammock-type sling was found most suitable, for he was a big heavy man and was having severe spasms. It was felt that a gas-powered flexor-hinge splint might improve his manual dexterity. He had a large and distended abdomen and was suffering from constipation, so an abdominal corset was made for him and an improved bowel routine was initiated.

A gas-powered flexor-hinge splint for the right hand was made and fitted during the first admission, and during the weeks of training there was some improvement in the passive range of movement in the fingers and thumb. A portable hoist was provided by the local authority soon after his discharge, he and his wife having decided that they would prefer this type rather than installing an electric hoist in their bungalow.

Six months after the first admission, they were readmitted to take delivery of the electrically powered chair. He was using the flexor-hinge splint for writing. At his request, the control valve for the carbon dioxide-powered McKibbon artificial muscle which operated the splint was altered, so that he could operate it by his chin. He could now use the splint for an hour continuously, writing or painting.

The electric chair was a great success and the added mobility it provided gave him considerable pleasure. His wife and mother were helped by the hoist and the electric chair since both these appliances reduced the physical effort demanded of them. This was fortunate because he had put on weight and would not bother to diet. However, because of his lack of education and his financial independence there was no incentive for him to change his mode of life, which he clearly enjoyed.

FLAIL ELBOW SPLINTS

A flail arm is a common result of brachial plexus injuries, poliomyelitis and chronic neurological disorders, and there are frequent requests for a functional arm brace to substitute for absent elbow flexion. It is rare for attempts to be made to provide a functional splint for the shoulder, as it is usually to the patient's advantage to leave this joint free and flail. The flail shoulders may tend to sublux and thus give rise to symptoms, but fixing the shoulder in a splint often imposes considerable restriction on the patient's ability to use the flail arm, or to manage it during everyday activities such as dressing. If it is necessary to fix the shoulder, surgical arthrodesis is usually reliable, and if the muscles acting on the scapula are functioning active movement of the arm can be achieved.

Dynamic support for the shoulder can be supplied by mobile arm-supports for wheelchair patients and, in certain circumstances, these supports can also be attached to chairs used by the ambulant disabled. Supportive mobile splinting for the shoulder during walking is virtually impossible. The amount of harness needed to obtain the mechanical advantage necessary to support the weight of the arm in a functional position is too much to be tolerated.

Elbow flexion is necessary to bring the hand into a position of function in front of the body, and it is to substitute for or assist this action that some arm braces are designed. Elbow extension can be assisted by the use of gravity.

To substitute for absent elbow flexion, springs, elastic or external power may be employed, but simple elbow flexion and extension are of little functional value without associated supination and pronation. For feeding, for example, pronation is necessary to reach food and partial supination to present it to the mouth. Thus, there is a tendency to provide linked movements in flail arm splints, elbow extension being coupled with pronation and elbow flexion with supination. This linkage is mechanically simple to achieve, but it has only a limited application in clinical practice.

The functions of the upper limb depend upon the activities of the hand, and the placing of the hand within the space around the body so as to enable it to reach the head, face, front and back of the trunk and perineum. No functional splint has yet been devised which can achieve this placing of the hand. Furthermore, if hand function is deficient, the orthotic devices currently available can only supply a few simple activities, such as the pinch grip of the flexor-hinge splint. Apart from this, the flail hand is merely useful as a prop or weight for steadying things while the other hand functions.

During the recovery phase of, for example, a brachial plexus lesion, an elbow splint may help to preserve passive range of joint actions, and to assist the muscles of the upper arm and forearm in their active movements.

If the flail arm is going to be used as a prop or subsidiary to the other arm, most patients will find that a splint providing stability of the elbow in several positions will give them added useful function. An elbow-locking device will enable them to carry bags and parcels, or to transmit trunk movements to provide pressure at the hand, to hold paper still while writing with the other hand, for example.

Devices providing active flexion and extension at the elbow must be balanced at the shoulder. Forced extension of the elbow must be balanced by an equal flexion force at the shoulder and flexion at the elbow requires balanced shoulder extension. Thus, devices required to flex and extend the elbow require an active shoulder or a stabilized shoulder. In the presence of a flail shoulder, elbow-flexion devices can only position the forearm, and an elbow-locking device is needed to stabilize the elbow for functional activities.

Multiple-axis splints are complex in design, cumbersome in construction, poor in mechanical efficiency and costly to provide. Their acceptance rate is low because they provide little direct functional advantage to the mobile patient. In the future, powered exo-skeletal devices with small but efficient power-packs may well become available; but at present simple, light, stabilizing splints are often of more direct functional value (case history No. 1154).

For the wheelchair patient, however, complex orthotic devices based on the mobile arm-supports are acceptable and provide a functional advantage (*see below*).

M.M.L. No. 1154 born 1946 female

Diagnosis: Anterior poliomyelitis

At the age of 3 years, this patient had a generalized attack of acute poliomyelitis, which resulted in widespread muscle weakness and a flail left arm. She achieved normal education and eventually qualified as a school-teacher, but at the age of 22 years, she enquired whether the function of her left arm could be improved. At this time, she was completely independent, and her function was so good that she swam and played tennis. However, she was unable to cut up her own food, and had difficulty with some daily activities because of the lack of bi-manual function.

The left arm was completely flail with subluxation at the shoulder. Furthermore, the shoulder-girdle muscles were also paralysed or very weak except for the upper fibres of the trapezius and the levator scapulae.

In the hands, she had activity of the finger flexors to M.R.C. Grade 3 and the flexor carpi ulnaris to M.R.C. Grade 3+.

Simple lightweight plaster and plastic splints were made for her to assess the effect of arthrodesis of the elbow and wrist, individually or together, but she preferred the flail mobility to a fixed position.

A commercially available gas-powered flail-arm splint was tried, but its size made it clumsy and inconvenient to wear, and its action was too slow for useful function. It was firmly rejected by the patient after reasonable trial.

A simple splint was made with quick-release elbow-lock. It was supported from a waistband, thus preventing any drag on the subluxed shoulder. A detachable lively splint for the finger and thumb was also made, allowing her to pinch the thumb and two fingers together, and providing active opening of this grip (*Figure 7.7*).

After a period of trial, this splint was also rejected, although it provided some functional advantage, because the patient preferred to continue with her accomplished trick movements and could not tolerate the restriction which any splint imposed.

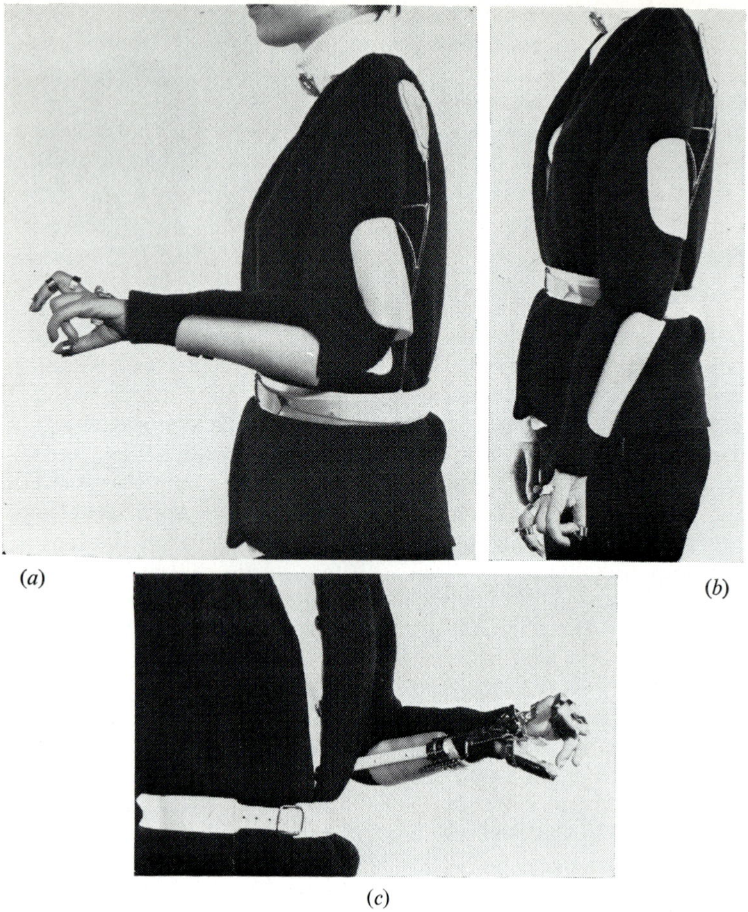

(a) (b) (c)

Figure 7.7. Patient No. 1154 showing the flail arm splint (a) with the elbow flexed and locked; (b) with the elbow extended; (c) the attachment of the lively finger splint

MOBILE ARM-SUPPORTS

Weakness of the shoulder girdle is a frequent disability of patients with muscular dystrophy and poliomyelitis. This weakness is very frustrating and incapacitating, as it may mean that a patient with useful function in the hands cannot use that function, because of inability to put the hands in a suitable position in space. Such patients develop trick movements, for example, 'crawling' with their fingers to reach out, or supporitng one arm with the other, but these manoeuvres have their limitations, and are little compensation for weak shoulders.

Various attempts have been made to support the arm with the hands in a functional position, and various types of gantries and slings have been employed for this purpose, either fixed to a table or workbench, or fixed to the back of a wheelchair. But slings and gantries have several disadvantages. They are usually cumbersome, and when fixed to a wheelchair may cause severe obstruction to mobility, and the range of movement which they produce tends to be limited.

Mobile arm-supports were introduced in an attempt to overcome these disadvantages. Various systems were devised and were given different names depending on the centres exploiting the idea. They were variously called balanced forearm orthoses; balance linkage feeders; ball-bearing arm-supports; and mobile arm-supports which is the name now commonly used.

Mobile arm-supports provide support for the forearm in a horizontal position, with a system of linked ball-races which allow the hands to be placed in an arc in front and at the side of the body, with a minimum of effort. It is usual to fix the apparatus to a suitable wheelchair, but they can equally well be attached to other chairs (*Figure 7.8*). An adjustable clamp is fixed to the back members of the chair, and into this are fitted the linkages with their ball-races. Careful adjustment and judicious tilting will determine whether gravity assists the movement of the forearm towards the body or away from the body, and in this way the system can assist whichever movement is weakest. The trough accommodating the forearm is also carefully balanced, and by tilting the forearm about its point of balance, effective internal and external rotation of the shoulder can be obtained. Once again, the adjustments will determine which of these movements is to be assisted by gravity. All these movements can be restricted by suitable stops fitted and adjusted during practical testing.

Thus, the basic appliance provides support for the arm (assisting or replacing shoulder abduction and flexion and extension), assistance for horizontal abduction and adduction of the arm (elbow flexion and extension with the shoulder semi-abducted) assistance for internal and external rotation of the shoulder with the arm semi-abducted (achieving elevation and depression of the hand). The combination of the movements assisted are those primarily used in feeding, hence the common reference to these appliances as 'feeders'.

The basic appliance does not influence hand function, but an extension of the forearm trough, such as a T-bar, with attachments to carry feeding or writing implements, may increase the manual competence of a severely disabled patient (*Figure 7.9*).

The functional activities which such appliances can assist are those associated with feedings, washing, shaving, making-up, typing and

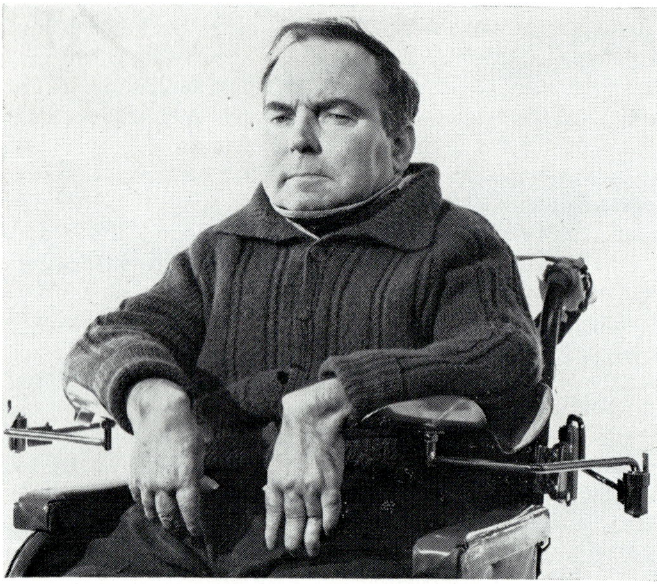

Figure 7.8. Patient No. 1158 in a standard wheelchair with standard mobile arm supports

writing. Furthermore, the hands are supported in the best position for controlling the steering handlebars of certain types of electrically powered indoor chairs.

Functional mobile arm-supports not only provide a more compact appliance than overhead slings, but the range of movement they provide for the hand is greater. *Figure 7.10* shows the range of mobility afforded to a patient with weak arms using a conventional overhead sling, and a mobile arm-support. These pictures were taken in the dark with a small torch-bulb attached to the ring-finger.

Criteria

For these appliances to function efficiently, the patient must sit upright and not transmit trunk weight on to the arm-supports. If they are unable to sit up straight themselves, the trunk must be supported, as the transfer of bodyweight through the arms on to the arm-supports will mitigate against the free movement provided

(*a*)

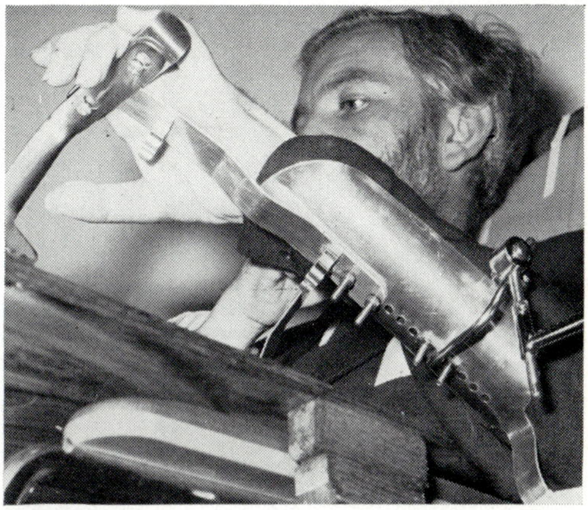

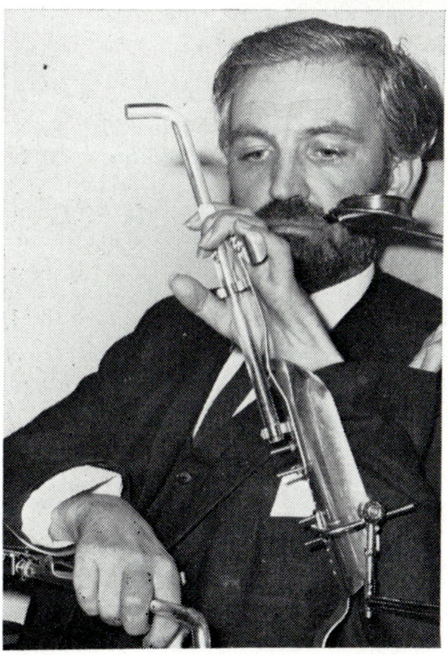

(*b*)

Figure 7.9. Patient No. 662 (a) extended T-bar attachment for mobile arm supports; note offset swivel attachment; (b) removable perspex typing stick fitted into clips on underside of T-bar attachment to mobile arm-supports

by the ball-race linkages. This problem tends to arise more frequently now that poliomyelitis is less common, and more patients with muscular dystrophy are being provided with this type of appliance.

A stable sitting position in good alignment is often the key to success or failure of the mobile arm-supports. Sometimes, mobile arm-supports can be successfully fitted for patients in a reclining

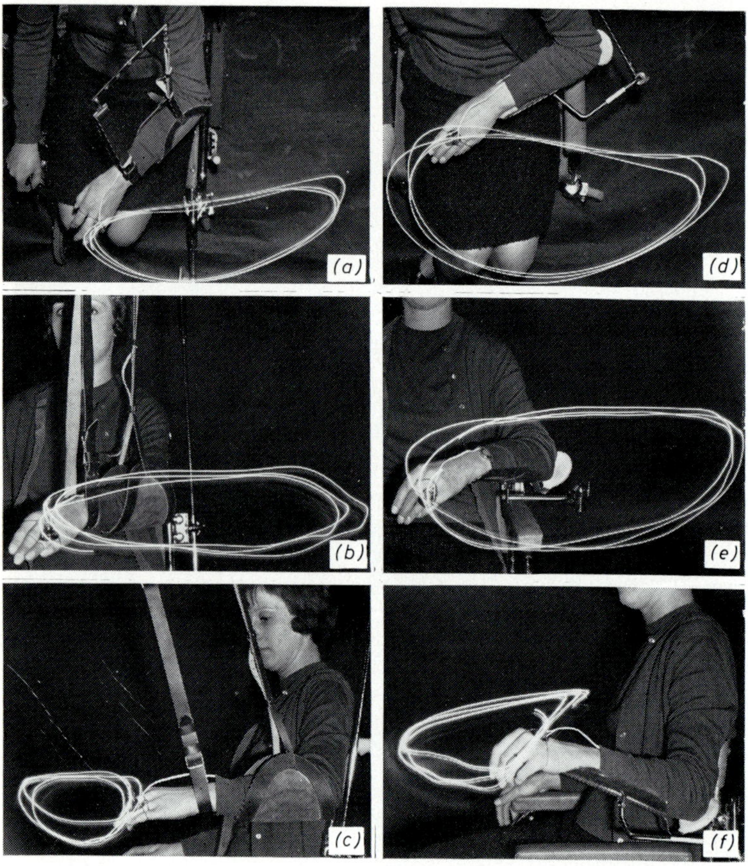

Figure 7.10. Patient using (*a*), (*b*), (*c*) *a conventional sling;* (*d*), (*e*), (*f*) *a mobile arm-support* ((*a*) *and* (*d*) *reproduced by kind permission of* '*Exerpta Medica*')

position, but usually the best results are obtained when the patients are seated in an almost upright position. Patients with progressive collapsing scoliosis may not tolerate extensive spinal bracing (for example, Milwaukee brace), and for these patients, special trunk supports can be made relatively simply, employing polyurethane foam on a plywood backing fitted to the armrests of the wheelchairs, either as permanent fixtures or on adjustable brackets.

Patients must have a good passive range of movement in the shoulders and elbows to achieve useful function with the arm-supports.

Adjustments

The siting of the supporting brackets on the uprights of the wheelchair back is critical to the functioning of the mobile arm-supports. Adjustments include alterations to the height of the bracket which will determine the over-all height of the arm-supports. Rotation of the bracket will bias the movement in favour either of abduction or adduction of the shoulder. The tilt of the bracket will determine whether flexion or extension of the elbow is assisted by gravity. Once adjusted, these brackets should only be altered by therapists experienced in adjusting them, as the adjustments are vitally important and wrongly adjusted mobile arm-supports can be a positive impedance to the production of optimal arm and hand function.

If the patient needs detachable armrests, such as for sideways transfers, then it may be necessary to supply armrests specially shaped to enable them to be removed without disturbing the brackets.

The setting of the trough will control internal and external rotation of the shoulder, and by altering the position of the fulcrum, it can either assist the elevation or depression of the hand. Other variations can be obtained by altering the shape of the proximal or distal linkage, and specially strong linkages may be necessary for heavily-built men. The supporting swivel for the forearm trough can be offset to the side of the trough, rather than placed below the trough. This allows the axis of rotation of the forearm to be moved closer to the elbow, and thus achieve a greater vertical range for the hand. From a practical point of view, this tends to bring the forearm back to the horizontal, and is thus particularly useful for working at a desk.

A further linkage can be attached to the forearm trough, so that when the forearm is tilted the movement is combined with supination and pronation. This assists in the feeding-movement pattern, and is particularly helpful when there is considerable weakness of the forearm and hand.

Elevating mobile arm-supports

A more complex accessory provides an assistance to elevation. By means of parallel linkages on the proximal part of the orthosis, the whole appliance can be elevated or depressed, bringing the forearms higher or lower, and enabling the patient to undertake activities at different levels when the degree of weakness is such that they are unable to achieve adequate function otherwise (case history No. 465).

M.M.L. No. 465 born 1956 female

Diagnosis: Anterior poliomyelitis

An acute attack of anterior poliomyelitis at the age of 5 years affected all this child's limbs, trunk and respiratory muscles. She was nursed in a respirator but was able to be weaned out of this using a permanent tracheostomy. With a Milwaukee brace and bilateral long-leg calipers, she could stand and walk for a few yards holding on to someone's hand, and propel a wheelchair slowly on level floors.

She was thin, fragile and underdeveloped, and at the age of 10 years she was admitted to the Disabled Living Unit to assess her suitability for mobile arm-supports.

At this time, her vital capacity was 400 ml. Her legs were flail below the hips, her hip-power in all movements was M.R.C. grade 3–4. The power of her arms was as follows.

	Grade	
	Left	*Right*
Shoulder elevation	4	3
Shoulder abduction	3	2+
Shoulder flexion	3	2
Pectorals	4	2
Elbow flexion	4	4
Elbow extension	0	0
Wrist flexion	3	3
Wrist extension	3+	3+
Hand—all groups	5	5

Once again, the initial approach to the improvement of independence was directed towards the wheelchair, and it was decided to give her an electrically powered chair as this was the only chance of increasing her mobility enough to enable her to attend a school. Having done this, attention was directed towards enabling her to get in and out of the chair independently. The provision of attachments to the locking mechanism of the swinging detachable footrests enabled her to swing them herself. Adaptations to the calipers enabled her to lock and unlock these herself. She could now achieve independence for toilet purposes.

The Milwaukee brace prevented her from looking down and interfered with reading and writing, but prismatic glasses solved this problem, enabling her to read more easily and also to see her food. She achieved these activities by resting her elbows on a table, provided that this was at the correct height and distance in front of her.

On her first admission, she was reluctant to use mobile arm-supports, but was encouraged when the provision of a simple fixed elbow-support ('flying saucer') improved her ability to type, and prevented her arm from getting so tired in the process.

On further admission, when she had gained confidence and mobility, she persevered with mobile arm-supports. Although these were a help, particularly when supplied with offset swivels, they were changed for elevating mobile arm-supports. On the left side, an elastic band was used and she had enough power to depress the trough. On the right, she did not have enough power to lift or depress, so a 'McKibben' Artificial CO_2-powered muscle was used to give necessary power to elevate. This she operated by a nudge switch controlled by the left knee.

With these elevating mobile arm-supports, she at last was able to reach her mouth for feeding, her chair for combing, and her face for washing.

Her gradually increasing confidence and functional competence, and in particular her independence in mobility, enabled her to leave hospital and be admitted to a School for Handicapped Children. When followed up two years later, she was making considerable use of the electrically powered chair and the elevating arm-supports (*Figure 7.11*).

Requirements for mobile arm-supports

Mobile arm-supports can be used as a therapeutic device. For example, in patients with rheumatoid arthritis who have had reconstructive surgery or synovectomy performed on elbows or shoulders, the arm supports can encourage active movement of these joints with gravity eliminated (*see* case history No. 99, Chapter 3, page 96).

These devices are primarily assistive for very weak muscle groups, and depend for their function on low-friction ball-races and accurate balancing. Consequently, any tremor or ataxia of the patient will tend to be exaggerated by the system. Attempts have been made to use similar systems with high-friction linkages for use by patients with inco-ordination. A 'friction feeder' will dampen down gross tremor, but the device has little value in the general management of patients with muscular inco-ordination.

The 6 basic requisites for satisfactory use of mobile arm-supports are as follows.

Weakness

Weakness severe enough to require assistance or substitution of either elbow or shoulder M.R.C. Grade 0 to 3 or M.R.C. Grade 3 to 3+ in patients with a very limited endurance.

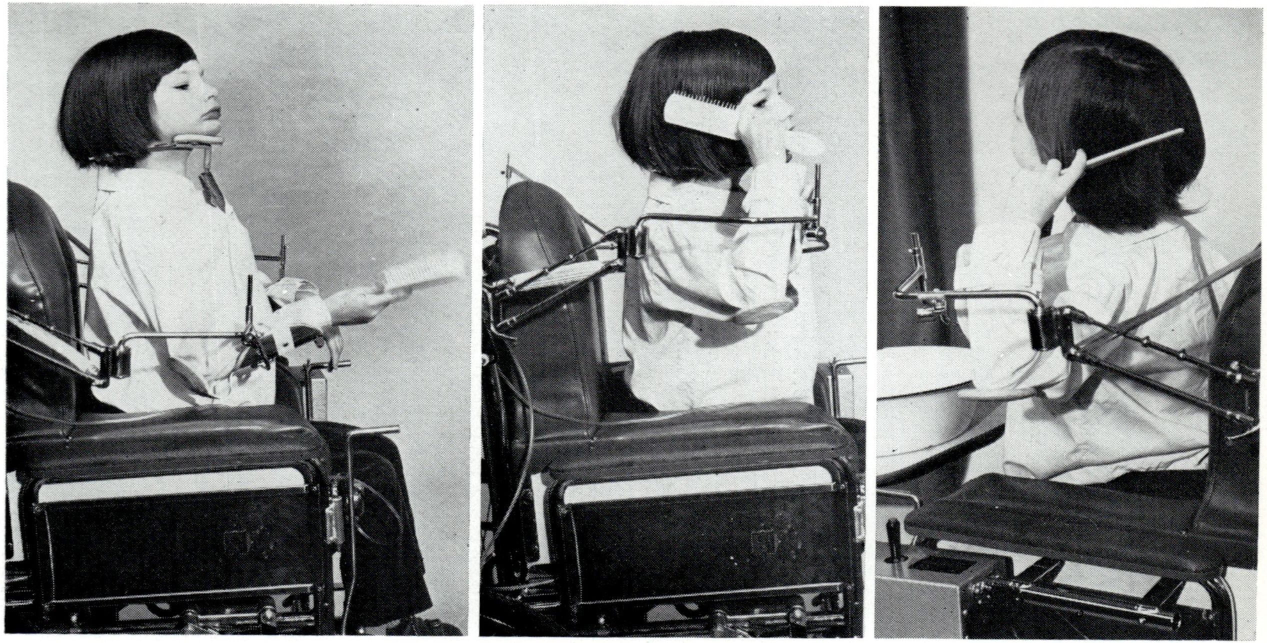

(a) (b) (c)

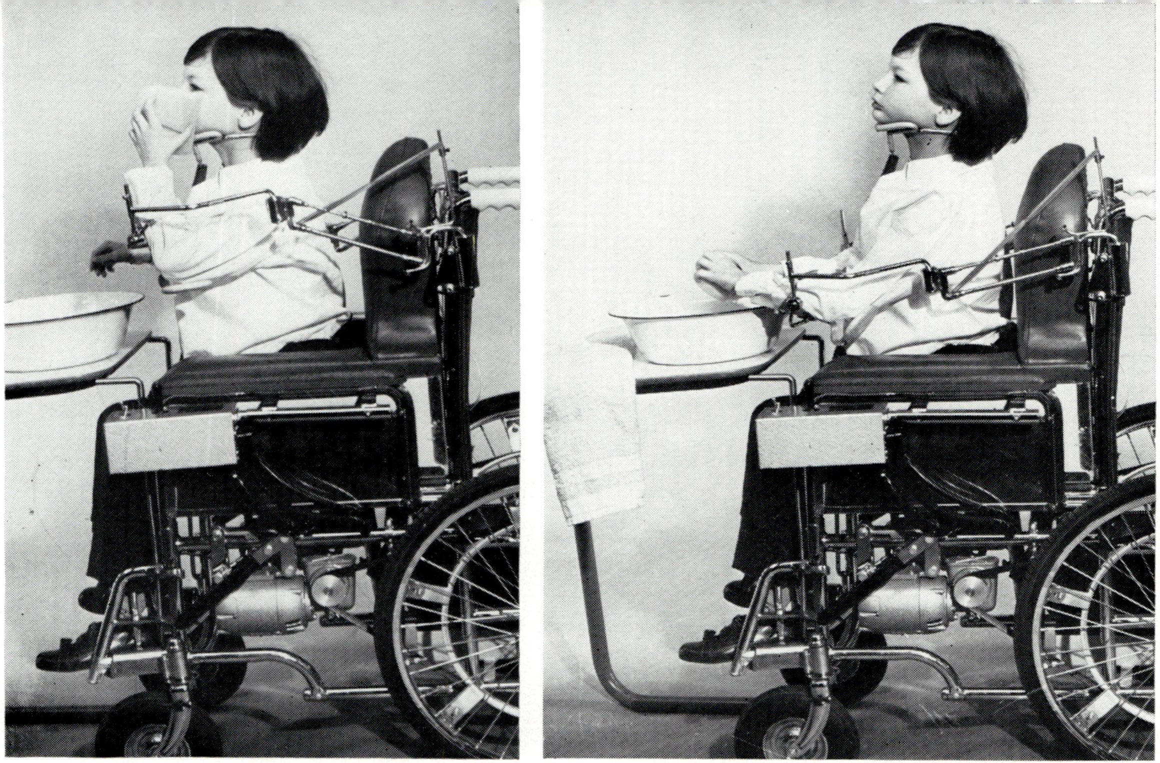

(d) (e)

Figure 7.11. Patient No. 465 using gas-powered right elevating mobile arm-support (a) depressed; (b) elevated; (c) using left elastic assisted elevating mobile arm-support showing the use of an offset swivel to achieve a greater vertical range; (d) elevated; (e) depressed

Power

Power needed to drive the mobile arm-supports is
elbow flexion or shoulder abduction 3+ to 4;
neck or trunk power to shift centre of gravity of the trunk.

Passive range

To achieve a useful functional range of hand movements, the patient needs adequate ranges of passive joint-motion to enable the hand to be placed in functional positions.

Co-ordination

Good co-ordination in muscle groups controlling the movements.

Sitting endurance

Patient must be able to sit upright for several hours (lateral trunk-supports may be needed).

Training

There must be adequate available training facilities and patient's motivation to accept training must be sufficient to tide him over the early stages of fitting and using the supports.

The 4 stages of adjustment of mobile arm-supports are as follows.

Position in wheelchair.—Comfort and stability.

Height of mobile arm-support.—Forearm at 45–55 degrees to the horizontal when hand is at the mouth.

Trough balance.—Pivot adjusted for optimal range of vertical motion (*a*) standard pivot, hand 'heavy'; (*b*) offset swivel, elbow 'heavy'.

Pitch and roll.—Adjustment at the bracket, (*a*) vertical position of bracket, (*b*) rotation of bracket.

M.M.L. No. 1158 born 1922 male

Diagnosis: Rheumatoid arthritis

In 1953, at the age of 31 years, this man developed rheumatoid arthritis, the progress of the disease was rapid and within a year he was unable to continue to work as a labourer.

He was looked after at home for several years, but despite the administration of prednisolone and bilateral knee synovectomy, his ability gradually diminished, and in 1963 he was admitted to a local authority Welfare Home.

On admission to this home, he complained of a recent alteration in feeling in his legs and arms. His neck was radiographed and he was found to have subluxation of the cervical vertebrae at different levels; C3 on C4, C4 on C5 and C5 on C6. A leather supportive collar was prescribed and brought about considerable relief of symptoms.

He was referred to the Disabled Living Unit for advice on independent living.

On admission to the Unit, he had very little movement in the shoulder, and dislocation of the wrists, but had retained a useful range of movement at the elbows. The hands were severely disorganized. His hips were grossly limited in range of movement. The

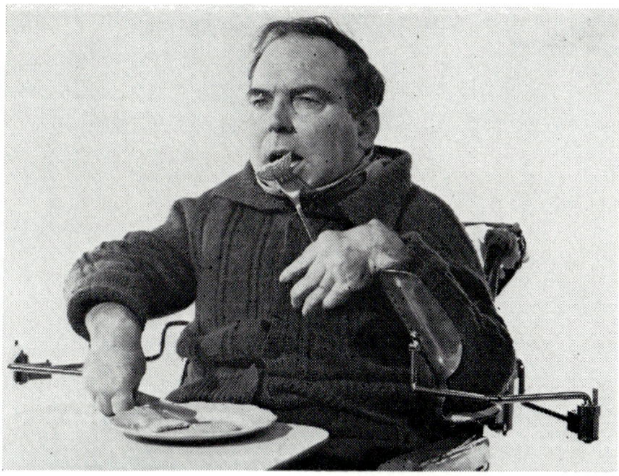

Figure 7.12. Patient No. 1158 using mobile arm-supports with extension to raise trough, enabling him to feed himself

knees could be fully extended but flexion was limited to 80 degrees. The ankles were fixed and the feet were in fixed eversion. However, he was able to stand and take a few steps using a walking aid, and he was able to propel himself backwards in a standard wheelchair by using his feet. He was quite unable to use his arms for wheelchair propulsion.

He was also completely dependent on assistants for dressing, washing, toilet and bathing. He was unable to feed himself because of weakness, stiffness and pain in the shoulders, coupled with the palmar dislocation of the hands and loss of pronation and supination of the forearms. However, the provision of a standard set of mobile arm-supports with a vertical extension to raise the trough, enabled him to feed himself (*Figure 7.12*). He was supplied with a lightweight plastic mug which he could lift with both hands, and thus became independent for drinking. For hot fluids, a plastic straw was found to be more suitable.

His mobility was considerably improved by the substitution of an electrically-powered indoor chair, but the only type of control which he could manage was the simple joystick control of the Powerdrive chair, with a T-bar extension. This enabled him to move around in the local authority home independently, and was a considerable pleasure to him. He could manage to stand and turn for transfers, and thus avoid having to be lifted.

Comments

This case history illustrates once again the use of a suitable electrically-powered indoor chair to give added independence. It also illustrates the use of mobile arm-supports in severe rheumatoid arthritis to give added function, particularly for feeding.

8—Architectural Problems

INTRODUCTION

Many of the day-to-day problems of the disabled are associated with architectural design of their houses, the buildings they want to visit or the roads and pavements they need to use. Some of these difficulties have already been discussed in relation to specific activities, but in this chapter, they are gathered together under the general heading of architectural problems. Often they are so fundamental to a patient's independence that they bear repeating. Furthermore, those concerned with the rehabilitation of the severely disabled may find it convenient to refer to these problems as a group, although their presentation must, of necessity, be somewhat fragmentary.

GENERAL PROBLEMS

In the general management of the physically disabled it is often as important to treat the environment as the patient himself. The cause of disability is often incurable and the disability is, therefore, not significantly alterable, but functional improvement of the patient's surroundings is often possible. Until recently, the special needs of the physically disabled have received scant attention. Nowadays, however, increasing attention is paid to design criteria related to the physically disabled, and to the many experiments demonstrating the major handicaps imposed on them by minor architectural features. Architects, social workers and others interested in the welfare of the physically disabled are now devoting much time and effort to the recognition, analysis and elimination of such architectural barriers to the participation of these members of the community in the normal activities of everyday life.

Minor variations in design can render private dwellings negotiable to the disabled, both ambulant and wheelchair patients alike.

The British Standards Institution has now published the first part of the new Code of Practice (C.P. 96), dealing with the general consideration of access for the disabled to public buildings, and this gives the lead for future developments. With these standards and with the active influence of voluntary organizations, now most public buildings incorporate some modifications to facilitate their use by disabled people, a distinct contrast to the situation 5–10 years ago, but the problem of altering existing public buildings appears to be virtually insoluble.

Some disabled and elderly people compensate for the architectural barriers and restrictions which they meet, by developing new skills and techniques to overcome or circumvent them. But many are frustrated and become more and more restricted, giving up, rather than trying to overcome the difficulties occasioned by venturing out into the general community. In surveys relating to the use made of public buildings by the disabled, it is difficult to differentiate between real lack of interest and the deadening effect of physical frustration which has built up over the years. Little reliable data exists to indicate the nature or extent of the need to provide facilities for disabled people, either in private dwellings or public buildings, and there seems little possibility of such data becoming available in the near future.

However, from the data available, it is clear that the main buildings which the disabled might like to use, and indeed should be actively encouraged to use, are often the most inaccessible. Churches, libraries, and cinemas are renowned for their steps, which are indeed often an architectural feature to the able, but an insurmountable obstacle to the disabled. The most important public building for many is the public lavatory, which is almost deliberately inaccessible in its traditional form. Typical situations chosen for the construction of these essential amenities may be underground, reached by narrow winding steps, or above ground on islands in the middle of busy roads, or in remote corners of market squares or railway stations. The conventional segregation of the sexes in public lavatories presents a further complication, since many disabled require some assistance in the toilet, and this is denied to them if the entry of a companion of the opposite sex is forbidden, although this companion may be their usual attendant at home.

Often it is the lack of information about the available facilities, rather than the lack of the facilities themselves, which constitutes such a handicap to disabled people. Appropriate sign-posting can help considerably and is being more widely used during recent years. More and more guidebooks for the disabled are being published, dealing with particular cities and towns, and are extremely helpful, since they permit the advance planning of route and activity, which is essential to eliminate wasteful digression from the programme of the disabled.

A further lack, less easily implemented, is that of space. In general, the physically disabled, whether ambulant or chair-bound, require more space for manoeuvring and for access than do the able-bodied. It is this extra space which is so difficult to provide, since extra space is almost synonymous with extra cost as far as building is concerned, and extra cost is an anathema to the private citizen, local authority and public corporation alike.

Local authorities have the power to make appropriate provision for housing the disabled, but these powers are permissive, and it may be difficult to justify extra expenditure on accommodation for the disabled, in the face of social pressures arising from long housing lists of economically productive able people.

Design of accommodation for the disabled

When faced with the prospect of advising on design of accommodation for the disabled, the first questions should be (1) what are the disabilities, (2) what is the patient like as a person, and (3) what are the circumstances regarding education, work, social background and so forth.

For individual patients, the answers to these questions can either be deduced or derived from simple trials. But to plan accommodation for disabled people *en masse*, without knowing their individual requirements, is almost impossible. Even so, local authorities tend to allocate and plan a certain number of dwellings which they classify as suitable for the disabled. The needs of a disabled bachelor differ from those of a disabled married man with a wife who is willing to care for him. The problems of a disabled housewife differ from those of a disabled man who has retired from work. Disabled children and disabled adults have different problems, and the problems of the ambulant are very different from the problems of those who are confined to wheelchairs. Arthritics have different problems from amputees and hemiplegics have problems not shared by paraplegics.

If a general approach is unavoidable, it must leave considerable freedom for final alteration to supply individual needs, an adaptable design with features capable of accepting constraints later (and this is likely to be expensive in space and material). It is, when possible, preferable to define the individual disabled user (or disability group), within fairly close limits.

The wheelchair creates major design problems. There are, of

course, many different types of wheelchairs (*see* Chapter 6), self-propelling, electrically propelled, front-wheel propellers and rear-wheel propellers. Each has features suitable for different activities and different disabilities. Even though the chairs may fold up, they are still awkward and take up considerable space. Designers tend to regard a wheelchair as a means of progressing from one place to another, and often suggest that the patient should have more than one chair for use in the home. But extra transfers for a disabled patient are to be avoided whenever possible, as a patient often comes to regard the chair as part of himself and resents frequent chair changes; each additional transfer represents an additional hazard; the use of two chairs may entail a loss of independence if help is needed for transfer from one to the other; and some wheelchairs are very expensive.

The features of general-purpose house design are largely determined by money. Disabled people require more than the average amount of space allotted for circulation and access, particularly in bathrooms, lavatories and kitchens. To compensate for the additional space allowed in these situations, houses for disabled people may be built with less garden space, or with fewer bedrooms.

Broadly speaking, authorities planning to construct private or municipal buildings likely to be used by the disabled must provide three main features: (1) ease of access outside; (2) ease of manoeuvrability inside; and (3) flexibility for fitments and furnishing.

When discussing details of design criteria imposed by disability, it is necessary to differentiate clearly between the requirements of private and public buildings.

Public buildings

As far as public buildings are concerned, there is likely to be considerable argument, of both political and sentimental nature, regarding designs for the disabled. There are those who maintain that all public buildings should be designed with the physically disabled in mind. These extreme views overplay the extent of the need, and offer a simplified solution which assumes that making public buildings more accessible to wheelchair-users will automatically make them more convenient for the able-bodied. This view has yet to be substantiated, and it certainly places an unwarranted constraint on architects and on the able-bodied population. It also refutes the contention that the disabled have, at some stage, to accept certain limitations imposed by their handicap. Such an approach also involves an unrealistic optimism about the amount of use which the elderly and disabled are likely to make of the buildings concerned.

Ideally, a consideration of the needs of the disabled should influence but not dominate the architectural plan of a public building. Such a plan would compromise between the imposition of additional expensive features on all buildings to make them accessible to the disabled, and the concession of complete artistic freedom to their designers, enabling them to create buildings with architectural barriers which might prevent their use by the disabled members of the community.

PRIVATE DWELLINGS

When a house does not fulfil the needs of the disabled person who lives in it, there are five possible courses of corrective action open to him:

(1) he can move house;

(2) he can have his house altered structurally;

(3) he can have an extension built on;

(4) he can have new equipment installed to facilitate his use of the existing architectural structure;

(5) he can be supplied with aids and appliances to mitigate the house's disadvantages.

All too frequently, when a disabled patient is being assessed, it is found that he lives in entirely unsuitable surroundings. His house is on a hilly site a long way from the shops, and there are no near neighbours. The staircase is narrow, dark, steep, and without a handrail. The kitchen sink is deep and at the wrong height. The oven is in an awkward corner and cannot be cleaned without imitating a contortionist. The cupboards can only be reached by standing on a chair, and recharging the gas-meter involves crawling in a cupboard under the stairs. All the electric plug sockets are too low to reach from a wheelchair, whereas the windows and lights are too high. The bath is difficult to get into and out of and there is no room for a wheelchair in the bathroom. The lavatory is often outside, and when it is indoors it is so small that not only is it inaccessible by wheelchair, but there is no room for an attendant to help the patient in and out. So frequently are these problems encountered that it is remarkable how so many elderly and disabled have managed for so long. Furthermore, these problems cannot be solved by simple measures, nor is it feasible or acceptable to contemplate rehousing all the disabled.

When private accommodation for the disabled is to be designed *ab initio* or to be extensively redesigned, it is essential that the problems at issue should be clearly defined for both patient and architect.

Stairs are almost invariably contra-indicated for the severely disabled, and prove a considerable barrier for the less severely disabled and for the elderly. An obvious solution to the problem offered by stair climbing to the disabled would seem to be a lift or a moving staircase. The large amount of space necessary to accommodate lifts and moving staircases, and the large amounts of money necessary to pay for them, combine to make their installation unrealistic in the average house. Added to this, they may not necessarily best fulfil a patient's requirements.

It is usually cheaper and more efficient to plan a purpose-built extension to the ground floor, when a disabled person is unable to move from a 2-storey house. With the many versions of the single-storey extension (sun-room or conservatory), available in prefabricated modular form, such a venture no longer calls for a prohibitive outlay of money, and may often provide a suitable and attractive room for a severely disabled patient.

Accessibility

The divergence of the needs of ambulant and wheelchair disabled patients is emphasized by a consideration of the accessibility of any house for the two groups.

For the wheelchair disabled, the approach to a house above ground-level should be by way of a gently sloping ramp, with a non-slip surface. Between the end of the ramp and the front door there should be a level area, to permit opening and shutting the door by the patient, and to enable his chair to await admission on other occasions. The door itself should be overhung by a protective canopy.

Ambulant disabled, however, may find that shallow steps are preferable to a ramp of unsuitable surface, as this may become slippery or treacherous under inclement weather conditions. For such patients, suitable handrails are essential. If one rail is fastened to a wall, it is essential that sufficient space be allowed between the rail and the wall to enable the patient's hand to grasp the rail firmly, without difficulty or trauma.

When access for both ambulant and wheelchair disabled is needed to the same house, a combined ramp and flight of shallow steps should be provided.

If conversion rather than construction is being considered, and there are front and back doorsteps in a house, both providing major barriers to access, the construction of front and back ramps is again indicated, from ground-level to the level of the steps. A gap between ramp and door-sill should be left in each case, to prevent rising damp, and should be covered with a fine-mesh grating. A canopy over each door and a level area in front of it are also necessary.

If possible, the path should be continued all round the house, and from the house to the garage. The path needs to be level and made of well-laid paving stones, roughed-up concrete or tar macadam; but crazy paving, loose aggregate and random bricks laid as paths are liable to separate and leave dangerous gaps. Paths should be at least 3 ft 6 in (107 cm) wide for ambulant disabled and wheelchair users, but if an electric tricycle is used, then 4 ft (122 cm) width is necessary. Turning areas may also be necessary for manoeuvring the powered chairs.

Garage

For disabled patients who use a car, either a carport or an outsize garage should be provided. Sufficient space is needed to transfer between wheelchair and car, and uncertain or bad weather-conditions make it preferable for this to be done under cover. Less space is needed by the ambulant disabled but transfers may be almost as difficult and time-consuming for them as they are for the chair-bound, and cover is a great advantage.

Garage doors are often heavy and difficult to operate, but counter-balanced ones are readily available, easily operable, and generally are more suitable for the disabled than side-hung doors. The area between garage and house should be covered whenever possible. A covered area giving access from door to garage can also be used to house the dustbin, fuel store, tool-shed and so forth, thus allowing the disabled person to carry out many of the tasks of running a house without being exposed unnecessarily to inclement weather.

Doors

General

In general, all doors should have a minimum width of 2 ft 9 in (84 cm) and should be without a raised threshold of any kind. Wheelchair-users usually require a space between the opening edge of the door and the 'return' wall of about 15 in (38 cm) so that they can operate the door handle. Door handles of the lever type are usually preferable for the disabled, and the bigger the better.

Outside doors

Front doors, and preferably back doors too, should have their fittings sited so as to be accessible to the wheelchair user. Thus door-locks both internal and external and a letter-box with retaining cage or tray should be within easy reach. The light switches for inside and outside lights should be immediately inside the front door at a convenient level, and the lights themselves should provide clear illumination of the door, and the hall and the front approach to the house. For wheelchair users, sufficient space for a 180-degree turn is needed both inside and outside the door.

Inside doors

Although side-hung doors of adequate width, opening from and into an unobstructed area are probably easier to manipulate, where a door serves a small room in which circulation space is required, it may be necessary to install a sliding door. Contrary to custom, it is advisable that bathroom and lavatory doors open outwards, not only to give more space inside these rooms, but also to provide easier access in case of accident. A pass-key should always be available to override any internal lock, and any internal bolts should be capable of being released from the outside.

Rising-butt hinges are of use, but mechanical closers are contra-indicated in most doors, since they are often inconvenient and sometimes dangerous for the elderly, fragile or ataxic patient.

Some protection against trauma from wheelchairs may be fixed to the bottom edges of doors, corners of corridors and door-jambs, made either from metal or plastic; some are available, which can be fitted to irregular shapes.

Grab or Grip rails

The position and location of grab rails or grip rails depends on many factors that need time and trial to assess. In certain situations, such as round the toilet pedestal and bath, and in the kitchen area, in the case of a disabled housewife, their siting is fairly constant; but in other situations, this will depend on the activities and habits of the individual patient concerned.

In general, the best type of rail is made of nylon-coated steel, but these rails are expensive. Vertical and horizontal bars are more useful than sloping rails. Patients either tend to pull up using a vertical bar, or to push up from a horizontal bar, but the heights and positions must be accurately assessed individually. Rails may also be required behind the patient, as well as at his side, and this particularly applies to the lavatory. When possible, it is a wise precaution to have additional rails fixed across the front of all wash-basins. Patients with poor balance who tend to grab fixed objects to steady themselves may otherwise grab the wash-basins, pulling them from the wall, or else losing their grip on the smooth wet sides. Heated towel rails should be avoided, as patients with diminished sensation may use them as grab rails, and thus run the risk of severe burns.

Circulation space

The internal circulation space required for any building depends on the purpose of the building and on the number of people using it. Thus a residential home for physically handicapped people will need a large amount of space for the comings and goings of its inmates many of whom will be chairbound. All wheelchair patients have three wants in common, a manoeuvrable chair, the strength or mechanical power to manoeuvre it, and sufficient space for manoeuvring within the building where they live. Yet while attempting to create the necessary space for wheelchair existence, either in a private or a residential home, it is important to remember that everyone, able or disabled, needs and wants a certain amount of privacy. The chief disadvantage of the open-plan family dwelling place is this lack of privacy. The combined noise-value of the television, the washing machine, the extractor fan and the transistor radio are likely to combine with the voices of various members of the family, until the chairbound patient may long for escape and will only find circulation space instead.

Once again, however, there is a striking difference between the needs and preferences of the wheelchair disabled and the ambulant disabled, for while a wheelchair requires plenty of space, many of the ambulant disabled, particularly patients with rheumatoid arthritis, strokes or multiple sclerosis, use the furniture and fittings as aids to movement. They prefer small spaces and narrow rooms, so that a wall or a solid fitting is always within reach, to give them stability should they need it.

Space heating

Many severely disabled have poor peripheral circulation, and are subject to chilblains and oedema of the feet. Many have respiratory deficiency, and have a greater susceptibility and a lower resistance to respiratory infections, than able-bodied people. Consequently, the maintenance of a reasonable background temperature and the elimination of draughts is important to their health as well as to their comfort.

Underfloor heating is unobtrusive. There are no cables, pipes or radiators to obstruct mobility or to give rise to unnecessary risks from contact. But such a system cannot be boosted or reduced quickly, to cope with the rapid alterations in weather characteristics of the British Isles. Probably ducted warm air is the most suitable form of central heating, but this can only be economically installed in a new building. Free-standing oil-fired radiators and electric fires are a positive danger to the disabled, particularly if they are ataxic or their sight is impaired. Night storage heaters, unobtrusively situated are a form of central heating which can be installed in most houses without much difficulty. They are economical to run, difficult to overturn, and effective in producing background heat.

Kitchen

The over-all design of the kitchen for a disabled housewife once again emphasizes the marked difference in the requirements of the ambulant disabled and the wheelchair-disabled patient. The ambulant disabled housewife prefers the galley-type of kitchen, where everything is close to her, and she can use the fittings for support and stability. The wheelchair user, however, needs circulation space in the middle, about 5 ft (1·5 m) diameter in which to manoeuvre.

Unfortunately, local authority dwellings might have to be used by an ambulant disabled patient for a while, and later by a wheelchair user. Or, indeed, it is not an infrequent occurrence that an ambulant disabled patient slowly deteriorates and has to accept a wheelchair existence. The double problem can be partially solved with careful initial planning and the use of demountable standard units. If the basic space requirements are determined by the wheelchair user, then the more restricted design can be fitted in, but if the appropriate space is not available, it is much more difficult to rearrange the accommodation for a change from ambulant to wheelchair use.

The combination of cooking and dining areas is usually convenient for the disabled housewife, as it reduces the carrying distance for food and crockery, whereas provision of a dining recess off the living room makes little concession to easing the problems of housework. Thus the most universally acceptable solution involves the provision of a kitchen-dining room, in which are interchangeable units capable of several rearrangements, and some variation in working heights, and the only constant features are the fixed plumbing, windows and doors.

Although the basic idea of a kitchen-dining room is a good one for a disabled housewife, the conventional planning of such a room is often unsuitable for the handicapped. The usual siting of the sink beneath a window means that the disabled housewife cannot reach the window to open or close it. Also although the units used within the room should ideally be interchangeable, in fact the size, shape and inter-relationships between sink, worktops and doors are usually predetermined and unchangeable. It is only by the introduction of modern fitments and the use of careful planning that variations of working-space can be provided within such a fixed framework.

An adequate work surface of the correct height is even more

important to the disabled housewife than to the able. Often a sturdy table will provide the necessary additional work surface and will reduce journeys within the kitchen area. A table, however, may not be practical for the wheelchair user, who may prefer a removable tray, with low rims to be fitted when necessary to her chair. Small trolleys, usually higher than normal, are often found to be an indispensable additional aid.

Efficient layout of the kitchen is essential to minimize problems of manoeuvring, lifting, carrying, reaching, stooping, and handling.

Storage space

Storage space is usually the most unsatisfactory factor in existing kitchens, and fixed or mobile storage areas may have to be specially designed. Much of the storage accommodation in kitchens is unsuitable for the disabled housewife by reason of siting, height, depth or design. Storage space is often too high, too deep and awkward of access for those with restricted function, and, it is often, therefore, a source of danger, since the disabled patient must make such physical effort to reach it, that she frequently falls or injures herself.

When planning or redesigning, allowance has to be made not only for reaching the shelf but for getting hold of the article safely. For ambulant housewives, the optimum height for shelves is between 2 ft 6 in and 4 ft (76–122 cm) whereas for those in wheelchairs, the preferred height is between 1 ft 6 in and 3 ft 6 in (46–107 cm). Long, open, narrow (shallow) shelves are more easily accessible and the objects on them are reached more easily than those in deep cupboards.

Storage cupboards are often awkward, but by careful organization entailing the separation of items used regularly from those only used occasionally, and the separation of those only used by non-disabled members of the household from items used by everyone, the storage system can be rationalized. Although the wheelchair user can only reach those cupboards which are within his limited height range, other members of the household can use the high and the low ones. Maximal and minimal heights of shelves which can be used from the wheelchair and the depth of shelf which is accessible, can only be determined by trial. Both will depend upon the degree of access available to the storage area.

General relationship of accommodation

Open-plan designs have certain distinct advantages. The simplified plan economizes in construction time and cost, and makes it easier and cheaper to maintain an even temperature throughout. When space available is strictly limited, then that saved by eliminating corridors can be utilized in areas where additional space is required, particularly the bathroom and lavatory. For the disabled, an open-plan house gives easier manoeuvrability, and for the severely disabled, it enables them to be more closely integrated into the family life than if they were restricted to a bedroom. A sleeping recess of reasonable size off the living space and a recess to house the dining table and chairs, with the kitchen-galley adjoining, will eliminate all corridors between these three areas. A sliding door or folding door can be used to open up or close off a part or all of the opening between living and sleeping areas. However, integrating the bedroom area with the living area has some distinct disadvantages. Beds and bedclothes are always highly productive of fluff and dust and this is no longer isolated to the bedroom but will spread to the whole of the open area. Furthermore, either the disabled member or other members of the family may require privacy for medical or personal reasons and privacy will often be difficult to obtain in a fully open-plan dwelling.

Thus, once again, it is necessary either to plan for a specific patient or to have a design which incorporates considerable flexibility.

Bathroom and lavatory

In designing the bathroom and lavatory, there is the customary discrepancy between the requirements of the ambulant disabled and those of the wheelchair users, the latter patients, requiring extra space for manoeuvring. However, by combining the bathroom and lavatory, a room with adequate additional space can be provided either for the wheelchair, or for attendants to help the patient in and out of the bath. For the severely disabled, having toilet and bathing facilities in the same room can reduce the transfer problems for the attendants, whether the transfers are by manual handling or by means of portable or fixed ceiling hoists (*Figure 8.1*).

For the severely physically disabled patient who needs considerable help, a free-standing bath is usually the most suitable. This allows attendants to obtain access from either side. Portable hoists can only gain access to a bath which is 10 in (25 cm) off the floor, and does not have solid side-panels. A fitted bench-type transfer seat may be of considerable help.

Some people prefer to use a shower, and for some disabled, the shower is the only satisfactory method of obtaining an all-over wash. Some patients have evolved techniques of using a flexible shower while sitting on a bath seat with their feet in the bath, and others of combining the use of the water-closet with the use of the hand shower.

Wherever possible, practical trials in a Functional Assessment Unit are the only means of establishing a suitable technique of washing, both for the patient and for the relative or other attendants.

The position of the pedestal or flushing-pan, the height of the seat and the position of the toilet-paper holders are all often critical, if a severely disabled person is to be independent, or if the patient

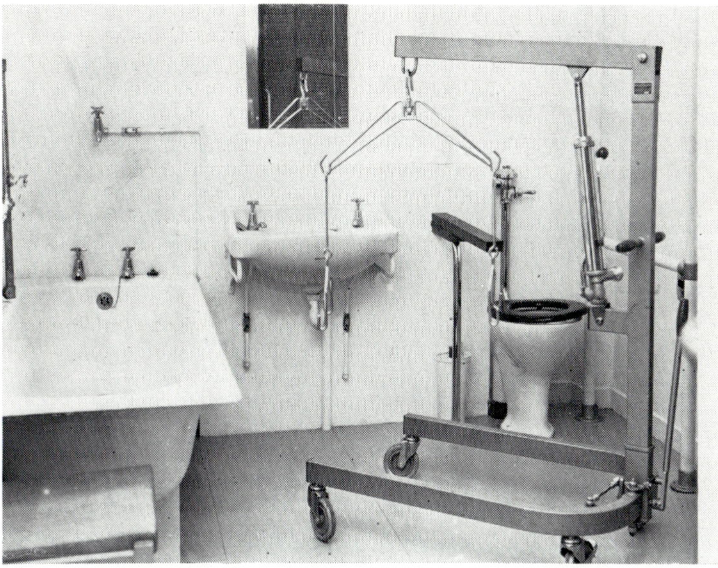

Figure 8.1. General view of combined bathroom and toilet indicating the problem of space when a portable hoist is necessary

is to be looked after at home by relatives, visiting attendants or neighbours.

For wheelchair users, transfers from chair to lavatory-seat may be accomplished in various ways and the correct access to the seat is essential for a patient's independence. Most severely disabled, and even the elderly with lesser disabilities involving stiffness of the hips, need considerable space around the lavatory pedestal, particularly behind it. Also the attendants who may have to help lift the patient on and off the seat, and the wheelchair-user who performs a true sideways transfer needs space to the side and behind the pedestal. In general, it is advisable to have a high-level cistern (waste-water preventer) in preference to the usual low-level modern suite, and thus leave the space behind and above the pedestal free (*Figure 8.2*).

Modern lavatory-seats are made of plastic and are small. The Victorian type of wooden seat is often the most suitable for the disabled. They are more stable, less likely to break, and can be extended sideways or behind the pedestal. The bidet is even less

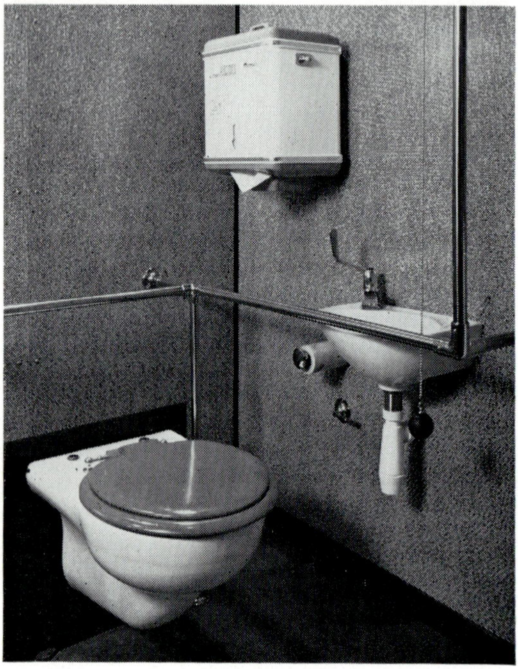

Figure 8.2. Part of a toilet compartment for the disabled

generally acceptable than the shower. Yet this apparatus can be shown to give considerable independence for some disabled patients who are otherwise unable to cleanse themselves. Once again, the correct height for transfers is critical, and the siting of the bidet in relation to the bath and flushing-bowl should be worked out by practical trials.

Components and fittings

Door handles, light-switches, taps, window-catches, cupboard doors and control-switches for kitchen equipment are the main fittings which the majority of people need to use frequently. The features to be considered include position and design. If a component which the patient can operate is not available, then some additional device may have to be used.

Most disabled people can operate lever door-handles when at the correct height. If they are not available or cannot be installed, then other gadgets or extensions to the existing handle may need to be devised.

Many window-catches are out of reach of the disabled, and the usual peg-stays are difficult to manipulate. Remote-control gear is usually expensive and awkward to install, but there are many different forms of fitments which can be tried. A built-in safety device to prevent the window blowing open and out of reach while a patient is attempting to open or close it, is incorporated in some fixtures.

The common problems with electrical installations concern the convenient siting of switches and outlet sockets, and the selection of switches with a simple positive action which the disabled person can operate. Once again, practical trials may save a lot of unnecessary time and expense. In general, switches should be adjacent to the door-handles and should therefore be sited between 3 ft and 3 ft 6 in (90–105 cm) from the floor, and the outlet sockets between 2 ft 4 in and 3 ft (70–90 cm) from the ground.

The fuse box and isolating switches, gas-meter and main water inlet control-valve should all be easily accessible and such controls should be regularly tested and operated to ensure their smooth function. Without such precautions, the chances of an emergency occurring are greatly increased, and the dangers to a slowly-moving disabled person in any emergency need no emphasis. Malfunction of some equipment leading to a minor accident for an able person, may lead to a tragedy for a disabled one.

The apparatus to deal with an emergency should be available to every disabled person, together with the means of summoning help. An emergency call system, telephone or intercom is therefore an essential installation, also easily manipulated fire extinguishers and a well-stocked first-aid box.

M.M.L. No. 907 born 1959 female

Diagnosis: Juvenile rheumatoid arthritis

When 2 years old, this girl had an acute polyarthritis. The steroids prescribed to control it were eventually withdrawn at the age of 8 years.

When referred to the Disabled Living Unit for assessment in 1967, she had considerable residual physical disability, with very marked limitation of movement of the cervical spine, hips and knees, and restricted movement of all other joints. She was very dwarfed, had flexion contractures of hips and knees and was unable to walk. Wheelchair-bound, she was unable to propel herself because of limitation of upper-limb movement, and might therefore be eligible for a powered indoor chair.

As part of the assessment for provision of a powered indoor chair, an inspection of the house is naturally carried out to assess, among other things, whether the chair can be manoeuvred around the house and thus provide additional mobility for the patient. She lived with her parents and sister in a council house with outside toilet, no bathroom and of such a size and construction that it appeared that an electrically-powered indoor chair would provide little additional independence to the child. At the instigation of the paediatric social worker, the local authority were apparently considering whether to undertake structural alteration to improve the bathroom and toilet facilities. However, it was pointed out that these alterations would not add to the suitability of the house for a powered indoor chair, and a strong recommendation for rehousing was made. The provision of the electrically-powered wheelchair was deferred until rehousing could be carried out.

About 6 months later, the local authority allocated to the family a most suitable bungalow, but they turned it down on the grounds that it was in a district away from all their friends and relations. The local authority then offered a less suitable bungalow in their own area and the family accepted it.

A meeting was held at the bungalow with a representative of the housing committee, a therapist from the Disabled Living Unit and a technical officer, and a detailed survey of the bungalow was undertaken and a series of minor alterations agreed upon.

In its original form, the bungalow consisted of a large sitting-room, 2 bedrooms (one at the front and one at the back), kitchen, bathroom and toilet in one, a hallway and a garden back and front.

Approach

There was one door for exit and entry at the side of the bungalow with a 4 in high step. It was suggested that this step should be made into a ramp 44 in (111 cm) wide and 6 ft (183 cm) long, continuous with a concrete path which should go straight over the grass and join up with the back access to the garages. This would involve making an entrance in the wire fencing which ran along the side of the garden, but would eliminate the awkward right-angle turn which would otherwise have to be made by a wheelchair patient attempting to go down the path.

Hallway

Once through the front door, which was 27 in (68 cm) wide, there was a hallway 46 in (116 cm) wide, with the door leading to the rest of the house situated directly opposite the front door, and a bathroom and toilet on the right. The door to the rest of the house opened onto the right towards the front door, and consequently when it was opened, it covered the entrance to the bathroom, making a very awkward turn into the bathroom. It was suggested that this be rehung on the left-hand side to eliminate the awkward turn.

The technical officer felt that negotiating the draught excluder in the wheelchair should not present a problem, but that if in practice this proved difficult to accomplish, then the draught excluder should be removed.

Bathroom and toilet

The doorway to the bathroom was 27 in (68 cm) wide and opened into the bathroom. As it opened back against the bath the distance between the door-jamb and the sink was 22 in (56 cm), and when closing the door the distance between the door-jamb and the toilet pedestal was 17 in (43 cm). This would make it impossible to close the door once the patient was in the bathroom in her wheelchair. Therefore, it was recommended that a sliding door be installed.

Going through the doorway from the hall to the rest of the bungalow, the kitchen was on the right, the door to the small bedroom at the back was straight opposite, the opening to the sitting-room was on the left, and the door to the large front bedroom opened out of the sitting-room on the left.

The kitchen was very small. If the patient went in while in her chair, she would be unable to turn round, and would have to back out. Once in the kitchen, the surfaces were at a reasonable height for her. The door hung on the left side opening out into the main room, and when it opened, it covered the entrance to the small bedroom. It was felt that this, in fact, would not present a problem, as the patient could easily push it to, if it was blocking her way when she came out of the bedroom. The smallness of the kitchen was no disadvantage from the patient's point of view, since for the moment she was unlikely to be very interested in helping her mother with the cooking, although there would be just enough room for her if she did feel so inclined!

Small bedroom

This was about 7 ft × 8 ft (2·1 m × 2·4 m), and because there was a main drain 4 ft (1·2 m) from the wall the building of an extension to this room was not possible. At first, the parents felt that the two girls would have to have the large front bedroom. But the small bedroom would clearly be too small for the parents and so the idea of having 2 bunk beds in the small room was suggested to the mother, with the patient having the lower one. This would leave enough space in the room for the wheelchair. The door to this room needed to be rehung as it was on the right, opening inwards, and this might prove awkward when the patient tried to turn into the room. If the door was rehung on the left, opening inwards, it would give more space for the patient to negotiate the turn into the room.

Sitting-room and large bedroom

There was a very pleasant, large sitting-room in the front, with plenty of room for the patient to drive around in, despite the usual amount of furniture. The large front bedroom which opened off the sitting-room was about 10 ft × 11 ft (3 m × 3·3 m) and would be very suitable for the parents.

Although not ideal, the bungalow was better than their previous home, and the electrically-powered indoor chair was ordered and the family moved in.

When reviewed 6 months later (a year after the original referral for assessment for a powered chair), the alterations to the bungalow had not been carried out, although the powered chair had been delivered. However, after a telephone call to the local authority, the work was put in hand and was completed within a matter of weeks.

Comment

This case history illustrates many of the problems which arise when a physically disabled patient has to be accommodated in an ordinary house. The key to the achievement of increased independence may well be the domestic architecture, since some of the techniques involved in attempting to achieve independent living demand architectural provisions rarely provided.

This case history also illustrates the need for a domiciliary visit to be made, in order to assess the particular problems which a patient faces in his own home. Such a visit should be made in the company of the family doctor, the domiciliary occupational therapist, the housing officer, and the builder concerned with the proposed alterations.

This happy collaboration between clinician, therapist, technician and local authority is rarely obtained, but can clearly lead to results which are a credit to those concerned and of considerable advantage to the patient.

9—Domestic and Social Independence

INTRODUCTION

For any disabled person, independence can only be reached by efficient organization and integration of the resources at his disposal. This means that any plan to assist a disabled patient to regain his independence must consist of 4 main parts.

(1) A review of his ability to perform the activities with which he currently needs help.

(2) Reorganization or retraining the resources of his body and deploying them with maximal efficiency.

(3) Supplying the necessary implements or equipment to subsidize his own achievements to enable him to complete these activities unaided by human help.

(4) A review of his physical condition after completion of each activity, to enable him to decide whether independence in that particular activity is a realistic aim or whether it demands too great an expenditure of time and effort to justify the advantage obtained.

It is important that any such plan takes note of the usual pattern in which the activities of daily life are accomplished, so that this pattern may be reduplicated as far as possible in the organized sequence of activities recommended as a daily living routine. For the establishment of this routine is an essential feature in regaining independence. A seriously disabled person has far less latitude for varying his behaviour than has an able person. For a disabled person, there comes a stage in the progress of his disability where every movement counts. It has a significance not only in itself, but as a means of producing a further movement. Therefore, it must be exactly performed, in the right way and at the right time, or else it jeopardizes the achievement of the movement which usually follows it. In short, beyond a certain degree of disablement, organization must subsidize disability.

With this in mind, the main activities of daily life must be considered, sleeping and working, drinking and micturition, dressing and undressing, eating and defaecation, personal soiling and cleansing, together with the mobility needed to enable the patient to undertake them in their usual domestic situations. They must be considered in that order in which they are usually performed, but also thought must be given to inter-relationships other than the obvious spatial and temporal ones, for example, drinking necessitates voiding a corresponding amount of fluid by micturition, and should be considered in this context, as well as an accompaniment of eating or as a means of quenching thirst. In other words, the consequence of any action has an importance, as well as the action itself, and its relationship to the actions immediately preceding and following it. When each activity is considered as part of the total activity, in these various ways, it finally becomes possible to achieve a meaningful pattern of daily living for any disabled person, with the maximal amount of independence which is advantageous to his total needs.

DOMESTIC FURNITURE

Introduction

As the ambulant disabled patient is likely to spend a considerable proportion of his life in the sitting position, it is important that due consideration be given to the selection of the chairs on which he sits. This applies to the easy chair which he uses for certain leisure activities, and to the functional chair which he uses to eat at table or to work at a working surface.

Easy chairs

The ambulant disabled frequently find that conventional fireside chairs are too low for comfort, and once in them, they are unable to get out of them. Often they are more comfortable in a dining-room chair, but these seldom have adequate padding for prolonged sitting. For the majority of the elderly and ambulant disabled, a robust chair, stable, well padded with firm armrests, high seat and high back and head-support is what is needed. There are several so-called 'geriatric chairs' on the market which attempt to combine these qualities.

Many disabled patients tend to drop on to the chair, and they sometimes have to rock themselves up from it. Thus, stability is essential, and the front legs must be straight and well forward to take the downward thrust, and the back legs slightly splayed to take the thrust when the patient rises from the chair. Non-slip ferrules are an aid to stability but may detract from its manoeuvrability. One type of geriatric chair combines stable rear legs with castors enabling an attendant to move the chair while the patient is still sitting on it.

Chair covering is important in cleaning if the disabled housewife has to clean the chair herself. Simple design with clear-cut lines, removable cushions and absence of seams makes this chore easier. For the more seriously disabled, the problem of incontinence or the likelihood of food being spilt on the chair demands plain, spongeable covers of the expanded Vinyl or leather cloth type.

Although the usual recommended seat height for the elderly is 17 in (43 cm) most elderly and arthritic patients prefer the seat height to be between 18 and 21 in (46–66 cm). Hand-grips well positioned for grasping and pushing up are essential. Many prefer a footrest on which to rest a leg when there is stiffness of the hip or knee. For wheelchair users, the method of transfer will determine the seat height for those patients who like to get out of their wheelchairs and use normal chairs.

Patients who have had strokes tend to lean towards the paralysed side when seated, unless that side is especially supported and the back of the chair is slightly more reclined than usual. High armrests help to prevent the lateral collapse. For the patients with neurological disorders associated with incontinence, a chair without arms makes the arrangement of urinary incontinence apparatus more manageable. Elderly women patients who like to knit, also prefer chairs without arms.

The problems are complex and comfort is such a subjective feature that whenever possible, practical trials should be arranged before purchase.

Dining and working chairs

The selection of suitable dining and working chairs is mainly the problem of the ambulant disabled patient, since the chairbound patient will usually eat and work from his wheelchair.

In selecting dining or working chairs, the same general principles apply as in the selection of easy chairs. Both dining and working chairs are, however, functional, and the need to combine stability, mobility and accessibility in the smallest possible chair must determine their over-all structure. Comfort for long periods of sitting in a relaxed position is not a dominant consideration.

Since a patient will need to make frequent transfers to and from these chairs throughout the day, the height of the seat is important. It should above all, permit the patient to get in and out of the chair without assistance. If possible, it should also permit him to sit comfortably upon the chair with his back supported by the chair back, and his feet resting comfortably on the ground. An over-long seat should be avoided, as it may prevent a short patient from sitting in this manner, even when its height is correct.

The back of a functional chair does not need to be as long as that of an easy chair, as head support is usually unnecessary. Back and seat alike are best padded lightly and covered with a spongeable material.

The legs must be strong and sited to give maximal stability. Castors are contra-indicated, because although they give the chair mobility, they tend to slip away from the slow, weak or stiff patient during transfers. Non-slip rubber cups are useful for the feet of chairs standing on uncarpeted surfaces, as they minimize slipping.

Unlike the conventional dining or working chairs, those for disabled people should have arm frames, topped with handgrips for grasping or pushing up. The heights of the handgrips are important factors in determining ease of access and exit.

Tables and chairs

For those who use wheelchairs, the requisite height of table or work-top depends on the style of the chair, the depth of the cushioning, and the disability or deformity of the patient himself. Particularly when profound muscular weakness or limitation of joint mobility restricts the range of positions in which a patient can sit and use the working surface, it is most important that practical trials are carried out to determine the optimal relationship between the heights of sitting and working surfaces.

Such trials are equally important for the ambulant disabled patient, who may need two levels of working-surface, one to be used in the standing and one in the sitting position. In the former position, the relationship between floor-level and working-surface is critical, and the standing height rather than the actual height of the patient is one of the determining factors in its ascertainment. Other factors are the ranges of movement of the spine and upper limbs—a patient with stiff, painful shoulders may need a lower working-surface than someone with normal shoulders. In the sitting position, the same determining factors operate for both the ambulant and the wheelchair patient.

British Standards recommend a height of 28 in (70 cm) for non-adjustable tables, and 17 in (43 cm) for chair seats, with armrests $8\frac{1}{2}$ in (21·5 cm) from the seat, and an allowance of 2 in (5–6 cm) for the table top and chair underframe.

But for many disabled these measurements are not suitable. Many arthritics and hemiplegics require chairs (and therefore tables) to be higher. A seat height of between 18 and 22 in (46–56 cm) is usually more comfortable. This demands a table or work-surface of between 29 and 33 in (73–91 cm). The elderly generally prefer chairs with a seat height of 77–18 in (43–46 cm) and a table height of 28–30 in (70–75 cm).

Beds and beddings

Although rehabilitation aims at enabling severely disabled patients to get out of bed and live as active a life as possible, the bed is an important piece of equipment, and requires as careful assessment and selection as any other item of equipment or any other appliance which is used by the patient. If the patient requires nursing attention, then a high (hospital type) bed will be most suitable for the attendant's sake. Unfortunately, it is rarely possible to find a bed which is the correct height both for nursing and for the patient's individual transferring. If the patient transfers himself to a wheelchair, then the bed needs to be lower than the usual hospital bed, but higher than the average domestic divan bed. If the patient is very stiff in hips and trunk, then a bed somewhat higher than a standard hospital bed may be necessary. If the patient is hoisted, then height can be related to the convenience of the attendant who has to provide attention.

In most cases, there will be a need to compromise, and practical trials in a special unit can determine the most satisfactory type of bed to use, unless an adjustable bed, for example, a King Edward Hospital Fund Bed, is available. In addition to the various mechanical beds, there are two particularly useful electrically-powered beds currently available. One of these tilts the patient laterally, and thus redistributes the pressure-bearing areas, and the other changes him from the horizontal to a sitting position.

Mattress

Most disabled patients are better on a firm mattress. It is easier for them to turn or to be turned. When transferring from bed to chair or chair to bed, a firm mattress enables the patient to traverse the gap from one firm appliance to another with less difficulty and effort. Modern interior-sprung mattresses are usually comfortable and functional, but only when on a firm base. Similarly, a Dunlopillo mattress on a firm base is usually satisfactory, but mattresses made from polyurethane foam are inclined to be hot and to induce sweating and thus increase the risk of pressure-sores.

Pillows

Firmly-packed feather pillows can be moulded to body shape and thus help maintain a good sleeping or sitting position, but they require frequent attention. Dunlopillo pillows are not so easy to mould, but retain their shape and do not ruck so easily. They are particularly useful for supporting and separating the legs and preventing localized pressure areas on knees and ankles. Used in conjunction with bed cradles and footboards, they are probably the most generally useful.

Butterfly pillows are often indicated for the use of patients with stiff, painful necks, who do not wear supporting collars during the night. These are best made to measure and can be carved out of blocks of polyurethane foam, and covered with washable nylon or cotton covers. Their use prevents the head from dropping down as the neck flexes with the relaxation of the cervical muscles during sleep, and also prevents side-to-side head movement.

Sheets

Fitted bottom sheets are recommended as they are less likely to wrinkle up and become untucked. Nylon sheets are helpful for patients who have difficulty turning over as they are more slippery. However, some patients do not like their feel and they do not absorb moisture so easily as cotton sheets. Protective undersheets are necessary for incontinent patients, and also for patients who are very weak or ataxic and thus likely to spill food in bed.

Blankets

Modern cellular blankets are light and warm, and may be obtained in wool, nylon and wool, nylon, wool and cotton, or cotton. They are all easy to maintain, and may be washed by hand or in a machine, or dry-cleaned. Cotton cellular blankets stand up to frequent washes best and may also be boiled.

The lightness of cellular blankets is particularly valuable to disabled patients who are very weak, or who have painful joints, as it facilitates movement in bed and prevents undue pressure or painful areas.

A simpler form of bedcover which does away with the need for sheets and blankets is the continental-style eiderdown with a washable cover which does duty as a top sheet. As well as being light and warm, they need little upkeep, and their use also reduces the daily effort demanded of a disabled person by conventional bedmaking.

DOMESTIC INDEPENDENCE

For the able-bodied, independence usually means independence of speech, of thought, of work and leisure activities. To the physically disabled, independence has a special meaning and significance, starting with the problems of personal care and daily living activities.

If the physically disabled man is to achieve wider independence, the narrow spectrum of problems must first be overcome. Most severely physically disabled patients rely considerably upon their family for both physical and financial support. Consequently, it may be more important to arrange the appropriate help for the family as a whole, than for the disabled member in particular. When family support is not available, or the family situation is unfavourable or unsympathetic then it may be necessary to advise that the disabled person enters a residential institution for the physically disabled.

Any assessment of a patient's ability to live outside an institution entails an assessment of the abode where he intends to live and the availability of essential services and possible sources of help in that particular area, in addition to an assessment of the patient's capabilities.

Thus, it is essential to know the advantages or disadvantages of the place where he means to be independent, its dimensions and the possibility of converting unsuitable parts of it to suit his requirements. A patient who can be independent in a ground-floor flat with a telephone, may well fail to be independent in a two-storied house without a telephone.

Much will depend on the availability of additional support such as district nursing, home help, meals-on-wheels, friendly neighbours, local voluntary organizations, nearby relatives and regular supervision from the local authority. For rarely will a seriously disabled patient achieve complete and permanent independence.

His increased susceptibility to infection and the risk that minor injury might prejudice his remaining functional capability, makes domestic independence a tight-rope existence.

In this chapter, a thumb-nail sketch of pertinent factors influencing the attainment of independence within the home is given, followed by several case histories of patients who have been referred to the Disabled Living Unit with precisely this aim in view. The difficulties they encountered, and the means which were employed to overcome them, illustrate how many things, people and authorities, apart from the patient himself, are concerned in the production of the final independent existence of one disabled individual, and emphasize the necessity for the integration of the efforts of each and every one of them.

The first activity to assess is that of getting up from bed, transferring to a wheelchair, if necessary, or walking with aids and appliances. Some disabled can be independent once they have been helped out of bed, but this places considerable responsibility on the helpers for initiating the daily routine, and unless helpers are forthcoming, even this degree of dependence can prove a bar to independent living in a private home.

Different beds of different heights, mechanical or electrically operated, can all be tried in an effort to assist getting up from bed. The combination of an electrically operated hoist and an electrically operated bed can solve the problem for some very severely disabled people. By pulling the slings of the hoist around themselves, operating the hoist and the bed together, they may be able to lift themselves up, dress, transfer to toilet or commode and onto an electrically propelled wheelchair.

Washing, toilet and dressing follow in sequence and are usually all linked to the technique employed for transferring in and out of bed.

Mobility in the home is partly dependent on the patient's means of moving around (whether he walks with walking aids and appliances, or whether he uses a wheelchair) and partly on the architectural features of the home. For assessment purposes, it is first reasonable to work in ideal surroundings with smooth floors and good accessibility. Then it is necessary to have detailed plans of the actual or proposed home. If necessary, the home situation can be simulated with portable screens and items of furniture, in order to establish realistic trials of the patient's likelihood of achieving independence. A visit to the home by a therapist, accompanied by the patient if possible, provides an even better method of assessment.

Sometimes the questions posed are theoretical and thus only theoretical and speculative answers can be given, but when the Disabled Living Unit has a kitchen and rooms resembling those likely to be occupied by the patient, realistic answers can be given.

Safety within the home, not only involves mobility, but the ability to control lighting and heating in at least one room. The patient must be able to provide himself with a hot drink, get a simple meal and clear up afterwards. Thus, he must be competent to manoeuvre in the kitchen. He must be able to carry food and drink for short distances and undertake simple household chores, making the bed, light dusting and cleaning and washing of personal undergarments and night wear. Above all, he must be able to operate an alarm of some kind, preferably the telephone, as this can also be used for ordering food and fuel and for social contact during inclement weather.

Achieving and maintaining this level of independence, involves a combination of physical ability and determination on the part of the patient; considerable preparation and forethought regarding the furniture, fittings and architecture of the home; the availability of family, friends and supporters for those inevitable occasions when things go wrong; and an understanding and co-operative local authority to loan necessary equipment such as electric beds and hoists, to install ramps and handrails as necessary, and to undertake any internal architectural alterations which are necessary.

A careful consideration of all these factors must form part of a total assessment before firm recommendations are made. Two of the most important factors are the patient's own personality and the attitude of the local authority. If the patient is well-motivated and determined, almost anything is possible, and provided he has the backing of an enlightened and co-operative local authority, he can produce remarkable results.

However, some local authorities are positively opposed to attempting to make severely disabled patients independent in their own homes, and should this be the case, the exercise may be doomed to failure. There are bound to be occasions when the patient will need help and if the situation is suddenly dependent upon extra but unforthcoming help from the local authority, then the total plan may be in jeopardy. An unco-operative local authority can soon precipitate a situation of impasse and it is unwise to try to force the issue in such a case, this situation luckily is a rarity.

There is no real reason why many severely disabled patients, even those with progressive disorders, should not live an independent life and contribute to the community as long as their physical condition allows.

M.M.L. No. 69 born 1924 female

Diagnosis: Juvenile rheumatoid arthritis

This patient developed rheumatoid arthritis during childhood and was left with fixed flexion deformities of hips, knees and feet, and with contractures and deformities of shoulders, elbows and hands. She had not walked since late childhood, nor had she been able to reach her face with her hands for the same period of time. Her mother looked after her with devotion, washing her, dressing her and helping her to the toilet. Then her mother had a stroke and was

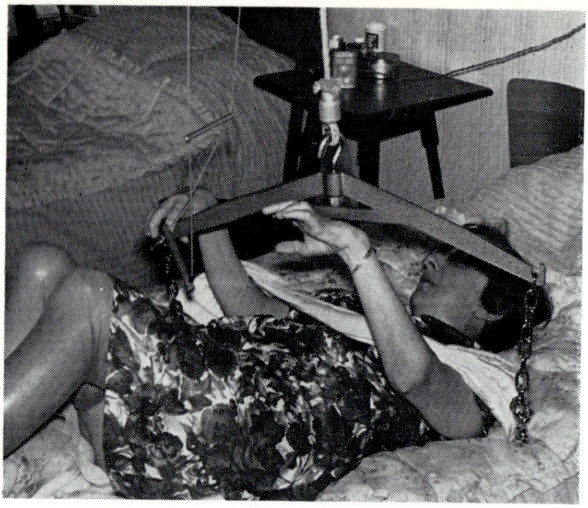

(a)

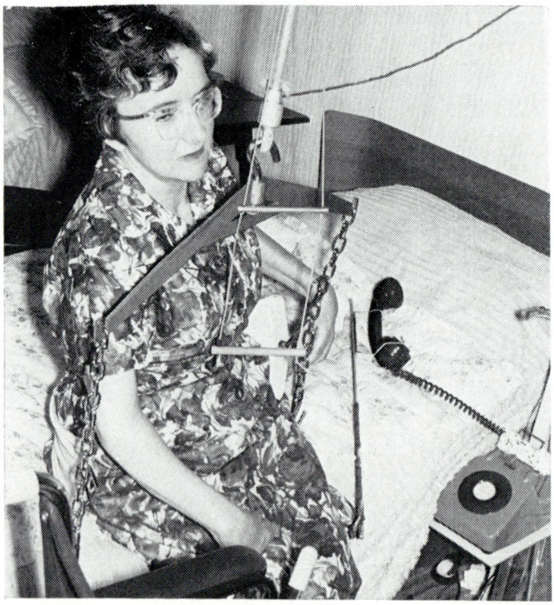

(b)

Figure 9.1. Patient No. 69 (a) arranging slings of electric hoist preparatory to sitting up; (b) sitting up. Note the flexion contractures of the knees and the long-handled stick for the telephone. (Reproduced by kind permission of the Editor, 'Orthopaedics': Oxford) no longer able to look after her, and it seemed likely that both of them would have to be admitted to a welfare home or similar institution.

The patient was admitted to the Disabled Living Unit for assessment, and, apart from refusing to undergo any form of surgery, she was most co-operative and eager to achieve added independence. Luckily, her clinical condition had been static for many years and she suffered little joint pain.

With a small car-transit wheelchair she was able to move around using her feet to propel herself along. From this chair, she could undertake a limited amount of cooking, enough for simple meals for herself and her mother, providing they were supplemented by meals-on-wheels.

Various long-handled aids enabled her to manage her own feeding, washing and toilet quite independently. She could transfer herself from bed to wheelchair and on and off the lavatory-seat with an electric hoist. The local authority were, therefore, persuaded to install this in her bedroom and also arranged for the track to run to the lavatory. She could thus put the slings on, transfer to the lavatory-seat and back to the bedroom. She could support herself in the slings while dressing (*Figure 9.1*).

She had remained at home looking after her mother for several years, and with her hoist, wheelchair and long-handled aids, is more mobile and independent than she had been in the preceding 30 years.

M.M.L. No. 107 born 1927 male

Diagnosis: Muscular dystrophy

This man had an unhappy school life as he was diagnosed as having 'lazy muscles' and consequently the boys at school and his family thought that he was lazy.

At the age of 14 years, he was diagnosed as having muscular dystrophy and by the time he was 18 years old he was wheelchair-bound. He was looked after at home, but in his efforts to get around, he developed a septic arthritis following trauma consequent upon crawling on his hands and knees. This led to admission to hospital.

From there, he was admitted to a private nursing home, then to a voluntary home for the disabled, and then to a geriatric ward of a general hospital. He had been in a geriatric ward for 11 years when he was first referred to the Disabled Living Unit for assessment for a wheelchair. He had managed to get friends to make him a wheelchair from a tub and bicycle wheels.

On admision at the age of 37 years, he had almost flail lower limbs with flexion contractures of the hips and knees, and severe weakness of the shoulder girdle with marked weakness of the forearm and hands.

The provision of an electrically-powered wheelchair, with mobile arm-supports attached was the initial step towards independence for this patient. After functional assessment, it was demonstrated that with appropriate equipment and assistance, he had the determination to achieve some degree of domestic independence. The local authority in collaboration with the social workers from the referring hospital, working on the assessment findings, converted a council flat for him. He eventually moved into this flat, which was adapted specifically for him.

He had an electric bed, electric hoist, a sani-chair which was used for showering as well as toilet purposes, and an adapted toilet.

The entrance to the house was ramped, and he was able to drive out into the garden in his chair and even do some shopping in a general store which was almost next door. With this equipment, using mobile arm-supports, adapted clothing, pick-up sticks and other simple aids, he became completely independent for dressing, washing and even cooking and shopping.

After a settling-in period, he was able to develop his natural artistic talents and eventually he became a talented and successful artist, holding several public exhibitions. He had over three years of independence in this flat, then he married and he and his wife were rehoused in a specially adapted bungalow. They are both happy and contented, and the patient has achieved a level of intellectual activity and artistic output which he had previously regarded as impossible. He has described his independence as a ‘reincarnation’.

He had problems. During his period of independence before he married, he was prone to knock his feet during transferring. He suffered considerably from blue, swollen feet and a tendency to chilblains. The skin of his feet was fragile and on several occasions, he developed painful ulcers on his feet. These could only be healed by admission to hospital or the Disabled Living Unit where he was given full nursing care for a few weeks, once or twice a year.

The tightrope organization leading to the initially complete and currently partial independence of this patient seems completely justified. His own personal satisfaction is great. The inspiration, interest and help which he has dispensed to other people, able and disabled, is not inconsiderable. His pictures contribute beauty of form and idea to an ugly world. Few able people can show so much return for the effort which others make on their behalf.

M.M.L. No. 1076 born 1926 female

Diagnosis: Multiple sclerosis

In 1948, at the age of 22 years, this lady had some visual hallucinations, then in 1953 she noticed the onset of left-sided weakness. This rapidly extended to involve both legs, and her vision became blurred. She managed as a housewife and a mother until she was 43 years of age, when she had to resort to using a wheelchair.

On examination, she had evidence of some optic atrophy, a left internal strabismus and a generalized increase in muscle tone with brisk tendon reflexes. Her legs were weak and spastic and subject to spasms. Her upper limbs were weak, spastic with diminished coordination and an intention tremor. Although not incontinent she had some difficulty in initiating micturition, particularly when her bladder was full. She could walk short distances using a walking-aid, but was very ataxic and unable to stand upright, and in addition, had difficulty getting up from a wheelchair.

She lived in a three-bedroomed council house which had been fitted with handrails in the toilets and on the stairs. However, there were steps at the front door and back door and into the downstairs toilet, so she could not get out of the house or to the toilet unaided. She and her husband shared a bedroom downstairs, while her married daughter and son-in-law and her 7-year-old son had bedrooms upstairs. The family all left the house between 7 and 8 a.m. in the morning, the schoolboy returning about 4 p.m. and the rest of the family at about 5–6 p.m.

The patient spent all day on her own sitting in her wheelchair and either reading or watching television. She was unable to do any cooking because the kitchen working-surfaces were at the wrong height, and the layout was difficult for her to manage.

She was admitted to the Disabled Living Unit for assessment when her daughter and son-in-law were about to leave her to move into their own house, and when it became therefore essential that she should achieve some increased independence. The particular objects of the admission was the improvement of her mobility and the provision of practical encouragement to undertake more domestic responsibility.

On admission, she was found to be depressed and ready to let her family do everything for her. Yet early in her assessment it was clearly demonstrated that she could improve her mobility by using a lighter wheelchair, and by improving her walking. She was independent for all domestic and personal activities, except for dressing when she wore dresses with long zips at the back. When the working surfaces were at a suitable height for her wheelchair she could manage many kitchen activities.

This patient was, therefore, discharged with a rather encouraging report to the general practitioner and the local authority. Her immediate family remained despondent and unconvinced, as there were other members of the family with multiple sclerosis. They still maintained that she was incapable of achieving any independence.

When she was seen again a few months later, she had reverted to the previous depressed state and made no effort to maintain any independence. The kitchen working-surfaces had been lowered for her and the steps ramped, but she made no effort to use the kitchen or to go outside to the toilet unaided.

Unfortunately, the lowering of the working surfaces made domestic work even more uncomfortable and tiring for the rest of the family. Thus, overconfident recommendations had made the over-all domestic situation worse.

The psychological assessment at this time was as follows:

(1) *Wechster adult intelligence scale.* Age-corrected scaled score on vocabulary: 11. This gives an estimate of the patient's premorbid intellectual level as good average.

(2) Verbal I.Q.: 92, that is, low end of average range.

(3) Age-corrected scaled score on Block Design: 7. This gives an estimate of the patient's level of spatial abilities to be currently in the borderline range.

(4) *Brody test.* Deterioration quotient 20. At the patient's age, this indicates the presence of mild to moderate intellectual impairment.

These tests indicated an over-all mild-to-moderate degree of intellectual loss. The different areas of cognitive functioning seemed to be affected unevenly. For example, her auditory retention was relatively severely impaired, whereas visual retention was probably unaffected. Over and above the organic loss, she showed signs of intellectual under-functioning, apathy, and loss of interest. She also had indications of a reactive depression.

Comment

It seems that patients with multiple sclerosis who have cerebellar signs are more likely to run a faster downhill course, and to show greater intellectual defects that those with the more slowly progressive paraplegic type of lesion. In this instance, if the psychological assessment had been available earlier, it is possible that the domestic situation would not have been disturbed. Interference, in this instance, tended to make the whole domestic situation worse than it had previously been.

The only recommendations which could be offered at the time of readmission were that the patient should attend the local day hospital, and the family were put in touch with the local branch of the Multiple Sclerosis Society.

M.M.L. No. 1021 born 1922 female

Diagnosis: Spastic paraplegia

After several years of symptoms in the left leg, this patient developed a spastic paraplegia, with complete loss of sensation below the waist, complete urinary incontinence and complete paralysis of both legs with exaggerated reflexes, extensor plantar responses and frequent painful spasm of the lower limbs.

She remained in a spinal injuries centre for just over six months and became quite independent for her personal care. She could manage her toilet (manual evacuation of bowels on alternate days) and her urinary appliance. She could wash, dress and transfer to wheelchair. She had purchased a car adapted for hand controls only, and was planning to return to her previous occupation as a schoolteacher. The local authority had been alerted and had agreed to provide her with a suitably adapted council flat in the area where she lived, so that she could be re-employed at the school where she had previously worked.

She was admitted to the Disabled Living Unit for a few weeks' practice at independent living, prior to moving into her own flat. As it transpired, she was in the unit for 10 weeks, since her council flat was not ready on schedule, and she needed considerable training and practice before she could attempt to manage on her own.

At each step, she was frustrated and some episode occurred which caused her to lose confidence. When she first tried to go home she discovered that the council had not started upon the conversion of her flat.

The next step was organizing outdoor transport. When she took her Disabled Driver's test, her car misbehaved mechanically and was difficult to handle. The examiner abandoned the test and her self-confidence was shattered. The car was not easy to handle even under normal conditions, and was awkward for her wheelchair. She sold it at a financial loss, and the Department of Health issued her with an invalid tricycle almost immediately. Once again, she had trouble because she was unable to lift her wheelchair into the tricycle, and once again she was upset. However, the technical staff very quickly made some alterations to the seating to enable her to transfer in stages, and also to lift the chair in and out of the tricycle. A lighter chair which was easier to handle was substituted for her older, heavier model.

After these various vicissitudes, she eventually regained confidence, but it took a considerable effort on the part of the technicians, the instructors, the therapists and the medical social workers to help her to do so.

Each set-back was reflected in the recurrence of severe muscular spasm in the legs. An anti-spasmodic drug (Diazepam) when given in doses sufficient to reduce spasm, made her drowsy, but withholding the drug was accompanied by an exacerbation of spasms. Spasticity also made her bladder management difficult, as she would eject the catheter from time to time when her spasms were severe. She had a persistent urinary infection for which she was prescribed various antibiotics and chemo-therapeutic agents, according to the sensitivity of the infecting organisms. She was eventually discharged on hexamine mandelate and methionine, and frequent self-administered bladder washouts. Because of difficulties with the catheter, this has to be changed weekly and she was given emepronium bromide (Ceteprin) 50 mg twice daily to reduce bladder irritability. The recurrent infection, the trouble with catheters (expulsion and leaking) also caused her considerable concern. Her bowels were a further problem. She had had no advice on diet, and was having considerable difficulty in attempting infrequent manual removal of hard stools. On a regimen of mucilaginous granules to produce a softer but bulkier stool, the time taken for manual removal was reduced from 60 to 15 minutes on alternate days. This was done sitting on the toilet. She tried using suppositories, but was unable to insert them high enough in the rectum to be effective. She rather resented the need to concern herself so much with her excretary mechanisms.

She was undoubtedly 'highly strung' and any set-back made her upset and depressed. Small doses of tranquillizers helped to maintain her on a more emotionally even keel, but considerable time and patience was required to enable her to establish a routine which could be realistically transferred to her own flat and enable her to return to work.

During her stay in the Disabled Living Unit, she established a morning routine which would be essential if she was to be independent and make her return to work. This regimen she carried out in the simulated flat with minimal supervision, progressing to complete independence. Her sequence was as follows: alarm—wake up; take mucilaginous granules; cup of tea (using bedside tea-making alarm clock); transfer to toilet; change urine bag, bladder washout; wash and dress top half while sitting on toilet; manual evacuation of bowels; wash hands; wash and dress lower half; transfer to wheelchair; make breakfast; complete make-up and so on; transfer to outdoor transport.

Continuous repetition of this sequence during the time in the Unit, enabled her to reduce the time to an hour and a half. Thus, awaking at 7 a.m., she was ready to drive off to work by 8.30 a.m., which was a reasonable programme. When she was first admitted, this sequence took almost all the morning.

When she was discharged to stay with members of the family for a week or two prior to returning to her own flat, there were 'crises' within a day or two and these entailed lengthy placatory discussions and advice dispensed over the telephone.

After a further short spell in the Disabled Living Unit and an assurance that all was at last ready for her to occupy her flat, she was finally discharged two weeks before she was due to start back at work.

The importance of good liaison is illustrated by the problem of the conversion of her flat. Although correspondence had been put in train by the spinal injuries unit several months previously, including setting out all the appropriate details regarding working heights, position of light switches, power points, cupboards, baths, gas points and so forth; no alterations were actually started until a short time before she was scheduled to start work. The knowledge that this was so, constituted a continual source of worry and tension to her. The alterations were only finally initiated when considerable pressure was exerted on the contractors by all the authorities concerned. This did not happen until many weeks after a member of the Health and Welfare Department and a local authority architect had visited the Disabled Living Unit and had there been able to review the patient's functional capabilities and to ascertain the final details of her requirements.

Unfortunately, in spite of assertions to the contrary by the local authority, the flat was not ready when she arrived there. There was still much minor work to be completed and there were several further teething problems during her early days of independent living within its confines (*Figure 9.2*).

Comments

In spite of long periods of rehabilitation, the final change-over from physical rehabilitation to practising for independent living takes

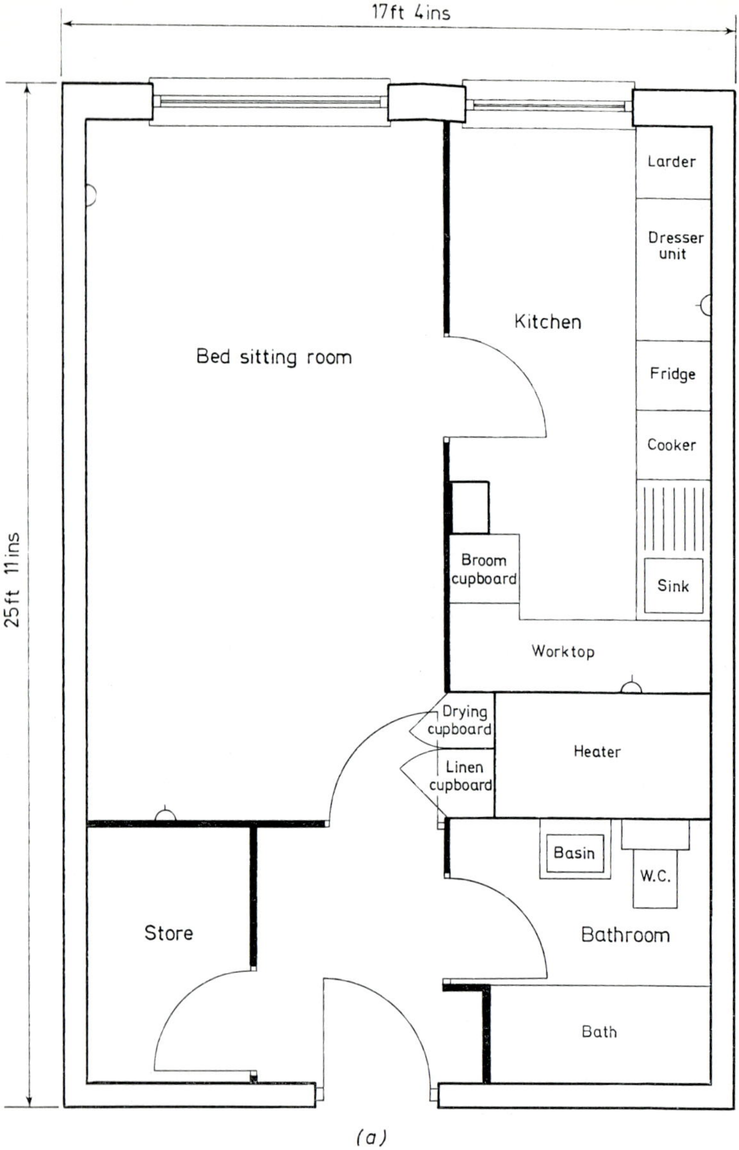

Figure 9.2. (a) Basic design of bed-sitter flat;

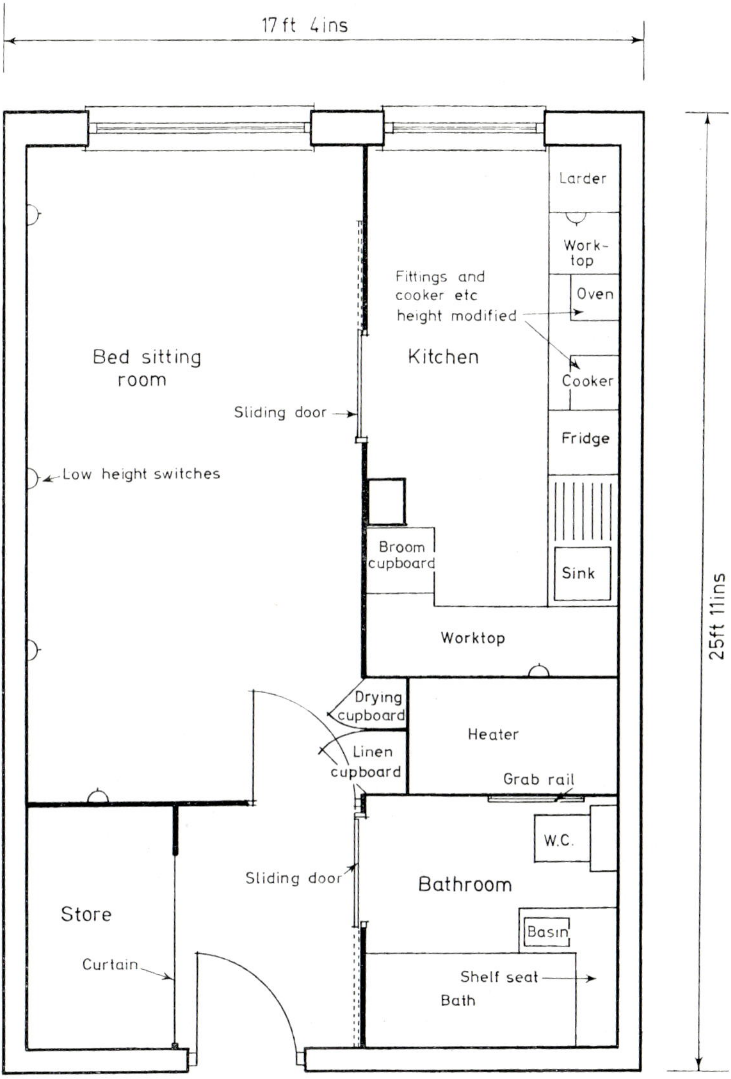

(*b*)

(*b*) *modified design for Patient No. 1021. All supports made bracket-type to move wheelchair in underneath* a long time. For a patient of nervous disposition, this period is often frustrating and difficult and she needs considerable help, understanding and patience to re-establish her self-confidence.

Minor set-backs are upsetting at this stage, and in the case in point, any one of the many set-backs experienced could have finally shaken her resolve to return to work had she not been given constant reassurance. It needed the skill and care of nurses, medical social workers, therapists and doctors to help her through each difficulty. Even so, on several occasions, she was tempted to give in and settle for institutional care.

Now, one year later, she is independent and working.

M.M.L. No. 241 born 1929 female

Diagnosis: Spina bifida cystica

This female patient was born with a lumbar meningomycelocoele, and the defect was closed operatively before she was a year old. She had an associated complete paralysis of the lower limbs, but with training, became continent of urine and faeces.

After the death of her father when she was aged 21, she was cared for by her mother alone. She was educated privately, and was encouraged to apply herself solely to academic work. She passed various examinations as an external student, and at the time when she was referred to the Disabled Living Unit at the age of 36, she had been granted a London Bachelor of Arts degree in English and was planning to write a thesis for a higher degree. All the domestic arrangements of the household had been carried out by her mother until her death, aged 87, in 1965, 3 months before the patient's first admission.

After an initial struggle to take over the running of the house, the patient found herself no longer able to cope with the extra physical effort entailed. Friends supported her, but without her mother's help with her personal care and the household tasks, her own academic work remained undone, and she became exhausted and despondent.

When referred to the Disabled Living Unit for advice on independent living, she was chair-bound, and able to propel herself in a rear-wheel propelling chair. She could transfer independently, using her powerful arms and dragging her flail legs after her. She seldom used her full-length calipers for walking even the short distances of which she was capable, as the effort of moving her heavy body and flail legs on axillary crutches was considerable.

Firstly, her wheelchair was changed from an old, rear-wheeled, self-propelling wheelchair with the footrests removed, to a front-wheel, self-propelled chair with an adapted footboard, which she could slide back under the seat herself, but which supported her legs with the calipers when in the forward position (*see Figure 9.3*).

As she had not walked since her mother died, she was given walking training, and her confidence slowly returned. She had had no previous experience of household activities and much time was necessarily spent in teaching her to plan, prepare and cook her own meals. Later during her stay, she was given practice in shopping.

She was very short and stout, and no off-the-peg clothes were of a

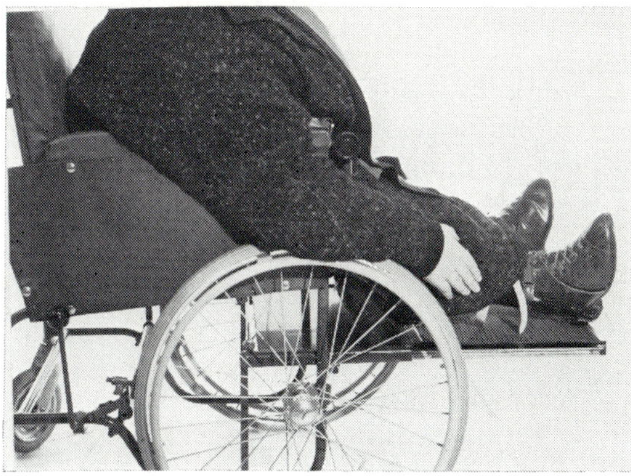

Figure 9.3. Patient No. 241 using a front-wheel self-propelling wheelchair with sliding leg-rest

suitable size. She was taught to adapt simple patterns and to make dresses and skirts as a relaxation from her studying, and as an alternative to interminable alterations of ready-made garments.

During her first admission, she was very tense following her mother's death, and she was found to have an essential hypertension with occasional attacks of angina pectoris and palpitations. She was obese, so part of her cooking training was directed towards planning a more suitable diet, but she would never adhere to the reducing diet advised. She had fair control of her bladder, but had stress incontinence and urgency, thus needing to wear incontinence pants. Her periods were heavy and she welcomed the hormonal suppression of these.

Various aids and alterations to her home were advised: bathseat; grab-rails in the lavatory; sliding-doors between various rooms; (to improve the accessibility of the various parts of the house); alteration of the heights of the working surfaces in the kitchen; and installation of storage heaters instead of coal fires to reduce housework.

All these alterations were carried out satisfactorily. The only gadget she needed was a pick-up stick.

Over the next 3 years, she was admitted on several occasions, usually to solve an additional practical problem, as she gradually regained confidence and established independence. She engaged a whole-time housekeeper, but her major problem was one of loneliness. Some 18 months after her first admission, she began to doubt her ability to continue independent living and arranged admission to a small institution. However, after a reasonable trial she decided that independence was more important to her and finally decided to remain in her own home with a housekeeper.

She is now still independent, is continuing her own private study, and is also tutoring for a correspondence course, marking examination papers and proof reading for a publisher.

Comment

This patient illustrates many features which the severely disabled hold in common. She first presented as a problem when her parents were no longer available to look after her, and because she had been cared for by her mother, her own training was sorely lacking. It took considerable persuasion, support and training to enable her to gain self-confidence and practical skills sufficient to enable her to retain independence. She still needed considerable support, both practical (from the housekeeper) and moral (from friends and neighbours); but having achieved this independence, she found it preferable to the alternative of admission to an institution. Finally, having come to terms with her disability, she then was able to concentrate on other things, her own intellectual activities, and the very real help she was giving to others. She thus achieved an interesting and satisfying life.

M.M.L. No. 106 born 1937 male

Diagnosis: Muscular dystrophy

At the age of 2 years, this patient was noted to be falling frequently, and was soon diagnosed as suffering from muscular dystrophy. He managed to attend a normal infants' school, and was soon transferred to a private school. By the age of 12 years, he was confined to a wheelchair. He was then admitted to a school for handicapped children, and on leaving it at the age of 16 years, he had a six months course on Accounts and Costing at a training centre. On leaving the centre, he was unable to obtain employment because of his disability, and, as his mother's health was failing, he was admitted to a residential home at the age of 17 years. After he had been resident for 10 years at the home, he was admitted to the Disabled Living Unit for reassessment of his ability to achieve independence.

The admission, in 1964, was largely at his own instigation. When first admitted, he was struggling to propel himself in a standard wheelchair, and the first step was to provide him with an electrically propelled indoor wheelchair and standard mobile arm-supports. Once he had achieved independence of mobility and the ability to use his hands without fatigue, there was no holding him. He clearly demonstrated that with an electric hoist and some domestic help, he had the will and the capability to achieve domestic independence.

The welfare officer of his local authority took a considerable personal interest in his case and the council eventually housed him in an adapted bungalow. The adaptations were worked out in detail in the flat of the Disabled Living Unit and in 1965 he set up house independently in this bungalow.

He had an electric elevating bed, with the electric hoist over it tracking across a room to a commode. A home-help came in each morning to help him get up and dress, and the District Nurse visited regularly for bathing and a general check-up. A local Men's Club undertook on a rota basis to come in every evening to help him to bed.

He had various adaptations to the house completed to his own design, made and installed either by friends, or the local authority. These included adaptations to the lavatory, wash-basins, bed-tables, telephone extensions and loudspeakers as well as adaptations to his typewriter. He was able to type, telephone, wash, shave and undertake minor domestic chores. But the major triumph was that within a year, he was so busy with real work that he was earning a surprising amount of money, and filling every day with activity. He acted as a telephone switchboard operator for two general practitioners; he was also the booking agent for two driving schools; he acted as a marketing agent for various sales organizations; he was actively involved in the local Boy Scouts troop; he was an active and enthusiastic radio 'ham', and in his spare time he typed manuscripts for an author.

He was readmitted to the Disabled Living Unit nearly a dozen times over the next 3 years, for short periods of assessment, for alterations or adaptations to his equipment, or to solve a new problem which had arisen. But as he achieved more independence and accrued more activities and work into his daily routine, he became happier and more contented than ever previously in his life.

Inevitably, he must deteriorate and his independence is limited, but while it lasts he is making a definite contribution to his local community, he has achieved a personal ambition and he is an inspiration to many who come into contact with him.

SPECIAL CONTROL APPLIANCES

During the autumn of 1966, the Department of Health and Social Security decided to make available a limited number of models of a type of special apparatus, designed to enable severely disabled patients to control such appliances as buzzers, lights, radios and typewriters and so to make life more tolerable and possibly enable some of them to leave institutional care and return home. The Department considered that eligibility for these pieces of special apparatus would be based on permanent severe paralysis or disability, or congenital defect, sufficiently severe so that the patient was unable to carry out simple tasks such as ringing bells or switching on lights and on condition that it could be certified medically as follows:

(1) they have the ability and will use the apparatus;

(2) they have passed the acute phase of the disabling illness and their chances of survival are judged to be reasonably good;

(3) they cannot be assisted as effectively by simpler or cheaper means.

The kind of patients likely to be eligible for such appliances are those who are severely paralysed (whether due to trauma, for example, fractured cervical spine or polio or neurological disease such as peripheral neuropathy), or those patients with severe arthritis, such as juvenile rheumatoid arthritis or severe ankylosing spondylitis, who have become so disabled as to be virtually bedridden. In most instances, they will have enough residual movement available to operate a simple control switch. A further group of patients likely to derive benefits from such appliances are those with advanced muscular dystrophy, or with severe Parkinson's disease; but in assessing these particular patients, there will need to be a careful appraisal of their rate of deterioration. There are many other groups of patients who have become virtually bedridden or chairridden and will remain so for many years. All these patients might be able to achieve some level of independence, even if only enough to render them more able to be left alone for periods, while their companions are free to leave the home. It might also enable them to be retrained to live in a home environment rather than be admitted to hospital, or indeed to be discharged from hospital to a home environment.

Perhaps a general definition of suitable patients might be 'Patients who are so severely disabled that they are completely unable to control their domestic environment, or who are so severely disabled (even though they may be able to control an electric wheelchair) that they would be materially helped to greater independence by means of a device which would enable them to operate selected pieces of equipment or apparatus.' Such patients are likely to come within the following classification:

(*a*) Tetraplegia—complete: { Fractured cervical spine; A.P.M.
Partial: { Disseminated sclerosis; Peripheral neuropathy.

(*b*) Severe multiple congenital limb defects.

(*c*) Severe generalized weakness, for example, muscular dystrophy.

(*d*) Severe generalized stiffness, for example, rheumatoid arthritis (especially juvenile form); ankylosing spondylitis; Parkinsonism; calcinosis universalis.

(*e*) Gross ataxia or intention tremor, for example, cerebral palsy; multiple sclerosis.

The control of the selector mechanism will be by means of 'minimal movement' (for example, microswitches) or 'pneumatic control' (that is, by sucking or blowing). In patients with minimal available movement, controls can be either operated by head movement, or by a 'nudge' finger or foot movement. The most likely control will be by means of a simple microswitch positioned wherever sufficient movement is available, such as head movement for high tetraplegia; for most others a simple finger control. Where there is no available limb movement, pneumatic (suck–blow) control can be used.

Many patients with neurological disorders (particularly cerebral palsy) have such gross movement disorders that they are incapable of performing simple manoeuvres. Many are completely confined to bed or pushchair. Such patients can be trained to give a repeated movement, providing that the target is large enough.

The apparatus will be concerned either with the input signal or the selecting mechanism and will switch on certain items of electrical equipment. In some instances, it may be possible to provide a simple control for these pieces of apparatus, the operation of which will raise an alarm in case of need, and will also control essential nursing apparatus. These items are likely to be:

Communication.—Alarm system (either bell or buzzer); disabled person's telephone.

Medical requirements.—Tilting (or other electrically motivated) bed; ripple mattress or cushion; cuirasse or similar respiratory apparatus required intermittently.

The next group of appliances are those concerned with controlling the patient's immediate environment: lights; heater; front-door intercommunication system; front-door opener; electric blankets; curtain opening and closing.

A third group of appliances are chosen for entertainment: radio; television; electric page-turner.

Finally, such an apparatus can be used to control appliances for hobbies and indeed work: electric typewriter; teaching machine; tape recorder.

Machines can be supplied by the Department of Health and Social Security, the Department of Employment and Productivity, local authorities or voluntary bodies. Sometimes, they may be provided as a joint project. However, the majority of patients can manage their immediate needs with a simple system of switches, and several mechanisms are now available in which such a system is incorporated in a compact piece of equipment.

Because of the multiple controls required for certain purposes, television, radio, tape-recorder, and typewriter, the individual requirements and capabilities of each patient must be carefully assessed. It may be easier to modify the peripheral apparatus rather than increase the complexity of the control system. Thus, the assessment must be made as a combined activity of clinician, therapist and engineer experienced in this type of work.

In the future, it is likely that multiple functions will be limited (that is, control will enable the television to be turned on and off but not tuned), and that the apparatus will be available in modular form, with some 4–6 switches available in each module. These modules can then be 'banked' to give progressively more available function. Most patients require 6–10 separate functions, mainly: alarm, lighting, heating and one or two items such as radio and television. Some patients have already achieved a working capacity with typewriter and telephone controlled by these systems.

However, this type of apparatus is very expensive (in the order of £300 to £400, plus the cost of the devices which it controls), because it has to be reliable and has to incorporate a 'fail–safe' system, it must also incorporate a secondary system to come into operation in case of power failure, and it entails the provision of complex multiple functions such as tuning a radio or television set.

By the end of 1968, about 100 patients were in possession of one of these sophisticated appliances supplied by the Department of

Health and Social Security, and the appliances are being supplied to about 10–20 patients per year. Even if the requirements doubled, the production rate would still not be enough to enable the cost to be significantly reduced.

The number of patients with electrically-powered indoor chairs at this time is nearly 2,000 and these are being supplied at a rate of about 300 per year. About one-third of these patients might well be helped by the provision of a much less sophisticated version of this type of apparatus. Such a version would control only five or six appliances, and the conditions would be such that there would be no need for the elaborate safety-factors necessary for the immobile severely-disabled.

MARRIAGE

Marriage for the severely disabled is a subject which provokes fierce and emotional comment. There are many who disapprove on financial or practical grounds, but the greatest disapproval seems to derive from some latent belief that marriage for the physically disabled is in some fashion 'wrong'. For those who are already married when one partner becomes disabled, the situation is acceptable to the community, but to deliberately marry a disabled person is usually only accomplished in the face of disapproval from the family and the neighbours.

Indeed the majority of homes and institutions for the physically disabled specifically prohibit the admission of married partners. In these circumstances, it is not unknown for residents of such a home to marry in order to escape from the institution by precipitating a situation which may lead to their being rehoused under more congenial circumstances.

The paraplegics have paved the way for many other disabled people by demonstrating that earlier prejudices and misconceptions regarding disability and marital competence were unfounded. Many paraplegics now marry; the male paraplegics are not necessarily impotent and the female paraplegic may be capable of childbearing.

It is possible that some disabled want to marry just for sex, or to have children or because they regard marriage as a symbol of normality. But most disabled desire the private and intimate companionship which makes up much of marriage. Certainly, as homes and institutions caring for the young permanently-disabled increase in number, and as the facilities for mobility, hobbies and training increase, so inevitably more and more young disabled will be thrown together. Their chance of meeting a compatible companion will increase and as a natural consequence the number of young disabled who fall in love and wish to marry will increase.

Their reasons for marrying may not be precisely similar to the able-bodied. Most realize that they cannot, or should not, produce children. Some are so physically disabled, that intercourse is an impossibility. Others suffer from conditions which are hereditary (haemophilia and muscular dystrophy are particularly relevant problems). But these conditions make up a relatively small proportion of the disabled population. Genetic counselling, however, is now becoming widely available.

The severely disabled are frequently naïve and have not been exposed to the usual introductions to sex and the normal processes of sexual education, particularly when disabled from birth or early childhood. Sexual matters are for them often theoretical concepts derived from the limited reading they have been able to obtain, and here one has to recollect that for many, even their reading matter has been effectively censored, and is usually only obtained through other people, and the sort of books which deal frankly with sexual matters may be the source of considerable embarrassment when a disabled person attempts to acquire them. Thus, often such people derive their knowledge from the television, films, novels and the more innocuous books dealing with the less practical aspects of marriage. Few doctors, social workers and others are able to discuss the problem openly and frankly with these young people. Once again, this reticence is a relic of an attitude that they should not be 'allowed to marry' or if they insist on doing so, then they should not consider having sexual intercourse.

The possible methods of sexual intercourse should be discussed unemotionally by a clinician who has understanding of the physical disabilities of the severely disabled. For example, the usual positions for intercourse are often precluded by deformities such as ankylosed hips, or adduction deformities, and the posterior approach may be the only one possible. When both partners are seriously affected by weakness or deformity, then it may be physically impossible to achieve normal intercourse by any method. In such situations, manual stimulation can be a satisfactory substitute. It is often necessary to impress upon the pair, that these practices are not abnormal, unnatural, or perverted, nor in any way harmful. Such counselling requires understanding, tact and an impartial and unemotional approach, which seems difficult to achieve for many of those who work closely with the disabled.

If intercourse is a possibility, it becomes a matter of urgency to discuss methods of contraception long before marriage.

The insertion of a vaginal cap is often completely impossible for a woman with weak upper limbs or stiff lower limbs. She may therefore have an intra-uterine device inserted; use hormonal suppression of ovulation, for example, by using oestrogen, progestrogen or the combined hormones; a radium or irradiation menopause; hysterectomy; or the fallopian tubes tied. A man wishing to prevent conception can use a condom, have his tubes (vas deferens) tied, or practice withdrawal.

The intra-uterine device can cause heavy periods initially, and this is not the ideal contraceptive technique in a disabled woman, whose perineal toilet may be difficult enough to perform during the normal menstrual flow. However, the increased flow usually settles down to a normal level.

Hormonal suppression of menstruation, itself a contraceptive technique, has already been discussed (Chapter 4). Commercial contraceptive tablets are now widely available and if care is taken to select the most suitable tablet, it can be most effective.

The disadvantages of any tablet containing oestrogen are weight gain; ankle swelling; breast swelling; exacerbation of spasms; headaches; nausea and/or vomiting; thrombo-embolic phenomena.

The nausea and vomiting can be relieved by taking perphanazine 4 mg with each daily dose of hormones.

The weight-gain frequently tends to right itself, but may also be offset by dieting. The thrombo-embolic phenomena may well be eventually shown to contra-indicate this method. Tablets only containing progestogen on the other hand, can cause nipple-discharge and vaginitis.

Understandably, hormone tablets vary greatly in their effect on the libido. It is particularly important that the balance of oestrogen and progestogen be adjusted to the sexual activity of the couple concerned. Certain tablets tend to increase the libido of the female, and may make difficulty if the male is disabled and his sexual activity is depressed in consequence. In such a situation, adjustment of the oestrogen/progestogen balance can avert a breakdown in sexual relations.

For many reasons, if the woman is certain that she does not wish to bear children, surgical intervention provides the surest and least-complicated method of contraception for the patient. The fallopian tubes can be cut and tied through a low transverse incision which carries little operative risk and little post-operative trouble. If menstruation is also a problem, then hysterectomy can be carried out during the same operation.

Surgical procedures for the woman may be precluded for clinical reasons. Perhaps the simplest other surgical procedure is the severing of the male vas deferens, an operation which can be carried out rapidly under local anaesthesia.

Marriage counselling for the disabled can be considerably more complex than for the able. For example, the effect on a marriage of the various drugs which the disabled partner is taking can be important. Men taking Aldomet have been reported to become impotent. Chlordiazepoxide on the other hand, often used to decrease spasm or relieve depression, appears to increase the sexual drive in some men. One patient habitually refers to his capsules of Chlordiazepoxide, he has 10 mg 3 times a day, as his 'sex pills'. He has multiple sclerosis and without the chlordiazepoxide tends to be morose and even violent. While taking them, he is cheerful and energetic, but has this remarkable upsurge in libido.

The sexual needs and capabilities of each partner should be taken into account in planning treatment of disabled married people, as it can be a decisive factor in wrecking a marriage. Thus, a marriage between a normal and a disabled partner can be very successful if each partner understands the other's needs, and is ready and able to meet them. The marriage between a paraplegic woman and a normal man can be a happy one, if the man is prepared to be more patient in his love-making, and conversely the marriage between a paraplegic man and a normal woman can be equally happy, as long as the woman is prepared to be the more active partner in love-making. For some women, this role is an impossible one. For the more masculine dominant woman, it is easy to assume.

When a man is impotent from disease or injury, if he is ready to adopt children and so give his wife a family to love, his marriage can still be a full and satisfying one.

It is easier for a marriage to succeed when it has occurred after injury or illness has brought disablement to one partner. The fit partner then goes into it with eyes open, and cannot feel trapped, because he knows the extent of the problems which he will have to face in advance, and does not have to take them on unless he feels ready to cope with them. While such a marriage can be deeply satisfying, it needs extremely careful consideration before it is entered into. The disabled partner will be a continual brake on the able partner's activities, and many pastimes will be denied to the latter partner because of disabilities which are not his own, for apart from the physical aspects of married life, there are all the other aspects of disabled living to consider.

There are 4 possibilities open to disabled people who marry each other.

(1) They can be married in name only and continue to meet whenever friends arrange it, living otherwise in their usual abodes.

(2) They can be married and live in a double room if the home in which they live can and will arrange this.

(3) They can live in a flat which is a part of the home or in the grounds of the home, receiving the same amount of help as they received prior to marriage.

(4) They can live in a council flat or purpose-built bungalow, with as much home-help as they need, and without any connection with an institution.

In all cases, there is an element of compromise and a need for sympathetic support from the local authority and other organizations. Wherever possible, integration into the normal community should be the aim and over-provision of support and aids should be avoided.

Unfortunately, facilities for a realistic assessment of the couple's mutual needs and mutual capabilities are very limited, but this is the only practical method of establishing the realities of the situation. The need for such assessment centres is almost a *sine qua non* if success is to be achieved in such marriages.

Practical trials to establish the feasibility of independent living are particularly important for the married severely disabled who are planning for domestic independence, and for the unmarried severely disabled who are contemplating marriage.

Engaged couples can attend holiday centres organized by charitable bodies, and there try out under supervised conditions some of the necessary activities of daily living, such as cooking, shopping, bed-making, house-cleaning and planning a day's activities.

In special disabled living units, they can practice more intimate activities, and practical trials can be made to see whether one can render sufficient assistance to the other, for transfers in and out of bed and on and off the lavatory-seat, for example. Frequently, the disabled are far less prudish about these matters than are their helpers. They have to accept indignities more readily, and they understand the needs of each other. But what is more important, they often only come to understand the stresses and strains of married life when they are made to carry out practical trials, and they are often surprised by the severity of the fatigue which follows their efforts to cope with simple routine activities. It is very difficult to balance the needs for practical help against the need to allow the couple to fend for themselves.

There is also no doubt that in caring for each other, they will make increased efforts at independence, and call for less help than

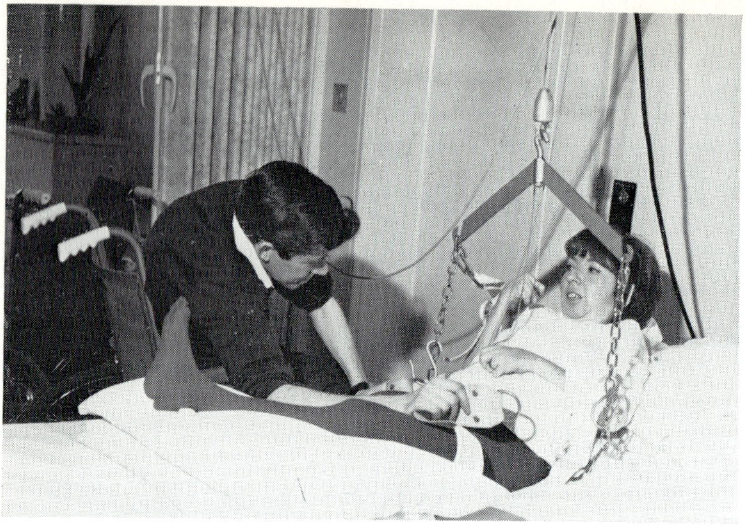

Figure 9.4 (a)

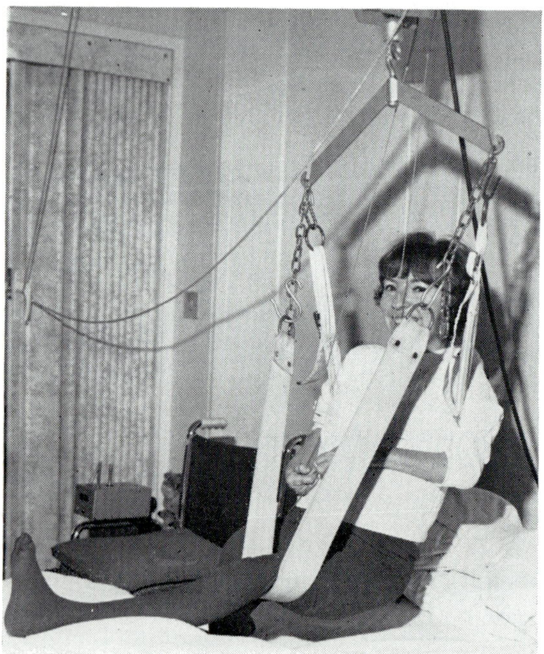

Figure 9.4 (b)

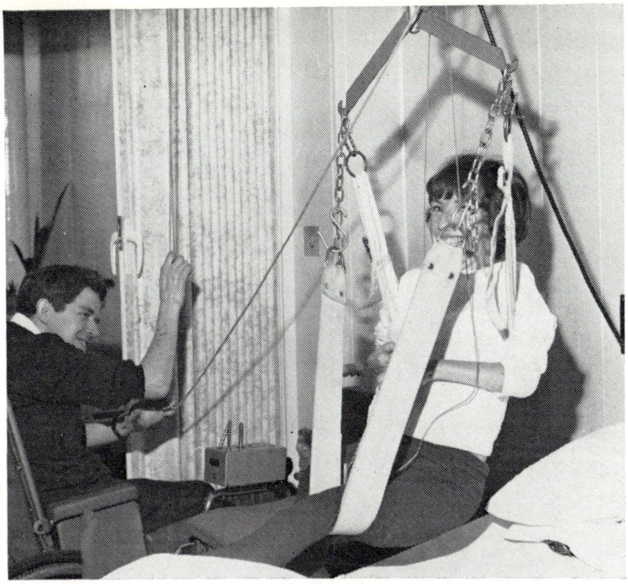

Figure 9.4 (c)

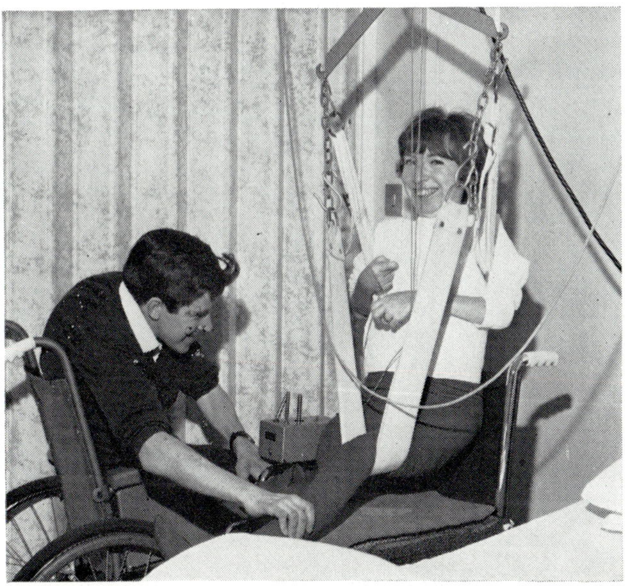

Figure 9.4 (d)

if they were single and being cared for inside an institution. They now have a purpose and an aim. Therefore, it is most important that the medical supervisors of disabled people should give them adequate help and advice about the physical side of marriage, and that the social and welfare workers approach the problems with similar sympathy, understanding and pragmatic practical help.

M.M.L. No. 1096	Partial tetraplegia	male
M.M.L. No. 356	Still's disease	female

A young man became a partial tetraplegic at the age of 19 years following the excision of a benign tumour of the cervical cord (C7).

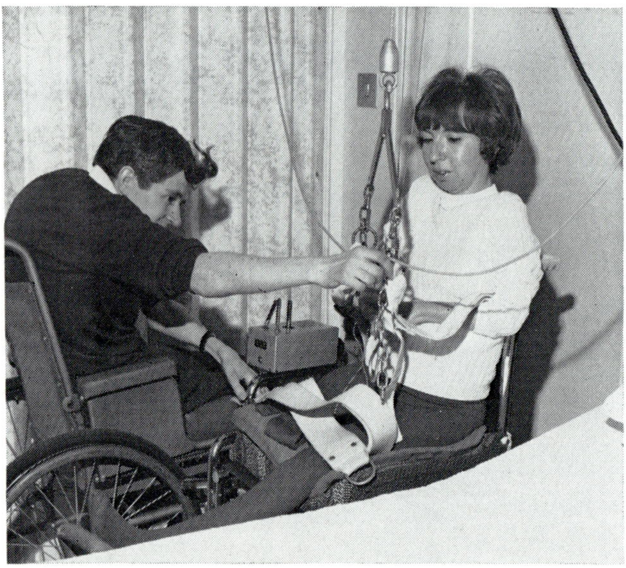

(*e*)

Figure 9.4. Patients No. 1096 and No. 356. Husband with partial tetraplegia organizing the transfer of the wife who has Still's disease: (*a*) *putting slings in position;* (*b*) *lifting off bed using electric hoist;* (*c*) *transferring from bed to chair;* (*d*) *settling onto chair;* (*e*) *removing slings*

He was admitted to a geriatric unit 3 years later (aged 22 years) as his parents were unable to look after him.

At the age of 24, he obtained a place in a residential institution and worked as a type-setter. His wife had Still's disease at the age of 6 years and eventually had involvement of most of her joints. Following complications of surgery, her right leg was amputated, and she had a Girdlestone arthoplasty of her left hip and an excision arthroplasty of both elbows. She was permanently wheelchair-bound and used an adapted electrically propelled indoor chair. She had been admitted to a Disabled Living Research Unit several times and eventually had been admitted to a home for the young chronic sick, where she was very happy and where she met her future husband.

These two were admitted together to the Disabled Living Research Unit and all their activities of daily living were reviewed and mutually discussed. They were both intelligent, very happy together and willing to practise techniques of daily living and to adapt themselves to their various needs. The man was able to cope with all his own and his wife's laundry, most of the routine light housework, including cooking, although he had never done any before.

He was able to cope with his wife's transfers, using an electric ceiling-hoist. Between them, they could cope with all the normal daily routine activities as well as his work as a type-setter (*Figure 9.4*).

They are awaiting admission into a purpose built, ground-floor flat or bungalow, where they hope to be able to live together with a minimum amount of outside help.

M.M.L. No. 977	born 1930	male
M.M.L. No. 975	born 1938	female

Diagnosis: Muscular dystrophy

Jack had muscular dystrophy developing early and had never walked. Since the age of 7, he had lived in institutions or hospitals. From 30 years of age, he had been living in a local authority home for the severely disabled, almost completely dependent for all personal care and transfers.

Margaret also had muscular dystrophy of early onset and had never walked. She was a resident in hospital until the age of 13 years. Since then she had always lived at home and spent most of her life in bed, cared for by her parents. She got up and dressed only at weekends, as this was the only time the family had time to get her up and dress her.

Some years ago, she began to attend the local authority centre for the disabled and there met her future husband. They married because they had mutual problems, mutual interests and a mutual need of companionship. After this marriage, they were admitted to the Disabled Living Unit to assess the possibility of their being able to manage in a purpose-built flat. Regulations did not allow for them both to be admitted to the institution where Jack lived.

They were a most self-contained and composed couple, making a desperate bid to achieve their aim of mutual, private companionship. Jack was so severely disabled that he was almost completely

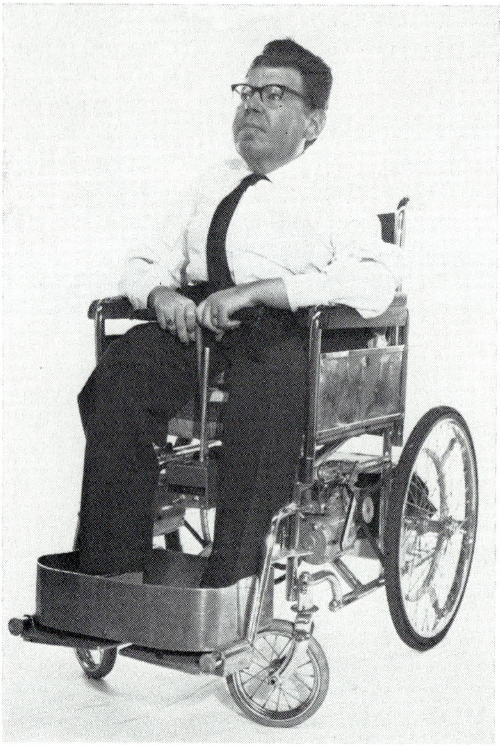

Figure 9.5. Patient No. 977 in his modified Powerdrive wheelchair

dependent, except for feeding and a few activities such as reading and playing chess. He was having increasing difficulty in controlling the tiller bar of his electric chair, the tiller bar was therefore changed for a different type easier to control (*Figure 9.5*). His arms were so weak that mobile arm-supports were found to be of no value. One of his major problems was coping with micturition. However, by adapting his clothing (extending the fly-front opening of his trousers), and using a urine-bottle with a long neck, his wife was able to give him a bottle during the day when necessary. Otherwise, he depended upon an able helper for dressing, washing, and giving him a bed-pan morning and evening.

Margaret was not so severely disabled, and although she had had

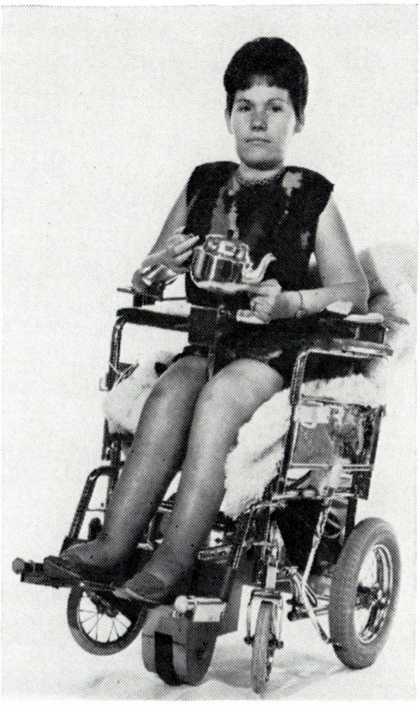

(*a*)

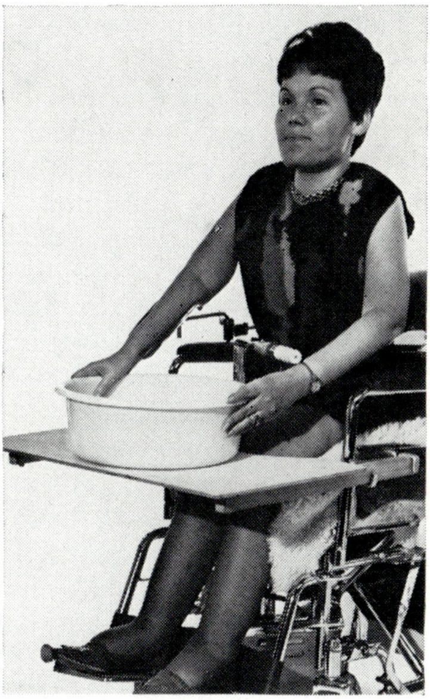

(*b*)

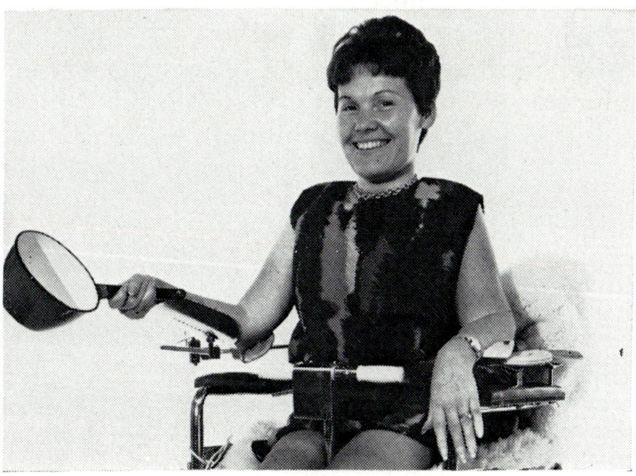

(*c*)

Figure 9.6. Patient No. 975 in her Monodrive unit (*a*) *with mobile arm-supports;* (*b*) *with tray;* (*c*) *showing range of movements* little practice, she rapidly became very competent in a powered wheelchair. Although she could manage many activities without mobile arm-supports, she found that these increased her range of reach and allowed her to work for much longer without tiring.

With the chair and mobile arm-supports, she was able to put into practice much of her theoretical knowledge of household activities. She and her husband were able to work out a programme of domestic activities, and also to plan more creative activities (*Figure 9.6*).

Margaret had written some stories and Jack had written songs. Between them they had hoped to create some independent life and interest. Proof-reading was one possibility of remunerative work.

The local authority were prepared to provide a purpose-built bungalow in association with their institution for the physically disabled, thus giving them close supervision and care.

The period of joint assessment in the Disabled Living Unit established:

(1) They would need help to get them up and dressed in the mornings, and to undress and put them to bed at night.

(2) They would need to have their shopping done for them, or else have all shopping delivered from orders by telephone.

(3) The wife could manage much of the cooking for both of them, and meals-on-wheels once or twice a week should give her a necessary break.

(4) They needed some help with toilet, morning and evening and possibly once midday.

(5) They could manage an alarm-call system on a disabled person's telephone.

The local authority are putting these recommendations into practice, and they are now living in purpose-built flat with warden supervision, associated with a local authority residential home for the disabled.

LESIURE ACTIVITIES

Introduction

Attitudes to leisure depend on personality and training, and are partly inherited and partly acquired. Leisure activities on the other hand, are often more closely related to personal idiosyncrasies and traits. They may be the deeply satisfying expression of a persons' inner self, uninfluenced by the constricting necessity of earning money in a competitive world. Certainly, they occupy a large and important part of able-bodied life, and an even larger and often more important part of the life of the disabled. Leisure activities must substitute for work in the case of such people, by providing the chance of participating in a creative occupation, and by bringing about changes in environment, increasing social contacts, introducing wider horizons of interest, and compensating for the lack of status which unemployment, whether through disablement or the state of the country's economy, carries with it.

In the case of those who have become suddenly disabled, by trauma or acute illness, leisure activities are a particularly important work-substitute, and during the initial months of readjustment. when life must be reorientated and reaccepted, satisfying leisure activities can help to compensate for the frustration which sudden deprivation of the ability to translate knowledge into action must entail. The sportsman who can suddenly no longer participate in his chosen sport, the breadwinner whose sudden disablement prevents him from earning his living and therefore denies him the right to be considered as a leader of the family, the mother who must suddenly employ another woman to take her place in the active running of the home, for them a compelling leisure activity is a necessity providing a source of interests, achievement and social contacts.

Previous training and conditioning must often influence the leisure activities of the disabled patient, but such activities are often the startling hybrid products of unknown, unexplored abilities and unwelcome physical disabilities.

For the disabled who are more intelligent and better educated, reading and serious study may become all-absorbing. But whereas the able-bodied man takes it for granted that he can attend an evening class to supplement his study, and to develop ideas by informal discussion with friends, all such activities pose extra problems for the disabled.

It is part of rehabilitation to explore the possibilities which are open to each patient and to lead him into appropriate leisure activities. Whenever possible, the aim should be to interest the patient in at least one hobby involving active participation and a positive contribution. Even when physical limitations are severe, it is a worthwhile aim to extend fields of knowledge and interest as a means to improving conversational powers, and this may mean a positive effort to watch a television programme or read up a subject of particular interest, later to provide a subject for discussion with friends, relatives or visitors.

While in an institution, group discussions led by a therapist can help to stimulate interest, but patients are often the most effective stimuli for other patients. A severely disabled patient arriving at a rehabilitation unit will often take more interest in another patient's successful hobby than in activities suggested by therapists

Severely disabled children are frustrated in their natural urge to explore and to learn, and consequently often become apathetic. Wide interests are quite as important as formal education, and friends of his own age are essential to a child's growth of personality.

It is important to assess leisure possibilities in context, and thus it is necessary to consider the area in which a patient lives and the facilities available to him, the patient's level of education and previous occupation, his temperament, whether social or solitary, and his home conditions. If the patient cannot go out then much will depend upon whether there are friends or relatives to visit him. Finally, the cost to be incurred and the capital outlay on equipment and subscriptions must be carefully considered. When embarking upon a new hobby, there are bound to be barriers to overcome; transport to club or to friends, architectural features at destination, and the need for mobility in new surroundings. An ability to cope with the toilet, if necessary, during a visit, may make a more social activity possible. The patient's fatigue-level and physical comfort may prevent active participation in many leisure activities. There may be special considerations, such as warmth or noise-level which have to be met.

Though many paraplegics take an active part in sports, for the more severely disabled the choice is limited, and where facilities and voluntary help is available, disabled clubs can be the best answer and provide the often much-needed physical exercise.

However, with encouragement and ingenuity, many severely disabled can take part in a wide variety of activities. Those taken up by patients of the Disabled Living Unit include:

Intellectual:	reading, writing, music, art
Collecting:	stamps, coins
Practical:	model-making, woodwork, radio, gardening, pets and aquaria, photography, sewing and dress-making, knitting, scouting and camping, bird-watching
Games:	snooker, bridge and cards, chess, draughts, darts
Non-participant interests:	television, radio, cinema, theatre, listening to records, following football, following horse racing
Social:	Visiting friends and relatives, entertaining friends and relatives, going for drives, visiting places of historic interest

Some of these require adapted or specially-made equipment. For example, there are playing-card holders, special billiard-cue rests, magnetic chessboards and electric scissors. For the very severely disabled, power-operated reading and writing aids are available, and special attachments for the complex appliances operated by a single microswitch or by sucking and blowing through a tube.

Holidays

The permanently disabled need holidays as do the able, and their relatives looking after them need a holiday break even more. Those who live in institutions also benefit from regular holidays which provide both a physical and intellectual change.

Many voluntary organizations are particularly anxious to co-operate in this activity, and will arrange individual or group holidays for the disabled.

As a matter of principle, institutions catering for the severely disabled patient should be encouraged to designate a few places for holiday admission, either taking patients from their own homes, or collaborating with other institutions to arrange suitable exchanges.

These arrangements are complex and require considerable collaboration between the institution, the voluntary bodies, local authority, general practitioner and the families. When well organized, the guaranteed relief for the relatives may help them to continue to undertake the major role in maintaining the disabled person at home. Periodic hospital admissions must also allow the patient's clinical and functional condition to be reviewed.

Gardening for the disabled

Gardening is probably the most widely pursued hobby in the United Kingdom, but the elderly and the disabled find many of the conventional garden activities increasingly difficult to manage. Cultivation is traditionally associated with heavy physical labour, but modern tools and techniques and careful planning can eliminate many of the more arduous activities, and different approaches to gardening can bring many aspects of this absorbing hobby within the capabilities of many disabled.

Accessibility

In the garden, accessibility is the major problem, as it is elsewhere for the severely disabled. Enabling a severely disabled person to get out of the house and into the garden may involve the provision of suitable doors and ramps. An adequate path all round the house is always an asset for the disabled, and naturally improves the access to the garden.

Paths in the garden should be wide enough to be usable by a patient in a standard wheelchair or on crutches (3 ft 6 in, 107 cm) or wider still (4 ft, 121 cm) if an electric tricycle is used. Many gardeners can manage quite large gardens from such a vehicle.

The paths should be made of non-slip paving or roughed-up concrete when the area is small. Tarmacadam may be more suitable for a large area. Crazy paving tends to separate and form dangerous gaps, and random bricks tend to break, crumble or separate and are, therefore, also unsuitable. Ordinary paving stones often have smooth surfaces and are also likely to be dangerous.

Cultivating

Cultivating, involving digging, hoeing and transporting earth, can be reduced in effort by the judicious selection of suitably designed tools. Many horticultural sundriesmen will now offer considerable help to the disabled gardener, both in advice and by permitting the gardener to try out the various appliances. In some cases, one design may be more suitable than another because of the set of the handle, or the size and angle of grip, or the weight. Others may be made more suitable by changing the style of grip, or by using specially adapted or altered handles. There are now many different types of long-handled tools which make reaching easier; some have the handle cranked and others have handles adjustable in length. Such variations make gardening from a wheelchair, or from a stool, or in a one-handed fashion, more easily managed. Current development is towards interchangeable tool heads.

Grass cutting presents problems, but modern motor mowers with electric motors (battery or mains) or modern petrol mowers with special easy-starting mechanisms may be managed by many disabled.

Chemical gardening, particularly the use of chemical spraying to control weeds and pests, has reduced much of the repetitive physical labour. The use of modern lightweight material for containers, and of lightweight composts for the planting media, can reduce the overall weight of a full 3-in pot to about 3 oz (80 g), thus bringing their use within the physical capability of many severely disabled.

Courtyard gardening

Courtyards and patios can be constructed with concrete or paving stones, and pergolas, car ports and similar constructions can form the basis of a sheltered accessible area which can be gardened by a disabled person all the year round. Access from kitchen or french windows makes the garden an extension of the house. Tubs, barrels, raised beds, sink gardens and similar containers enable the gardener

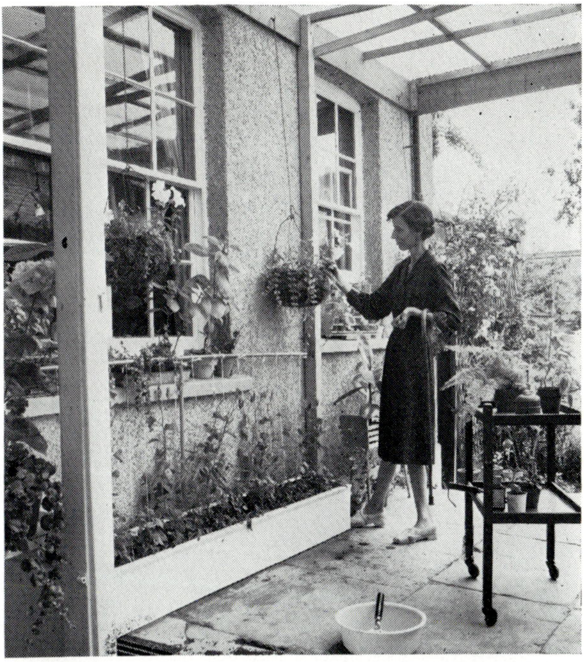

Figure 9.7. A disabled gardener in her courtyard garden

to produce a variety of miniature gardens with an all-the-year-round interest. Plastic tubs are more moveable, but larger, more stable containers can be created from old sinks. Sections of concrete sewage-pipes placed on top of each other make a circular garden of any height desired (*Figure 9.7*).

Raised beds

Raised beds can eliminate much of the labour of gardening and can bring the plants to a level suitable for the gardener whether ambulant or wheelchair-bound. Such beds are a logical extension of the tubs, sinks, and so on described for miniature gardens. A height of about 2 ft (61 cm) is generally suitable for the wheelchair gardener and 2 ft 10 in (86 cm) for ambulant disabled gardeners (*Figure 9.8*).

The width of the bed should not be more than 4 ft (122 cm), then a wheelchair user can adequately cultivate the whole bed, working from either side with suitable hand tools. A 4 ft (122 cm) path all round gives suitable access.

Raised bed can be made from paving-slabs 36 in × 24 in × 2 in (91 cm × 61 cm × 5 cm) mounted vertically and sunk 12 in (30 cm) into the ground. Precast concrete fencing slabs which are usually in

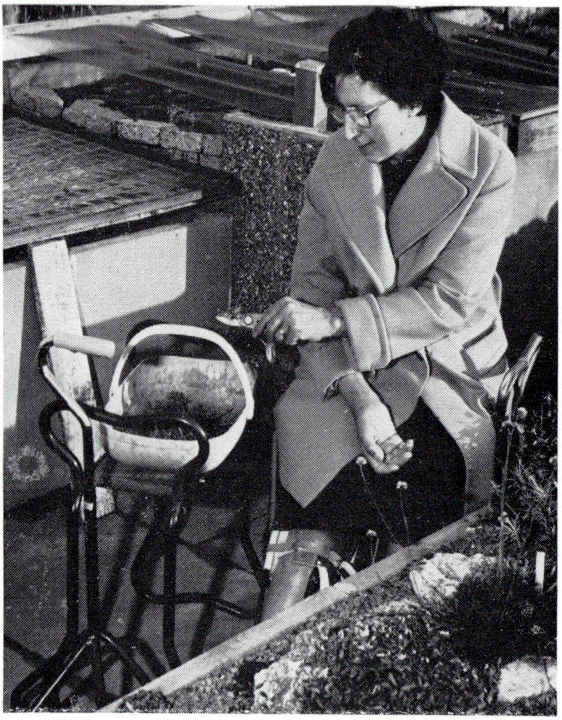

Figure 9.8. Gardening from a stool with raised garden beds

modular form 4 ft × 2 ft 4 in are particularly suitable. Most attractive raised beds are made up using natural stone, but these will also be the most expensive largely because of the labour involved.

Raised beds require 4 in (10 cm) of rubble or bricks for drainage at the bottom, and 2 in (5 cm) of sedge peat on top to reduce their tendency to dry out. Such beds are particularly suitable for alpine and rock plants, but can also be used as a vegetable garden and with careful intercropping can be very productive. The technique involved is similar to traditional cloche gardening.

Greenhouses

Greenhouses are relatively expensive, but for the ambulant and wheelchair gardener they can provide an all-the-year-round, productive, and sometimes lucrative hobby.

For the wheelchair user, the doors of a greenhouse need to be wider than usual, and care is needed to select a suitable greenhouse in this respect. Some are provided with single or double sliding-doors, the shelving heights and depth may be critical and width between the shelving may need to be greater than usual. All these features impose a great need for the potential customer to insist on a practical trial of the greenhouse. The central path will probably need to be paved or concreted and the greenhouse should be sited so as to permit adequate access and with the optimal exposure to the sun.

Automation is now available for those who can afford it; automatic watering, ventilating, and heating can be installed in a small greenhouse and can take much of the physical strain from this hobby and do away with the need for emergency trips to the greenhouse provoked by the unpredictable British weather. Complete automation of a medium-sized greenhouse can be achieved for under £100.

Indoor gardening

For those who are unable to manage outdoor gardening, either because of severity of their disability, or the inaccessibility of the garden, or because no garden is available, some of the varieties of indoor gardening may provide a hobby within their capabilities.

The simplest technique either for window-boxes or for window-sills or free-standing indoor troughs is to stand the plants in their original containers in a trough of sand or peat. This simplifies watering and obviates the need for planting out and repotting when flowering is over. It also enables the trough to be replanted without disturbing the other plants.

Shallow indoor containers are satisfactory for cacti, small alpine plants and Bonsai trees. Attractive miniature gardens can be constructed with a wide range of available plants giving varied colours, shape and foliage throughout the year.

Bottle gardens, developed from the Victorian Wardian cases, which were sealed glass cases or glass bell chambers, are currently very popular as decoration, or as decorative bases for table-lamps. Plastic miniature greenhouses are now available both for propagating or for growing small indoor plants, and can also be heated to overcome the more difficult problems of propagation and also to control the temperature and humidity for the more tender and exotic indoor

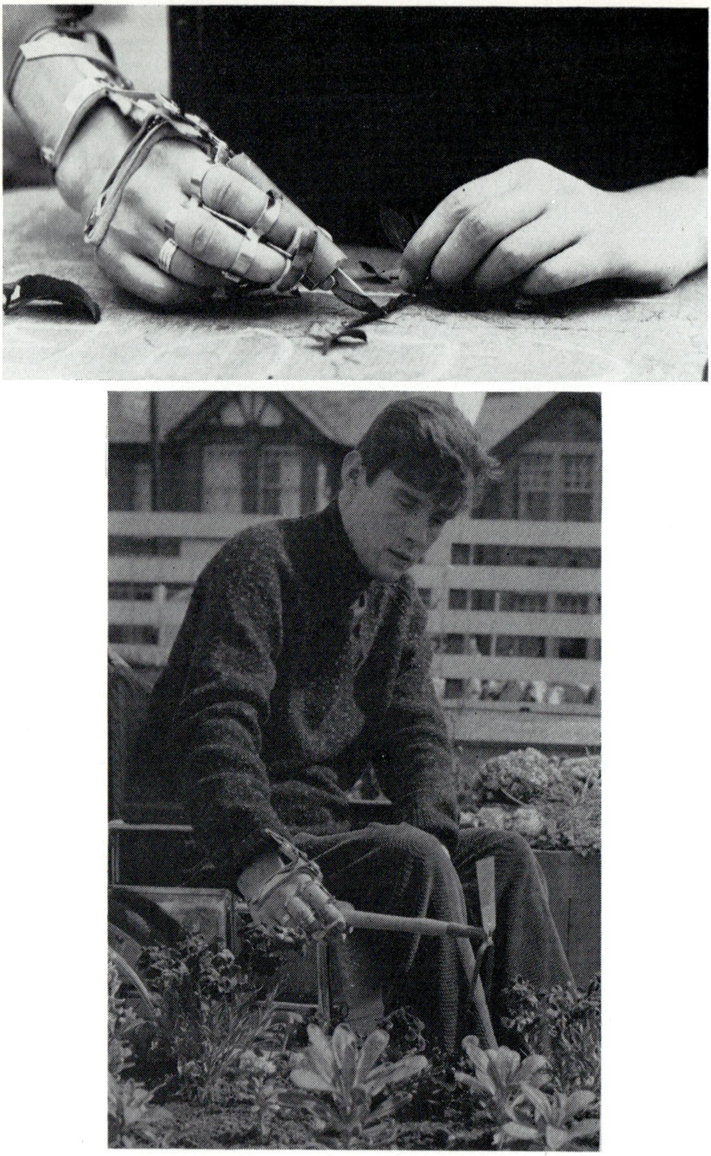

Figure 9.9. Patient No. 420 using flexor-hinge splint by making cuttings for the greenhouse and working at a raised garden bed (the lower photograph reproduced by kind permission of the Editor, 'Oxford Mail')

plants. Even rearing orchid seedlings need not be an expensive hobby.

Gardening is not only an absorbing hobby, but it can also supply valuable therapeutic exercise, ranging from finger exercise, for example, pricking out (*Figure 9.9*) to strong muscular exercise, as in digging. Modern horticulture and the popularity of indoor plants has brought much of the work involved in the industry within the capability of the disabled. Continuous indoor greenhouse work, however, or light activities for the permanent employment of a disabled person could only be achieved within a larger organization, or on a small individual basis, with the disabled person acting as a subcontractor and producing specific types of plants for a particular market. This is a field of resettlement for disabled patients which has not yet been fully explored.

EDUCATION AND TRAINING

For those who are physically handicapped, intellectual competence assumes an importance even greater than for the physically able. In early childhood the responsibility lies with the Health Service, but the local education authorities are empowered to provide facilities for children over the age of 2 years if they need special education. Unfortunately, many authorities do not do this, and often the special needs are not discovered or assessed until the normal age of entry to school is reached.

Between the ages of 5 and 16 years, the responsibility lies with the Department of Education and Science, except for children who are assessed as 'unsuitable for education in school'. These are usually those with I.Q. of below 50, and they are the responsibility of the Department of Health and Social Security.

Handicapped children over the age of 16 years are once more the responsibility of Health and Welfare rather than Education Authorities, except for the responsibilities of the Youth Employment officer who may represent the Department of Employment and Productivity or the Local Education Authority.

There is, thus, a division of responsibility between local health authorities, local education authorities and the central bodies (Department of Employment and Productivity, Department of Education and Science, and Department of Health and Social Security).

Frequently, the children fall into a limbo between the various bodies, particularly when they reach 16 years of age and are physically unable, or intellectually ill-equipped, to proceed to employment.

Voluntary bodies traditionally assume a considerable responsibility for covering the gaps in the mandatory and permissive provisions of the various authorities, and frequently act as a substitute for family, school, further educationist, and employer.

Assessment for special education

Assessment for special education is usually the responsibility of the school medical officer in collaboration with education psychologists. The decisions regarding the special education of any child depend upon the local influences and organizations and there is unfortunately, considerable variation from area to area. Furthermore, once a decision has been made it may be difficult to change the pattern of education for an individual child. Nevertheless, continuous assessment and reappraisal are essential as the child's reaction to his disability and to school often changes. Diagnosis and assessment in these children should be a continuous process and not a once-and-for-all decision.

Unfortunately, recommendations made for a child to change from normal school to special school, or special school to normal school, may be interpreted as failure on the one hand, or criticism of an earlier decision on the other. Frequently, however, it is only the acceptance and understanding of the natural development of the child and his disability. The assessment of a disabled child's function is more than simple appraisal of activities of daily living and of intelligence quotient; the assessment must be made in terms of real life, with the parents and teachers integrated into the decision-making assessment team. Physical fatigue is often also a feature for consideration when deciding to which school a child should go.

The early recognition and assessment of handicap is essential for forward planning, and for those children with established mental disability, an early assessment of their learning facilities is of equal value. For these reasons, the admission of disabled children to normal nursery schools can often lead to sensible decisions being reached regarding further schooling. Unfortunately, there are not enough nursery-school places for this to be a universal approach.

There are still those who believe that all handicapped children should be educated in special schools, and others who believe in educating practically all handicapped children, including the blind, in ordinary schools, as is done in some states in the United States of America.

Many children with physical disabilities are often better at a normal school near their home than a school for the physically handicapped located further away. Sitting in a bus for long journeys is tiring for able children, and may be particularly so for disabled children with severe deformity. It may be necessary to adapt the child's physical environment so that he is not penalized by architectural barriers and unsuitable classroom furniture.

In this country the approach is flexible. There is a variety of different types of special schools providing for different levels of intelligence, different types of handicap, and also for children with multiple handicaps. There are many children with a variety of handicaps in ordinary schools.

In recent years, teachers in special schools have shown increasing awareness of the need to extend their facilities and techniques, while yet exploring the advantages of specialization gained by the study of children of one type. At the same time, teachers in ordinary schools have become much more welcoming to exceptionally talented children, handicapped or not, but are aware that they could help such children more if they knew more about their difficulties.

In the last 10 to 15 years, such schools have accepted large numbers of children with severe multiple physical disabilities. Sometimes they are of borderline level intellectually and may not be able to reach sufficiently high levels of attainment, skill or social competence to permit them to be employed. The presence of such children in the special schools interferes with the level and quality of the education provided for the less severely disabled children.

Because the pace of schools for the handicapped often has to be adapted to the most severely disabled, the level of social and academic education reached does not often equip children to take their place in a normal work situation.

Probably, what is a more important conception is that there should be a freer movement of children from normal schools to special schools and from special schools to normal schools.

Some severely handicapped children would be better advised to start in normal schools, transferring later to special schools when they required a quieter and less physically demanding atmosphere in which to pursue their scholastic careers further, possibly even to university entrance standard.

The disadvantages of handicapped children attending ordinary schools and colleges are largely compensated for by the advantages they gain from the rough-and-tumble of ordinary life. There may be some practical disadvantages, such as exclusion from, say, the school library, certain common-rooms or laboratories. It is important, however, that each disabled person faces the realities of his disablement and comes to terms with life as he must live it, as soon as possible. Thus, those responsible for selecting their schools, have a heavy duty to try to choose the best school for each child, at each stage of their development.

There has been a remarkable change in the pattern of handicaps catered for by the special schools. In about 1930, the majority of the children in these schools were disabled by chronic rheumatic heart disease, many were suffering from the aftermath of poliomyelitis and a further high proportion from the end-results of various infections, particularly osteomyelitis. The situation now is that the majority of the children in the special schools are those with cerebral palsy, and the next largest groups are those with meningomyelocoele. Congenital heart defects, congenital deformities of the limbs and haemophilia are well represented and indicate the ability of the medical profession to save the lives of these children by antibiotics and modern surgical techniques.

It is the declared policy of the Department of Education and Science that, whenever possible, children should be educated in an ordinary school and that only those who for physical, intellectual or social reasons cannot be accommodated in ordinary schools and in their own homes, should be placed in special schools. This policy means that the children in these schools are likely to be predominantly those with some degree of backwardness, or disabilities which will inevitably make them slow learners. This will naturally tend to slow down the education of those who can proceed more quickly, unless a hierarchy of special schools is developed. There is already a trend in this direction, and certain special schools cater for children of grammar school calibre, and provide education to G.C.E. level.

It is to a large extent an expression of the magnitude of the problem of dealing with cerebral palsy, that it is this disease which determines the pattern of special-school education at the present time. These children are in the numerical majority, and about half of them are educationally subnormal. Furthermore, their physical disabilities are such that their ability to learn and partake in school activities is less than for many other disabilities. But as the numbers of children with other disabilities increase, particularly children with meningomyelocoele, it is likely that the educational pattern of the special schools will change accordingly.

The clinical problems engendered by these disabilities are much more complex than those which the special schools had to deal with a decade or so ago. The care of the doubly incontinent spina bifida, the management of an unstable haemophiliac and the care of a child with juvenile rheumatoid arthritis, for example, place a considerable responsibility upon the nursing staff and the attending medical staff of the special school. This also demands an increasingly efficient collaboration between the controlling hospital team and the special school. There must be a very close working relationship between all concerned including the parents, if the child is going to obtain the best possible treatment and education. The communication system is complicated by the fact that often the school doctor and the family doctor are two different people, and the parents may rarely meet the school staff, or the hospital doctors. The responsibility for the essential co-ordination may be taken on by the school, the hospital, the general practitioner or the parents, depending upon circumstances, but it behoves all who are concerned to ensure that the communication system is efficient and to contribute to it.

Questions to be answered when considering the most suitable school for the disabled child are:

(1) Can he get to school, and then can he get about within the school?

(2) Can he manage to use the toilet on his own, or does he need to have help from an adult?

(3) Can he feed himself?

(4) Does he need any special furniture (desk or table)?

(5) Does he need any special appliances (wheelchairs, crutches)?

(6) Does he need any special apparatus for classroom use (typewriter or tape-recorder, magnetic board)?

(7) Is he socially acceptable to staff and pupils (continence, communication)?

(8) Can he overcome his handicap and appearance when in the school community?

(9) Is he likely to need frequent attention which cannot easily be provided in an ordinary school?

(10) Is he likely to be frequently absent or need treatment which will seriously interfere with his education?

Universities

Admission of handicapped students to universities depends on scholastic achievements, as it does for non-handicapped students. Sympathy plays no part here, and this is important, because a combination of academic failure and a physical handicap could be disastrous. A university degree could be of greater importance to a handicapped student than to a non-handicapped, taking them into the professional classes where physical disability is less restricting than in the artisan classes. Some universities encourage the admission of disabled students, having created suitable facilities in all university buildings. Some of the newer ones have been designed to be accessible to the physically disabled, whereas others provide special, but segregated accommodation. The older universities, however, are bedevilled by architectural barriers to the physically handicapped.

Once again, information is not widely available, and too often inadequate or conflicting advice may be given when the schoolchild contemplates courses of further or higher education. This leads to frustration and wrecked hopes, and one more disabled person unable to obtain the type of employment to which he considers he is entitled, and indeed, suited.

M.M.L. No. 247 born 1946 male

Diagnosis: Acute anterior poliomyelitis

At the age of 3 years, this young man had poliomyelitis resulting in completely flail legs and weak arms and weak trunk. He wore a spinal brace and used a wheelchair. He was referred to the Disabled Living Unit when he was 18 years old as he had obtained a place at University, and an assessment had been requested by the University authorities, to determine his capability for independent living. While at school, he lived at home and had been transported by taxi, being lifted in and out by an attendant. He was also helped on and off the toilet, and was completely dependent for washing and dressing. When admitted to the Unit, his upper-limb muscle chart (M.R.C. Grade) was as follows.

Muscle group	*Right*	*Left*
Shoulder elevation and abduction	2	2
Elbow flexion	4	1
Elbow extension	1	1
Wrists and hands—all groups	5	5

Although he had never tried before, he rapidly became independent in dressing, including putting on his spinal brace. He also became independent for washing. The main problems were self-propelling the wheelchair and transfers to and from the wheelchair. His hands were good, but his arms were not strong enough for a conventional form of transfer. After practice, it was found that he could become independent for transfer using a sliding-board, providing the height of the bed, shower-seat, lavatory-seat and so on were at 17 in (43 cm) He could not transfer sideways, but could traverse the sliding-board forwards and backwards if he took his spinal brace off, or he could go backwards through the back of the wheelchair, if this had a zip-fastener in it to allow him to open the canvas back. The easiest technique for the toilet was to transfer forwards onto the lavatory-seat, using the pedestal back to front.

When at University, these manoeuvres were essential. At home, it was quicker and easier for his father to lift him.

He could self-propel a wheelchair on the flat, but he could not propel fast enough to get way on or to push himself up a slope. A pair of one-way brakes was made and fitted to his chair (*Figure 9.10*)

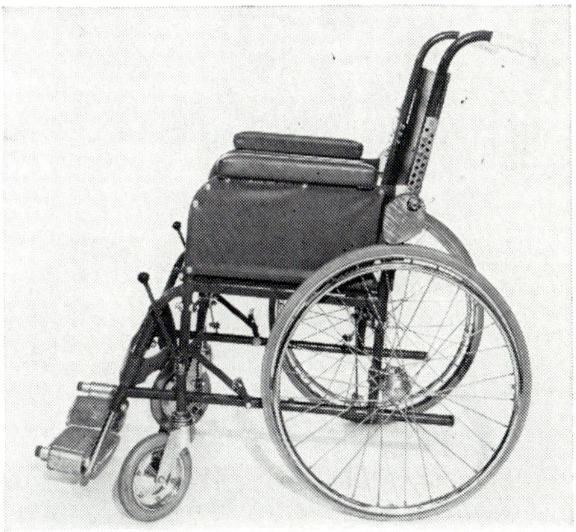

Figure 9.10. Wheelchair fitted with a one-way egg-shaped brake fitted above the wheel, which prevents the chair rolling backwards on a slope

which enabled the patient to propel up a slope since the chair no longer ran back between pushes.

This assessment indicated that he was capable of being almost independent at University, and on the strength of this, he was accepted. Two years later, he was completely integrated into University life, taking part in many social activities as well as coping successfully with the academic work. He had improved physically, functionally, and psychologically, and was obviously not requiring undue assistance from anybody. The only adaptations necessary at the University were the removal of some partitions between wash-basin, showers and toilets, to give his wheelchair access, and the provision of a shower seat and a bed of the correct height for transferring. In practice, he lived fairly near and went home each week for a bath.

The significance of the contribution of the Disabled Living Unit was most evident in convincing the patient and the authorities that he could be independent, rather than providing any technical help or advice. The wheelchair brakes and the zip-back for the wheelchair were important, but not so important as accepting a degree of responsibility for the decision to admit him to the University.

WORK

Introduction

It is unrewarding to proceed with any course of training without first attuning it to a realistic appraisal of likely work. This entails a detailed knowledge of likely outlets for the trained disabled. Unfortunately, in spite of a widespread organization, the chances of gainful employment of the severely disabled are negligible. It should be the aim to further the patient's education and training towards personal independence first, and then towards domestic independence, and finally towards other activities. These may be at best work, and at least such that they allow the disabled patient to achieve a continued interest and to maintain his self-respect.

The majority of the severely disabled are unable to achieve work, because of lack of training and lack of suitable employment near to their home or institution, as well as because they are physically unable to achieve a sufficiently high level of functional competence or endurance to become employable. A very high proportion, however, could achieve part-time employment of a limited nature in suitably sheltered surroundings. Unfortunately, these facilities are not readily available, although theoretically there is a very comprehensive organization for assessing, training and placing the disabled in work.

Assessing for work

Medical rehabilitation has as its aims the restoration of function after injury or illness and is the responsibility of the patient's doctor. Social rehabilitation is designed to enable the individual to resume his life in the family or community, despite a disability so severe in some instances that formerly he might well have been restricted to living in an institution throughout his life. This is largely a family or social-welfare responsibility. Industrial rehabilitation has as its aim the restoration to fitness for work after injury or illness, and ideally should overlap and follow medical rehabilitation without a break. As a natural prerequisite to industrial rehabilitation, a period of work assessment is usually necessary. This assessment is aimed at establishing patient's intellectual, educational and physical competence, his natural aptitude, his work tolerance, and physical and mental ensurance, and his capacity for further training.

The Department of Employment and Productivity is responsible for industrial rehabilitation, and directly administers 22 Industrial Rehabilitation Units, (IRU's), designed to accept almost every type of physical disability. There are also many industrial rehabilitation schemes run by voluntary organizations, and local authorities, for particular classes of disability. There are 8 agency schemes at present, 2 for the blind, 2 for the cerebral palsied and 4 for mentally handicapped persons. The Department's IRU's take some 12,7000 entrants annually.

The courses at the IRU last from 6 to 8 weeks but may, in exceptional cases, be extended up to 26 weeks. They are planned and controlled through the Unit Case Conference, comprising the rehabilitation officer, medical officer, occupational psychologist, social worker, occupational supervisor (in charge of the workshops) and disablement resettlement officer. The courses include an assessment by the psychologist, using a battery of psychological tests, direct observation in the workshop, and exposure to a simulated industrial environment in the workshop. Insistence is made on the completion, under normal production stresses, of work subcontracted from local firms. The workshops include facilities for woodwork, bench engineering and machine operation, and there is provision for gardening and heavy work, stores and kitchen experience, clerical and industrial records work and for brushing up educationally. IRU's do not set out to provide training, only to assess the disabled person's capabilities for training or work. They aim to make work attainable for those who have lost the habit through illness or injury. Any necessary tuition in industrial techniques or the use of machines is given by supervisors experienced in the industry and trained in instructional techniques, but this tuition is regarded as incidental to the rehabilitative purpose of the units. For those who prove apt at learning and need training, a full training course at a government training centre or a residential training centre may be recommended.

Currently, IRU's are equipped to deal with relatively unskilled technical work, manual labour, and clerical work. There are difficulties in the provision of rehabilitation facilities for people in higher grade office jobs, including those at managerial level, and there may be a case for instituting a small residential IRU for the professional man, or the business executive, who is unable to carry on with his existing job.

One in 6 of the attendances at IRU'S terminates prematurely, half of these for medical reasons. Of the remainder, 2 in 3 are at work or accepted for training, as recommended by the units, within 3 months of the termination of their courses.

There is a tendency for the handicapped school-leaver with several

'O' levels and perhaps 1 or 2 'A' levels to fail to be accommodated by the IRU–Government Training Centre organization. Disablement Resettlement Officers (DRO) and Youth Employment Officers are often unable to advise realistic placement for these patients.

The early referral of the schoolchild to the youth employment officer, the early consultation of the youth employment officer with the disablement resettlement officer, detailed consultations between the consultant and the youth employment officer and/or, the disablement resettlement officer, can prepare realistically for his appropriate training and employment. Unfortunately, it is more usual for the school or the family to consult the youth employment officer or the disablement resettlement officer only when employment problems arise. Children in special schools are almost invariably referred early to the youth employment services, because these schools often accept the responsibility for advising on and planning for the disabled school-leaver's placement.

It is not easy for the professionals, the doctor, the psychiatrist, the medical social worker, to communicate with the layman, for example, the patient, the patient's family, his priest, and other interested workers, professional or lay, paid or volunteer. It is essential that they not only communicate, but that they also understand one another, if the disabled are to be helped to maximal rehabilitation and optimal resettlement.

The Disabled Persons (Employment) Act, 1944, provides for the appropriation of certain occupations for registered disabled persons only. The only occupations so designated at present are those of car park attendant (which is particularly unsuitable because it involves being out in all weathers), and passenger lift attendant (which is of strictly limited appeal).

Techniques for assessing the potential abilities of young people and adults have advanced considerably in recent years. An adequate assessment of handicapped children and adults is the basis of realistic settlement.

Because of the limitations of the IRU system, many rehabilitation units undertake some degree of work assessment. They are finding an increasing need to do this and to plan retraining at a stage when the patient is unacceptable for the IRU. There is an urgent need to integrate the facilities for continued medical rehabilitation with those for work assessment and vocational training. One combined Unit has now started at Garston Manor, Watford, but too frequently there is an administrative and physical barrier to the integration of rehabilitation and the organization of assessment and training early in recovery and while medical rehabilitation is still proceeding.

Vocational training

There are over 40 government training centres which provide a variety of training courses. Disabled people may be accepted for these courses provided they are considered likely to benefit from the training given, and provided that they have reasonable prospects of securing a job in the occupation for which they have trained, on completion of the course.

In addition, there are a number of establishments run by voluntary organizations and providing training facilities. These are subsidized by the Department of Employment and Productivity.

In addition to training centres, there are facilities for the disabled to train in commercial and technical colleges, or partake in industrial training schemes. Disabled persons of suitable ability and educational background may be helped to undertake courses of training, including University degree courses. However, disablement resettlement officers often have difficulty in finding premises which, for example, a wheelchair can negotiate.

Another frequent complication is that the disabled student may well take longer to achieve the academic qualifications for higher education, and it is often difficult to persuade the authorities to accept the older student with the additional problems of physical disability.

Disabled young people frequently require additional general education and medical supervision, as well as practical training to fit them for eventual employment. Such preparation is usually only provided by prolonged courses at residential establishments run by voluntary organizations. Once again, it is often difficult to obtain continued medical rehabilitation and educational or vocational training.

National Advisory Council on the Employment of the Disabled and District Disablement Advisory Committees

Section 17 of the Disabled Persons (Employment) Act, 1944 requires the Secretary of State to establish a national advisory council on the employment of the disabled together with district advisory committees. The functions of the National Advisory Council are to advise and assist the Secretary of State in matters relating to the employment, self-employment or training of disabled persons generally. The Council has 4 constituent committees; there are the Sheltered Employment Committee, the Training and Employment Committee, the Blind Persons Committee and the Medical Committee. There are about 250 district Disablement Advisory Committees throughout the country, each serving the area of an employment exchange or group of exchanges. These committees (or in some cases their panels) are required to give advice on individual cases referred to them, and to make recommendations and reports on matters referred to them under the various provisions of the Act, namely:

(1) applications for entry into the register of disabled which are not approved in the first instance by the Secretary of State;

(2) removal of names from the register;

(3) application for a reduction in an employer's quota of disabled persons;

(4) application by employers for permits to engage able-bodied persons;

(5) allegations of discharge of disabled persons without reasonable cause.

The effectiveness of these Disablement Advisory Committees varies considerably. A good local committee can influence local employers, and the public in general, well beyond the letter of their terms of reference.

Employment agencies

The more intelligent and well-motivated disabled people often obtain work themselves, through private agencies, advertisements, direct application and friends. Furthermore, many voluntary organizations devoted to the disabled, or to particular disabilities, provide advice and help.

The Department of Employment and Productivity provides a special placement service for disabled persons seeking employment, as part of their general placement service. This is the primary function of the 1,000 or more Disablement Resettlement Officers (DRO's) employed by the Department of Employment and Productivity in Great Britain. DRO's will deal with all types of disability, including, of course, persons not on the register, but excluding blind persons. These men and women form part of the normal career structure of the executive grade of the civil service. Small employment exchanges usually employ a part-time DRO combining the duty of placing disabled persons with that of manager of the exchange. DRO's are recruited from the existing staff in the Department of Employment and Productivity. The Department's policy is not to transfer them to other work until they have served at least five years as DRO's; but in practice, this is difficult to achieve, and they may be transferred to other duties or promoted before the expiry of the period.

The DRO's task is not an easy one. He is essentially an employment officer and not a social worker. He should be an integral part of a team, ideally consisting of a medical consultant, a social worker, a psychologist or psychiatrist, a relative, the applicant and other specialists, if necessary. His function is to advise the team on the possibilities of local employment, mechanical aids which can be provided, transport, industrial rehabilitation and vocational training facilities and, where appropriate, on sheltered employment. However, the team is frequently more theoretical than practical and the DRO service is often blamed for what are really inadequacies in the education, training and medical services provided for disabled persons.

Some disabled persons are incapable of working either because of the severity of their disablement, their personality, or due to the locality of the district in which they live, their inability or unwillingness to move, or to a combination of features. In such instances, no matter how efficient or conscientious the social workers, DRO'S and others, failure is inevitable.

For the younger disabled, the Youth Employment or Careers Service, based on the Employment and Training Act, 1948 is available. For the most part, this is run by local education authorities and grant-aided by the Department of Employment and Productivity, and where a local education authority does not exercise its powers, the service is wholly undertaken by the Department of Employment and Productivity.

Many disabled persons are working in open employment side by side with non-disabled persons. They may have certain aids or facilities provided by the firm or the Department of Employment and Productivity, for example, provision of ramps, adjusting the access to work benches, widening lavatory doors.

Trade Unions

Although the Trades Union Congress is interested in the employment of disabled persons, Trade Unions on the shop floor vary considerably in attitude. Individually, they are usually sympathetic, but they are particularly concerned that disabled workers do not become a source of cheap or exploited labour. Furthermore, they are also very jealous of the rights of all their members and must be assured that the disabled are not receiving unfair, preferential treatment.

Private employers

There are 3 main types of employers; those who pity the disabled and are willing to make work available as a charity, those who take advantage of the disabled and regard them as a source of cheap labour, and those who treat the disabled on merit and pay a fair wage for good work. But there are problems outside the jurisdiction of the employer. For example, the Factory Inspectorate do not allow anyone in a wheelchair or on crutches to work other than on the ground floor; this is for safety reasons. Sometimes other workers object to working with a disabled person, and in particular they usually (wrongly) fear that the disabled are getting special favour; others object, for example, to the complex toilet arrangements for some disabled.

Central and local government and nationalized industries

Public bodies are usually conscientious employers of disabled persons and central government has undertaken to honour the requirements of the Act of 1944, although it is not bound by it.

Diversionary occupation

For those unable to achieve sheltered work, or for whom work is uneconomic, diversionary activities have an important part to play in maintaining a patient's alertness and motivation. Diversionary workshops provide employment for men and women who are too disabled to work in sheltered workshops and are often occupational therapy centres.

Facilities vary considerably, depending upon the local authority and voluntary bodies. In some areas, the organization is comprehensive and patients may progress from diversional occupational therapy to training and to sheltered work. But in too many areas, the facilities are inadequate and haphazard. Many of the residential homes for disabled people providing accommodation and social facilities also provide diversionary employment.

Homework

Work can be arranged for disabled persons to undertake at home, and this may well represent a large untapped source of skilled and semi-skilled labour. However, the training of the patients together with the organization of distribution and collection, presents many problems, and the system is open to exploitation. Unfortunately, several schemes have failed and thus produced more frustration for the disabled, and have earned this type of employment a bad reputation. For suitable patients, there are limited opportunities for professionally qualified, homebound, disabled people to be provided with work by government departments, and information on this can be obtained from the Department of Employment and Productivity.

Sheltered work

The major objective of obtaining employment is to earn a living, and work in open employment should be the first objective of any disabled person seeking employment. If this is not attainable, then the next alternative is sheltered employment. This is provided by a non-profit-making, distributing company set up by the Government in 1945 (Remploy) under the 1944 Act, by local authorities under the Disabled Persons (Employment) Act, 1958; or by voluntary associations or bodies, with a workshop or facilities of the required standard.

A sheltered workshop employs men and women too handicapped to be able to reach the average rate of production achieved by open industry. However, while working under sheltered conditions the process of rehabilitation continues and some workers proceed to open employment. The Department of Employment and Productivity has an inspectorate, one of whose functions is to advise on methods of improving the efficiency of the disabled. The advice of the Ministry of Technology is available to the Department of Employment and Productivity on all aspects of workshop management.

Unfortunately, there are not enough facilities for sheltered employment, and most sheltered workshops require standards of working capability which approach those of the non-disabled, particularly regarding the number of hours to be worked. For sheltered workshops run by voluntary bodies to qualify for deficiency grants from the Ministry of Labour, they have to provide employment for the disabled, under normal industrial conditions before wages and employment can reach an economic level. This means, in effect, that the employees have to accomplish an 8-hour day and approach a 40-hour week.

There is a considerable need for sheltered employment of a part-time nature, in conditions where more of the severely or progressively disabled can be accommodated, and where competent and sympathetic supervision is provided and both work and accommodation are available. The need for more sheltered work is mirrored in the need for more training facilities for the disabled. Preferably, the facilities should be linked so that training programmes are geared to available work, and regionalized so that patients are not unnecessarily moved from one area to another, with consequent changing of supervision as well as separation from friends and family to add to their difficulties.

Resettlement in work

Some of the problems are geographical, particularly in rural areas, and some are caused by the limitation of earnings imposed by the

Social Security regulations. Too frequently, facilities are fragmented, and closer co-operation between local authorities and voluntary bodies, grouping patients with different disabilities and different qualifications, might lead to improvement in the facilities which could be provided.

As the situation stands, it takes considerable time and organization for the rehabilitation team to establish an individual patient's work capabilities, and to find available training facilities to process his acceptance and provide active support during training to process his return to his original community and help him seek for employment. In order to get a disabled person to work, it is not uncommon for the co-ordinating social worker in a rehabilitation unit to have to co-ordinate the activities of 15–20 individuals, often each working to different sets of rules and within quite separate organizations. The actions of one often have to depend on decisions of another. The main actors in this complex drama usually are the following.

Hospital or Rehabilitation Unit

Clinicians; physiotherapists—mobility/transfer; occupational therapists—personal care and independence; medical social workers

Local authority

Educational psychologist; welfare officer; housing officer.

Department of Employment and Productivity

Disablement Resettlement Officer; Government Training Centre; Industrial Rehabilitation Unit.

Appliance centre

Medical officer/technical officer—for powered outdoor transport or wheelchairs and so on.

Employers

Personnel officer; Trades Union official; chargehand; welfare officer.

Accommodation and transport

The problem of providing accommodation for the severely disabled is closely integrated with the problem of work. Too frequently, the major factors preventing the disabled patient from working or partaking in diversionary activities, or enjoying other group activities, is the lack of suitable transport facilities.

The deficiency is usually both quantitative and qualitative. There is not enough transport available and the local authorities are unable to provide the service, and furthermore, what can be provided, frequently cannot cope with the peculiar and complex needs of many of the severely disabled. It is not infrequent that the patient can be transported from home to a diversionary occupational therapy centre, but it is not possible to take his electrically-powered wheelchair. Thus, when at the centre, he is more incapacitated than necessary. Furthermore, the duplication of the necessary appliance would constitute an unacceptable or unwarranted expense, and raises problems of supervision and maintenance.

The solution lies in the development of community areas with appropriate warden-supervised accommodation, and readily accessible to the work centres. If such an organization could be provided on a large enough scale, and if facilities could be pooled and grouped on a regional basis, with graded work facilities both in skill and endurance both for part-time and full-time employees, then a larger proportion of the disabled could partake in active productive employment.

Not infrequently, a sympathetic employer will offer a job to a disabled patient if he can obtain training. The patient could cope with the work if he could obtain accommodation, but the housing department of the local authority will only allocate priority when the patient has a definite job. In order to obtain training, the disabled person has to travel to a training centre, and both for this and for work he requires his own transport. Although entitled to a powered outdoor vehicle provided through the Appliance Centre, this cannot be issued until he has his own accommodation where a shed for the vehicle can be erected. Thus, a vicious circle is formed in which training is denied until accommodation is available, accommodation is denied until work is available and work is denied until training has been completed. Co-ordination and agreement between several Government departments, local authority departments, public, private and voluntary bodies has to be engineered, if this type of frustrating impasse is to be avoided.

Co-ordination of activity of the social and welfare services is a time-consuming activity, and it is often only within the medical rehabilitation centre organization that enough co-ordinated effort is available to carry the remaining services. The rehabilitation unit must provide the lead for resettlement, and must establish an organization for co-ordination. As disabilities change and patients grow up or deteriorate, the facilities and personnel alter. A central, co-ordinating body can provide a valuable regional service to clinicians, local authorities, welfare organizations and employers. For only through some such organizations can the necessarily changing concepts be progressed, and the changing conditions for each individual patient be assessed.

The problems arising from the employment of severely handicapped people are controversial and their solution often depends on the expenditure of public money, mainly in education, training and overcoming architectural barriers. One very important factor is the isolation of so many of the groups of people working in this field. There is a lack of co-ordination and a lack of effective liaison which cannot be solved by central legislation. There is a severe lack of any kind of reliable statistics regarding work, working efficiency and economic implications. Furthermore, the social benefits resulting from the full employment of disabled people do not lend themselves to measurement and have not been widely publicized in this country. Probably, the major current problem is the separation between medical rehabilitation, educational and work assessment, vocational and educational training and trial periods of sheltered or partially sheltered work.

Although each particular disability has its specific limiting effect on the range of suitable employment, general assumptions are misleading and each patient must be considered on his own merits. His disability, his personal capabilities, his domestic and family background, his ability to follow written, verbal and pictorial instructions, and the specific requirement of the job under consideration, all these factors influence the type of work which he can do, and the efficiency with which he will do it.

When considering the possibility of employment of a disabled patient, his disability and capabilities must be assessed in the context of:

(1) The area in which he lives or is likely to live with particular reference to available employment.

(2) His level of education, intelligence and his previous occupation.

(3) His family responsibilities and available family support.

(4) His personality, temperament and work record.

The degree of handicap resulting from a disability is affected by the age, sex, social class and financial position of the person concerned; but the most important factor is the patient's personality.

The most important environmental factor affecting the disabled person of any age is the family. There may be a tendency for overprotection on the one hand or rejection on the other, and there is often a tendency to concentrate on the financial hardships resulting from disability. In spite of the various provisions of the welfare services, the family has to bear the brunt of the problem of nursing and caring for the disabled.

The second stage is to assess the problems he is likely to meet, and the barriers which need to be overcome to enable him to go out to work; transport problems; working environment; mobility at work; toilet facilities and requirements; and fatigue-level and endurance under working conditions.

In order to help with these assessments, it is advisable to study the particular area of employment and analyse the necessary processes, study the grading and progression of the activities and devise realistic tests for the patient to attempt.

Many of the more severely disabled are unlikely to attempt work other than light assembly hand-work, or clerical and office work. Many activities within the occupational therapy department can be aligned to light hand-work; for example, carpentry, and other activities can be devised to give a realistic trial, such as assembly of hospital dressing-packs.

Within the occupational therapy department a very realistic trial of clerical and office work can be achieved with readily available equipment (*see* Appendix S).

Most modern occupational therapy departments have a training kitchen and the planning, preparing and cooking of a meal can be an excellent test of manual skill, endurance and concentration for both men and women. A complete cookery programme (Appendix T) over a period of time will often give an experienced staff a clear estimate of a patient's capabilities to be able to run their own home, to follow instructions and to achieve a working situation.

Similarly, gardening can be used as an activity to assess working capability under certain limited situations.

As a general principle, even for the severely disabled, rehabilitation should aim at achieving maximal activity whatever the disability and whatever the prognosis. The goal should be work or sheltered work, whichever is appropriate. If these cannot be achieved, then rehabilitation should aim at achieving, not only personal independence, but activities which can best be described as 'active leisure' which can provide the disabled person with a sense of achievement, even if no financial remuneration is forthcoming from them.

Friends and colleagues

The disabled need to make friends, and every facility should be offered to enable them to join associations and societies, both those societies specially catering for the disabled, and also those that are not specially for the disabled. Disabled children often prefer to meet non-disabled children, resenting being grouped as handicapped. However, disabled adults often seem to prefer to spend their leisure time with others similarly disabled.

Not infrequently, those working closely with the disabled have to cope with extra duties which the disabled person cannot do. This often is related to fetching and carrying. Conversely, the disabled person himself can sometimes render a service for non-disabled colleagues if he has a mind to. A difficult and often resented chore is lending some assistance to the disabled trying to cope with their personal toilet. Recognition by the disabled person of the extra assistance provided by colleagues, recognition of the fact that extra assistance can be given to non-disabled colleagues, and recognition that help given to disabled colleagues makes both sides—giver and receiver—more co-operative, helps to create a pleasant atmosphere in places of work.

These last 2 case histories exemplify much of the philosophy behind the comprehensive rehabilitation of the severely disabled. The schoolmaster by his own determination and effort got himself back to work after a severe injury. He has exploited various rehabilitation services, and he uses appropriate aids, appliances and equipment to achieve functional results for himself, and to relieve his wife of some of the physical strain of looking after him. With the support of his wife, family and colleagues he works full-time, and he achieves not only a personal satisfaction from his work but an adequate financial reward which enables him to retain independence.

M.M.L. No. 257 born 1934 male

Diagnosis: Traumatic tetraplegia (C5)

At the age of 25 years, this schoolteacher broke his neck playing rugby football. The lesion was at C4–C5 vertebrae and he was left with almost complete paralysis of muscles supplied by C6 and below. He was in a spinal injuries unit for 6 months, and was then discharged home in a wheelchair. In both arms he had good power in the deltoid, biceps, brachioradialis, supinators and extensor carpi radialis. He had an automatic bladder but intermittent urinary infections. Although he could manage to propel his wheelchair, he found this a considerable physical strain. He, therefore, bought himself an electrically propelled indoor chair, and with this was able to undertake many more activities. After a further 2 years, during which time he was struggling to cope, he was admitted to the Disabled Living Unit for provision of a flexor-hinge splint.

At this time, he was using a hand-strap to hold a fork for eating, and a pencil, but his school work was seriously impeded by an inability to write legibly. Flexor-hinge splints were originally made for both hands, but after practice he discarded that for the left hand.

The other main achievements of the Disabled Living Unit were to revise the lifting techniques used by the patient's wife, and to implement the installation of hoists in their home. This relieved the patient's wife of considerable physical strain. Further recommendations, including the use of an electric typewriter and other aids to facilitate his work, both at school and at home, were given.

After about 12 months, he became completely dependent upon the right-hand splint, and in the course of 4 years, has worn out four splints.

With the splint and simpler aids for the left hand, he has become very competent at school. He teaches whole-time and has not had a day off for nearly 4 years. He writes, corrects exercise books and marks examination papers. He writes on large sheets of paper which can then be put up on the wall instead of writing directly on the blackboard. With modern visual aids, teaching from an electrically-powered wheelchair presents surprisingly few disadvantages.

He is dependent upon his wife for considerable help with dressing, toilet and bathing, but skilful planned use of hoist with a track over the bed and bath reduced the physical strain considerably. An electrical hoist on the car-top has further reduced the need for manual lifting.

Comment

Originally a sports master, this patient has now become a whole-time teacher in a secondary-modern school. He has completed over 4 years whole-time work without absences. He attributes his ability to continue at work to the intelligent employment of aids, appliances and equipment which reduce the physical stress of severe disability on both himself and his wife.

M.M.L. No. 288 born 1940 female

Diagnosis: Anterior poliomyelitis

This young lady contracted anterior poliomyelitis when she was 15 years of age (1955). She had an almost complete tetraplegia, retaining some minimal movement in her feet and hands only.

She was in a tank respirator for 9 months and then was weaned out of it, using a cuirasse for some months more, and then abandoning all respiratory aids. She remained in hospital for 3 years, and then was admitted to a residential home for the severely disabled.

She was in a reclining wheelchair and spent her time reading and making jewellery.

She became steadily more listless and apathetic, her ability to concentrate deteriorated and she became slowly weaker.

On admission to hospital in 1962, 7 years after her acute illness and 6 years after discarding all respiratory aids, she was found to be in respiratory failure. After a period in a tank respirator, she was then weaned onto a rocking-bed and cuirasse. She slowly improved, and was transferred to the Disabled Living Unit. After 14 months in hospital and the Disabled Living Unit, she returned to the home able to type and write and feed herself by using mobile arm-supports, and using a cuirasse respirator at night. During the next few years, she lived in a residential home, spending her time eating, typing letters and getting more and more frustrated because she could not achieve a more active life either intellectually or physically.

Early in 1966, she was readmitted to the Disabled Living Unit again for reassessment and was readmitted at intervals of about 6 months for the succeeding few years.

In 1966, she was given an electrically-powered indoor chair adapted so that she could drive it with her foot and this immediately led her to extend her interests and activities (*Figure 9.11*) and enabled her to embark on training as a social worker.

In 1967, she was found to be suffering from mild pulmonary insufficiency—Arterial P_{CO_2} 78 mm Hg; arterial P_{CO_2} 41 mm Hg; vital capacity 900 ml. She was taught the glossopharyngeal method of breathing, and this increased her vital capacity from 900 to 1400 ml. However, frog breathing was not sufficient and it tired her, so she was given a portable intermittent positive-pressure respirator. This increased her vital capacity to 1,500 ml and produced a steady improvement. On readmission 6 months later, her vital capacity after frog breathing or using the respirator was up to 2,100 ml. She was using the respirator for 5–10 minutes every hour throughout the day. During this time, she continued her training as a social worker, and her admissions to the Disabled Living Unit were utilized for practical training in case work.

On one admission she was found to have an abdominal tumour, and laparotomy under spinal anaesthetic revealed a non-malignant dermoid cyst of the right ovary, which was removed. She was put into a tank respirator before the operation and immediately afterwards (the following day), and she then resumed use of the night cuirasse and the intermittent positive pressure respirator. Her post-operative recovery was quite uneventful.

She has now finished her training, qualified as a social worker, and

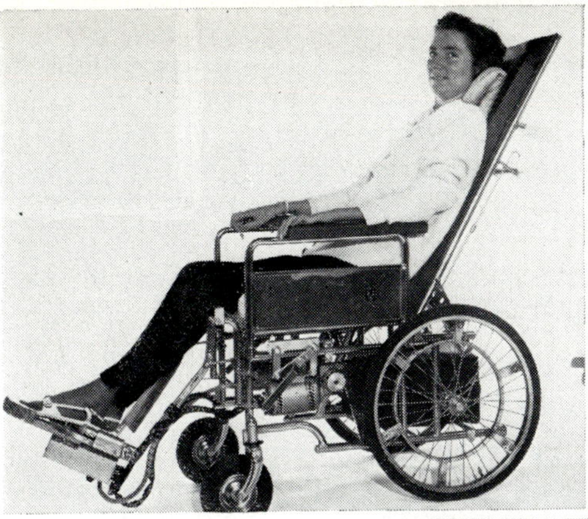

(*a*)

Figure 9.11. Patient No. 288 (a) comfortably reclined with the control box repositioned under the left foot-plate; (b) the foot control; (c) portable positive pressure respirator fixed to the back of the chair with plastic air delivery tube in her mouth

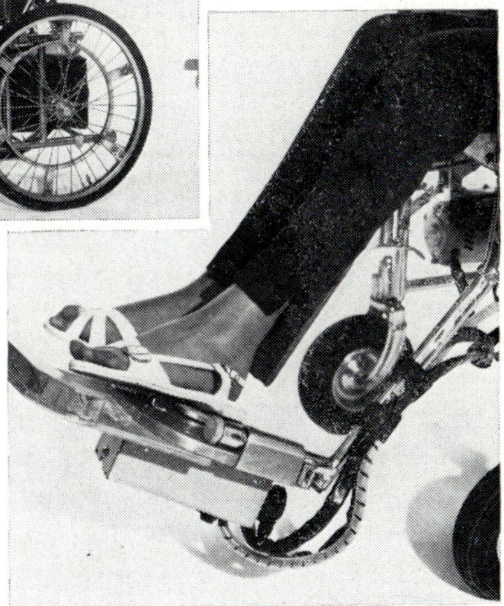

(*b*)

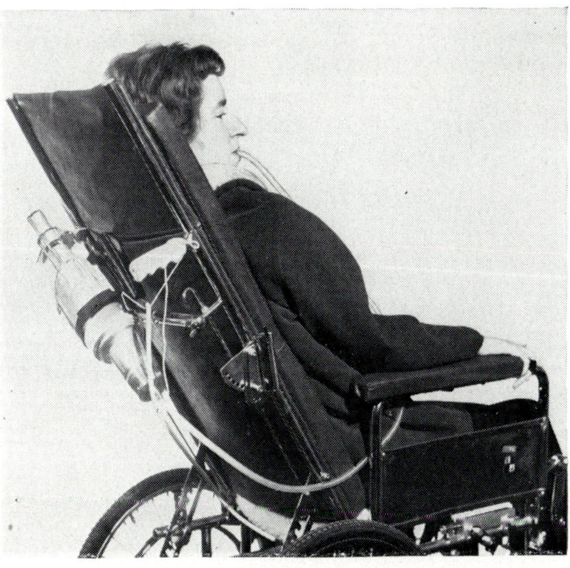

(*c*)

is working one day a week at her local hospital. Recently, she married another severely disabled patient (also suffering from paralyses after poliomyelitis) who is also working, although he too requires a portable positive-pressure respirator, and has had many admission to the Disabled Living Unit to sort out his various problems.

The couple are living in specially-adapted accommodation associated with a local authority residential home for the physically disabled.

Comment

This case history illustrates many problems and features of the rehabilitation of the severely disabled. Firstly, much of the success is due to the patient's own indomitable spirit and high motivation. Repeated assessment over many years was necessary to obtain maximal benefit from each new accomplishment. The dramatic effect of providing powered transport and so some independence of mobility, was the turning-point, as this enabled her to obtain further education and training. The diagnosis and treatment of her chronic respiratory insufficiency, which was probably accentuated by her increasing activity, was another marked step forward.

Although her vital capacity was under a litre, by careful preparation and anaesthesia she underwent major abdominal surgery with almost less disturbance and less complications than many normal patients.

Finally, she demonstrated that the severely disabled, when cared for by a sympathetic and far-sighted local authority, giving strong and sensitive backing and working in close collaboration with the Disabled Living Unit and the hospital, can achieve independence of spirit and personal dignity and happiness.

Appendices

List of Appendices

Appendix A

PRELIMINARY ASSESSMENT FORM

Name: Diagnosis:

Date: Age: Duration of disability:

Consultant
G.P.
M.S.W./W.O.
Physiotherapist
Occupational therapist
Equipment on admission
Chairbound/ambulant
Lives at home
- House
- Flat
- Bungalow

Housing difficulties
Hospital/residential home
Family consists of:

Home help
Person giving care
Nursing care needed
Schooling
Occupation
Last worked
Future occupation

Difficulties with:
- Transferring
- Dressing
- Washing
- Bathing
- Toilet
- Household
- Ironing
- Cooking
- Eating
- Shopping

Work centre
Hobbies/interests
Outdoor transport

Main objective

Secondary objective

Appendix B

THERAPIST'S DISCHARGE REPORT

Name: Age: Address:

Diagnosis: Reason for Admission: Referred by:

Date of Admission: Date of Discharge:

Home circumstances:
- Housing
- Wheelchair cushioning
- Outdoor transport
- Appliances

Physiotherapy:
- Treatment
- Future programme

Walking:

Transfers:
- Bed
- Chair
- Toilet
- Bath
- Car

Nursing report:

Personal care:
- Dressing
- Washing
- Bath
- Toilet

Cutting and eating food:

Drinking:

Household:

Hobbies:

Education:

Summary:

Re-admission plans:

Discharge report—copies to:
- G.P.
- Occupational therapist
- Physiotherapist
- Medical Social Worker
- Welfare Officer
- Technical Officer, Ministry of Health
- Artificial Limb and Appliance Centre

Appendix C

THERAPIST'S REPORT ON HOME CONDITIONS

Name: Age: Address

Diagnosis: Equipment:

Neighbourhood:
Rural; suburban; urban
Distance from shops
Transport available

Housing:
House; flat; bungalow
Owned; rented; tied
Council; private ownership
Pre-war; post-war
State of repair
Occupiers
Who gives care

Access:
From street to house
To front door (if used)
To back door (if used)

Circulation in house:
Adequate space
narrow passage; easy turn into rooms; awkward corners

Flooring:
Types—carpet; lino; polished surface
Condition
Level

Doors:
Widths
Thresholds

Stairs:
Straight; turned
State tread
Rise

Rails:
One side; both sides
Are they adequate?

Lighting:
Dark corners; passages

Alteration potential:
House structure
Furniture—heavy; light, too much

APPENDIX C

Details of rooms:

Kitchen

Surface heights—table
cooker
sink

Storage—larder; refrigerator; cupboards (doors, shelves)

Are facilities adequate?

Additional requirements:—

Bathroom

Up; down; none

Height of bath

Lavatory:

Up; down; outside

Height of seat

Patient's bedroom

Circulation space
adequate; insufficient

Height of bed

Attitude of family:

Flexible; understanding;
co-operative

Unco-operative; over-protective

Patient's activities:

Responsibilities
children
dependent relatives
business

Main problems:

To be done:

Garden:

Cultivated; otherwise used (*e.g.* children, washing)

Approximate size

Paths—level; steep; smooth; rough; firm; soft; wide; narrow

Is there a garage; shed; fuel store?

Occupational needs:

Hobby needs:

Being dealt with by:

Appendix D

SIMPLIFIED CHART FOR MUSCLE POWER
AND JOINT CONTRACTURES

Diagnosis:

		Power		*Contracture*	
		L	*R*	*L*	*R*
NECK	Flexion Extension				
UPPER TRUNK	Extension				
LOWER TRUNK	Flexion Extension Rotation *R* Rotation *L*				
HIP	Flexion Extension Abduction Adduction Internal rotation External rotation				
KNEE	Flexion Extension				
ANKLE	Dorsiflexion Plantar flexion Inversion Eversion				
FOOT	Flexion Extension				

		Power		*Contracture*	
		L	*R*	*L*	*R*
SCAPULA	Elevation Retraction Protraction Depression				
GLENOHUMERAL	Abduction Adduction Flexion Extension Internal rotation Lateral rotation				
ELBOW	Flexion Extension Pronation Supination				
WRIST	Flexion Extension				
HAND	Grip Finger extension Opposition				
	Vital capacity				

Appendix E

CHECK LIST OF ACTIVITIES OF DAILY LIVING

Bed activities:
Ring bell
Roll on to right side
Roll on to left side
Roll from back to stomach and back
Sit up from lying
Sit erect in bed
Sit erect with feet over edge of bed
Use bedpan or get out of bed to commode

Wheelchair activities:
Propel forward
Propel backward
Turn
Use brake
Propel chair on uneven ground
Mount kerb
Propel chair up slope
Propel chair down slope
Cross street at traffic lights
Wheelchair to bed
Bed to wheelchair
Wheelchair to toilet
Toilet to wheelchair
Wheelchair to bath or shower
Bath or shower to wheelchair
Open and close door
Reach floor
Wheelchair to car
Car to wheelchair

Standing and walking:
Bed to standing position
Standing position to bed

Standing and walking—(contd.)
Wheelchair to standing
Standing to wheelchair
Chair to standing (state height of chair)
Standing to chair
Toilet to standing
Standing to toilet
Bath or shower to standing
In and out of car
Walk less than 5 yd on even ground
Walk 5–10 yd on even ground
Walk more than 10 yd
Walk independently
Walk with sticks; crutches; aids
Walk on uneven ground
Walk up slope
Walk down slope

Personal care:
Blow nose
Wash face
Wash trunk and arms
Wash below the waist
Clean teeth
Brush or comb hair
Clean nails
Shave or make-up
Turn on taps
Manage bottle
Manage toilet
Use paper
Flush toilet
Get in and out of bath

Dressing:
Fastening Velcro
Fastening zips
Fastening buttons
Fastening press-studs or hooks
Put on clothes over head
Put on trousers or slacks
Brassiere
Roll-on or corset
Stockings or socks
Shoes
Jacket or cardigan
Tie
Orthopaedic appliances

Eating:
Use fork or spoon
Use both together
Cut own food
Drink with straw
Drink from cup
Reach and pick up plate

General activities:
Turn pages of book
Write name and address
Fold letter and seal envelope
Open envelope and remove letter
Type
Strike match and light cigarette
Switch light on and off
Use telephone
Wind watch
Handle money

Laundry:
Wash small clothes in sink
Rub clothes
Wring clothes

Laundry—(contd.)
Use washing machine
Use spin dryer
Peg clothes on to line
Carry laundry basket
Ironing
- Erect ironing board or prepare table for ironing
- Switch on iron
- Iron handkerchief, pillow-slip
- Iron shirt
- Refold ironing board

Kitchen:
Turn on gas/electric taps
Open oven door and move shelves
Lift cake trays in and out of oven
Lift kettle of water
Turn on tap
Fill saucepan/kettle at tap
Open tins
Cream fat and sugar
Rub in fat and flour
Roll out pastry
Cut loaf of bread
Carve meat
Spread butter
Peel vegetables
Wash up, wipe up
Open refrigerator door

Housecleaning:
Sweep floors
Vacuum-clean
Mop
Polish
Dust surfaces, high, low
Clean sink, basin, bath, toilet
Make beds

Appendix F

ASSESSMENT FORM FOR LOWER-LIMB DISABILITIES

Name: Age: Address:
Number: Date of Admission: Consultant:
Diagnosis: Occupation:
Lives in house; flat; bungalow. Family consists of:
Domiciliary care authority: Housing difficulties:
Home help needed: Nursing care needed:
Outdoor transport:

A.D.L. Check List and Progress Report

Activity	*Admission Date:*	*Progress Date:*	*Discharge Date:*	*Remarks*
Transfers				
On/off bed				
Domestic chair to standing				
Walking				
Independent				
with aid:				
sticks;				
crutches;				
calipers				
Walking distance in yards				
Stairs				
Steps				

Activity	*Admission Date:*	*Progress Date:*	*Discharge Date:*	*Remarks*
Self care				
Wash lower extremities				
Toilet, on/off				
clean self				
Bathing, in/out				
Dressing				
Stockings/socks				
Shoes				
Pants/trousers				
Calipers				
Household				
Clean floors				
Pick up from floor				
Clean grate				
Lift from oven				
Carry tray/saucepan				
Other difficulties and Summary				

Appendix G

WHEELCHAIR CLINIC QUESTIONNAIRE

Name: Hospital number:

Address:

Age: Height: Weight:

Can you walk? YES/NO
If Yes, (*a*) what distance?
(*b*) with what aids?
If No—when were you last able to?
When were you last out of the house?
Was this walking or in a chair?

Have you already got a chair or a tricycle? YES/NO
If so, is it privately owned, hired or on loan?
If on loan, from whom?

Do you want a chair for indoor use? YES/NO
If so, have you any steps indoors?
Where are these steps?
What is the width of your narrowest doorway, when measured with the door open as wide as possible?
What is the width of the passage outside this door?
What is the width of the narrowest part of the passage that the chair must go through?
How do you get about indoors now?

Do you want a chair for outdoor use? YES/NO
If so, are there steps at the front or back door?
What height are these steps?
Can you get up and down these steps?
Do you live at street level?
If not, is there a lift?
If so, what size is the lift?
If there is no lift can you get up and down the stairs?
How many flights of stairs must you climb?

Have you somewhere to keep the chair at street-level?
If not, who would take it up and down?
What is the width of the narrowest passage through which the chair must pass?
Is there someone at home to push you out?
Who is this?
What age is he/she?
If he/she in good health?
Do you live in a hilly district?
Would he/she be able to push you out of doors?

Do you want to take the chair in a car? YES/NO
If so, what make and model is the car?
Do you go regularly to a club or a day centre?
If so, is transport provided?

Appendix H

DISCHARGE REPORT FOR UPPER-LIMB AMPUTEES

Name: Date of birth: Site of amputation: *R* *L*

Cause of amputation and date:

Pre-amputation occupation: Relevant hobbies:

Dominant hand: Date of commencement of arm training:

Tolerance to prosthesis		Use of kitchen utensils	
Putting on prosthesis		Peeling vegetables	
Dressing		Washing up	
Toilet		Control of cooker	
Feeding		Baking	
Writing		Laundry	
Technical drawing		Housework	
Typing		Sewing	
Use of telephone		Knitting	
Metalwork		Ability to drive a car	
Woodwork		Conversion of car indicated	
Assembling electrical fitments			
Gardening—digging			
Gardening—long-handled tools			
Gardening shears			

Score: Excellent 4
Good 3
Fair 2
Poor 1

Special Comments:

Appliances ordered

Interviewed by D.R.O.

Ressettlement:

Completion of arm training date:

Appendix I

DISCHARGE REPORT FOR LOWER-LIMB AMPUTEES

LOWER-LIMB TRAINING REPORT

Type of prosthesis:

Flexion deformities: Knee: Hip:

Patient can put prosthesis on: Yes/No

Patient can take prosthesis off: Yes/No

Type of walking aid:

Walking ability—Flat ground
Slopes
Rough ground
Stairs

Wheelchair: Type:

Ordered/Issued/date..

Referred for outdoor transport: Yes/No

Transfers: Patient can—Stand up
Sit down
Manage lavatory
Get in and out of bed
Get in and out of bath

Social problems: Referred to:

Future walking training arrangement:

Comments:

Date:

Appendix J

SIMPLE ASSESSMENT FORM FOR HAND FUNCTION

Name:
Age:
Diagnosis:

Date:
Dominant hand:

Score for Tests: 1 = Normal
2 = Slow
3 = Not possible
P = Pain on movement

Tests for Pinch and Grasp

Type of pinch/grasp	*Objects used*	*Inner range*		*Objects used*	*Middle range*		*Objects used*	*Outer range*	
		Right	*Left*		*Right*	*Left*		*Right*	*Left*
Pulp to Pulp pinch	Pins			Pencil Tweezers			Marble		
Lateral pinch	Playing cards Key Hot water bottle			Plate			Book		
Spherical grasp	$\frac{3}{4}$-in nut and bolt Draughts			Tennis ball $2\frac{1}{2}$-in tin lid			4 in tin lid		
Cylindrical grasp	Wooden spoon			$1\frac{1}{2}$-lb hammer (*a*) grasp hammer (*b*) lift hammer (*c*) use hammer			Tumbler Full tumbler		

Strength of Pinch and Grasp

(Measured on Vigorimeter)

		Right	Left
Pulp to pulp pinch			
Lateral pinch			
Cylindrical grasp			
Sensation:	Identify—velvet		
	wool		
	rubber		
	sponge		
	metal		
	wood		
	glass paper		
Stereognosis:	Identify—buttons		
	coins		
	key		
	cigarettes		
	safety pin		
Flat hand:	Place hand flat on table		
Writing:	Time taken to write 75 words with dominant hand		

Comments

Appendix K

SOURCES OF INFORMATION IN THE UNITED KINGDOM

Information centres

Disabled Living Foundation,
346 Kensington High Street, London, W.14

The Hospital Centre,
24 Nutford Place, London W.1

Mary Marlborough Lodge,
Nuffield Orthopaedic Centre, Headington, Oxford

Organizations concerned with the disabled

Association of Occupational Therapists,
251 Brompton Road, London S.W.3

Association of Social Workers of Great Britain,
296 Vauxhall Bridge Road, London S.W.1

British Council for Rehabilitation of the Disabled,
Tavistock House South, Tavistock Square, London W.C.1

British Legion,
49 Pall Mall, London S.W.1

British Red Cross Society,
14 and 15 Grosvenor Crescent, London S.W.1

Central Council for the Disabled,
34 Accleston Square, London S.W.1

Cheshire Foundation Homes for the Sick,
7 Market Mews, London W.1

Church Army,
185 Marylebone Road, London N.W.1

Department of Education and Science,
Curzon Street, London W.1

Disabled Drivers Association,
Blue Star House, Highgate Hill, London N.6

Disabled Living Activities Group,
39 Victoria Street, London S.W.1

Disablement Income Group,
Rellen House, Bushbridge Lane, Godalming, Surrey.

Department of Health and Social Security,
Alexander Fleming House, Elephant and Castle, London S.E.1

Elderly Invalids Fund,
34 King Street, London E.C.2

Friends of the Poor and Gentlefolk's Help,
42 Ebury Street, London S.W.1

Greater London Association for the Disabled,
183 Queensway, London W.2

Institute of Welfare Officers,
56 Stamford Street, London S.E.1

Institute of Medical Social Workers,
42 Bedford Square, London W.C.1

Invalids at Home Trust,
23 Farm Avenue, London N.W.2

Joint Committee on Mobility for the Disabled,
c/o Spastics Society, 12 Park Cresent, London S.W.1

National Children's Home,
Highbury Park, London N.5

National Corporation for the Care of Old People,
Nuffield Lodge, Regents Park, London N.W.1

National Council of Social Service,
26 Bedford Square, London W.C.1

National Old People's Welfare Council,
26 Bedford Square, London W.C.1

Queens Institute of District Nursing,
57 Lower Belgrave Street, London S.W.1

Special Schools Association,
366 Yardley Wood Road, Birmingham 16

Specific disability groups

Association for Spina Bifida and Hydrocephalis Ltd.,
3 Hengist Close, Horsham, Sussex

British Epilepsy Association,
27 Nassau Street, London W.1.

British Limbless Ex-Servicemen's Association,
185–7 High Road, Chadwell Heath, Essex

British Polio Fellowship,
Clifton House, Euston Road, London N.W.1

British Rheumatism and Arthritis Association,
1 Devonshire Place, London W.1

British Association for the Hard of Hearing,
Briarfield, Syke Ings, Iver, Bucks.

British Deaf and Dumb Association,
3 Compton Street, Carlisle

British Diabetic Association,
3–6 Alfred Place, London W.C.1

British Migraine Association,
17 Bryanstone Road, Bournemouth, Hants

Chest and Heart Association,
Tavistock House North, Tavistock Square, London W.C.1

Deaf, Blind and Rubella Children's Association,
63 Horn Lane, Woodford Green, Essex

Haemophilia Society,
94 Southwark Bridge Road, London S.E.1

Ileostomy Association of Great Britain and Ireland,
Drove Cottage, Fuzzy Drove, Kempsholt, Basingstoke, Hants

Invalid Children's Aid Association,
4 Palace Gate, London W.8

Multiple Sclerosis Society,
10 Stratford Road, London W.8

Muscular Dystrophy Group,
26 Borough High Street, London S.E.1

National Society for Mentally Handicapped Children,
5 Bulstrode Street, London W.1.

National Society for Autistic Children,
100 Wise Lane, Mill Hill, London N.W.7

National Deaf Children's Society,
31 Gloucester Place, London W.1

College of Speech Therapists,
68 Queen's Gardens, London W.2

National Children's Home,
85 Highbury Park, London N.5

Royal National Institute for the Blind,
224 Great Portland Street, London W.1

Royal National Institute for the Deaf,
105 Gower Street, London W.C.1

The Responauts,
39 Essex Street, Newbury, Berks.

Society for the Aid of Thalidomide Children,
28 Four Acres Walk, Hemel Hempstead, Herts.

Shaftesbury Society,
112 Regency Street, London S.W.1

Spastic Society,
12 Park Crescent, London W.1

Select list of organizations holding information which may be of use to the disabled

British Standards Institution,
2 Park Street, London W.1

The Building Centre,
26 Store Street, London W.C.1

British Electrical Approval Board,
Mark House, 153 London Road, Kingston upon Thames

The Design Centre,
28 Haymarket, London S.W.1

Electrical Development Association (or Home Economist of local Electricity Board),
2 Savoy Hill, London W.C.2

Gas Council (or Home Adviser of local Gas Board),
4 Grosvenor Place, London S.W.1

The Heating Centre,
34 Mortimer Street, London W.1

Home Economists of Great Britain,
Kensington Square, London W.8.

International Wool Secretariat,
Wool House, Carlton House, London S.W.1

Royal Society for the Prevention of Accidents,
Terminal House, 52 Grosvenor Gardens, London S.W.1

Appendix L

SUMMARY OF REGULATIONS GOVERNING THE PROVISION OF MEDICAL AND SURGICAL APPLIANCES IN THE NATIONAL HEALTH SERVICE

The procedures for prescribing, ordering and supplying appliances are published from time to time by the Department of Health and Social Security. Details vary according to current legislation and arrangements.

The duty of the Minister under the National Health Service Act, 1946 is to promote the establishment of a comprehensive health service, including the provision of surgical, medical and other appliances. This provision is effected (1) through the general medical and pharmaceutical services; and (2) through the hospital and specialist services.

Local health authorities have wide discretionary powers under section 28 of the Act and local welfare authorities have permissive powers under section 29 of the National Assistance Act, 1948 to arrange for works of adaptation in the homes of the physically handicapped people and to provide some additional facilities.

A patient who wants a more expensive appliance than those normally provided through the hospital and specialist services must make his own arrangements and meet the whole cost, except for spectacles and dentures, when a patient may elect to pay the additional cost of more expensive types approved by the Minister.

It is for the consultant dealing with the patient to prescribe whatever appliance is considered necessary for the patient's condition.

If, however, the clinical needs of a patient can be met by the provision of a standard article such as may be worn as an item of normal clothing (for example, footwear, corsets or brassieres), or such an article suitably adapted, specially made appliances are not supplied under the National Health Service but the patient must purchase the item privately. Any adaptations considered clinically necessary by the consultant should be carried out free of charge to the patient either by the hospital or by firms in contract with the Ministry. Where garments are to be provided by the patient for adaptation, the hospital should give advice on the type of article considered most suitable.

The consultant is responsible for ensuring that each completed appliance conforms to the prescription and is satisfactory in manufacture, fit and function when fitted to the patient.

If a consultant prescribes for the treatment of a patient an appliance or article which is not available under the Ministry's central contracts (for example, crutches, oxygen equipment, tracheotomy equipment, low visual aids, and so on), then usually the hospitals should make their own arrangements for the purchase of the item and issue it to the patient on loan for as long as it is required. Hospital authorities are responsible for the installation and/or maintenance of such items where necessary.

Invalid chairs and tricycles

Invalid tricycles and wheelchairs can be provided through the hospital and specialist services in accordance with the following principles:

(1) Power-propelled tricycles can be provided by the Department on the recommendation of a consultant for:

(*a*) patients who have one leg amputated above the knee and the other amputated either above or below the knee;

(*b*) patients suffering from paraplegia or other defect of the locomotor system equivalent to the total or almost total loss of use of both legs so that the patient is to all intent and purposes unable to walk;

(*c*) patients slightly less severely disabled with very limited walking ability who because of the disability need a machine to get to and from work.

Note: Patients suffering from non-locomotor disabilities may now be included in this category.

(2) Hand-propelled tricycles can be similary provided for:

(*a*) patients in the above categories who are not recommended for a power-propelled tricycle;

(*b*) other patients with very limited walking ability for whom the consultant considers one necessary.

(3) Wheelchairs, including spinal carriages, can be provided for patients whose disabilities are such that the consultant considers such provision necessary. An indoor and/or transit chair can be supplied as well as motor- or hand-propelled tricycle when considered necessary. Where patients temporarily require a chair the local health authority should be asked if they can provide one; or one may be loaned from the hospital's own stock.

(4) Electrically-propelled indoor chairs can be provided for patients who are not only unable to walk because of some disability affecting their legs, but who, because of weakness in their arms, are also unable to propel themselves in a wheelchair if, but only if, this will help them to achieve some measure of independence in the home.

Recommendations for the provision of power-propelled tricycles should be forwarded to the nearest Ministry of Health Appliance Centre on Form A.O.F. 6. Each individual case is carefully considered by the Ministry's medical and technical officers who have special experience in this field. It is for the Ministry's officers to ascertain the facts about employment in the cases envisaged in paragraph 1(*c*) above and to determine by practical tests the patient's ability to drive. In cases of progressive nervous or neuro-muscular disease, a consultant physician's assurance that the patient is fit to control a power-propelled tricycle is necessary.

A patient who is eligible for a power-propelled tricycle, may, as an alternative, ask the Department to have the controls of his motor-car adapted to enable him to drive, but such conversions cannot be undertaken more than once in 5 years. Where patients for whom consultants would recommend a power-propelled tricycle are interested in this alternative, they should be referred to the Manager at the nearest Ministry of Health Appliance Centre, to whom the recommendation for a power-propelled tricycle should also be sent, and who can advise patients about firms doing this work.

Cars may be provided instead of power-propelled tricycles for:

(i) two related members of the same household both of whom are eligible for tricycles or where one is so eligible and the other blind;

(ii) a disabled widow or widower eligible for an invalid tricycle who has to care for a child.

It will be necessary to examine applicants to ensure that they are capable of controlling a car.

The patient with two leg amputations, one above the knee, receives special mention in category of paragraph 1(*a*) because there are some patients with these disabilities for whom walking, though possible, is such a strain that a tricycle should be provided to prevent damage. Some patients falling within category 1(*b*) are chronic invalids who could only make occasional use of a power-propelled machine and it is hoped that consultants will take this into account in their assessments and refrain from recommending a power-propelled machine. The Ministry is receiving an increasing number of recommendations for elderly patients where a locomotor disability is worsened by the general cumulative effects of old age; consultants are asked not to recommend power-propelled tricycles for the elderly unless their limitations in walking strikingly exceed the normal limitations due to advancing age and where a hand-propelled tricycle or wheelchair would not suffice.

Patients suffering from what may be termed non-locomotor disabilities (that is, vascular or respiratory ailments) with very limited walking ability, who are in full-time employment will qualify for a powered machine to get to work on the same terms as those with locomotor defects.

Before a patient can get a tricycle in category 1 (*c*) he must have a job or a firm promise of a job. Tricycles are not issued to enable patients to look for work. Eligibility in this category depends (if the medical case is accepted) on whether the particular journey to work is beyond the patient's capacity. The consultant need not delay, however, in recommending a patient who intends to seek work, if he considered that the patient is medically eligible; the Ministry will be glad to consider such cases. Because the difficulties of the journey to work cannot be established until the job is found, no promise of a tricycle can be given at this stage; but if the medical case is accepted, the patient (and the consultant) will be told that, if he obtains a job, and the journey to work is one which in the opinion of the Ministry he cannot be expected to make without a tricycle, one will be supplied quickly. The local offices of the Department of Employment and Productivity will see that the patient is enabled to attend for interview wherever there is a possible opening for employment, and can also sometimes help with temporary difficulties in getting to work.

In general, the Department's consideration is concerned with seeing that the patients recommended for the supply of a power-propelled tricycle do fall into one of the three categories of eligibility, as the Minister interprets them. Experience shows that most of the applications rejected by the Department (other than those rejected on non-medical grounds) fall into two groups:

(1) Patients recommended as being in category 1 (*c*) who may have difficulties with their journey to work but who cannot be said to have very limited walking ability. The Minister could not normally accept a patient who can walk several hundred yards as eligible for

supply of a tricycle under the National Health Service, whatever the effect on his employment.

(2) Patients recommended as being in category 1(*b*) with disabilities other than paraplegia where the effect of the disability on the locomotor system is not such that to all intents and purposes the patient can be said to be unable to walk.

Generally speaking, appliances which are required for the continued active treatment of out-patients and discharged in-patients should be supplied by the hospital. Articles required for home nursing are normally provided by local health authorities. Where there is any difficulty in determining for which of these purposes the appliance is mainly required, the hospital should assume responsibility for supply if the item has to be specially made for the individual patient. The permanence of the patient's need for the appliance can also justify supply by the hospital but only if it is impossible to apply the foregoing criteria.

If, in borderline cases, the hospital and local health authority should be unable to agree as to who should accept liability for supply, the patient should not be deprived of the use of an item of equipment while the question of financial responsibility is being explored. Whilst the local health authorities' powers under the National Health Service Act, 1946, section 28 are entirely discretionary, they are also very wide and the extent, therefore, to which authorities may be prepared to use them may well be found to vary from area to area. If agreement cannot be reached at once, the hospital should provide the equipment as a matter of expediency and the financial question should be settled later, in consultation, if necessary, with the Ministry of Health, Supply Division (S.5), 14 Russell Square, London, W.C.1.

It is important, however, that any necessary equipment should be made available to the patient as soon as he is discharged. Therefore, when a hospital is about to discharge an in-patient or is treating an out-patient, who in the opinion of the consultant, should be provided with some items of equipment for home care, the hospital should notify the requirements of the case to the local health authority in whose area the patient resides, as soon as possible.

When equipment is provided under section 28 of the Act, the local health authority may recover from patients such charges as are considered reasonable having regard to the means of the patient concerned.

Local welfare authorities have permissive powers under section 29 of the National Assistance Act, 1948 to assist substantially and permanently handicapped people in arranging for the carrying out of works of adaptation in their homes and the provision of additional facilities required for their comfort and convenience. These powers are wide in scope, but the following examples may serve to illustrate some of the ways in which many local welfare authorities are willing to assist physically-handicapped people resident in their areas.

The provision of ramped access to homes.

The widening of doors to allow the passage of wheelchairs.

The provision of bath and toilet facilities at ground-floor level.

Alterations to kitchen fittings to make them more convenient for the disabled user.

The re-location of taps or the substitution of lever handles for conventional fittings.

The provision of driveways for invalid tricycles.

The local welfare authority may recover from persons availing themselves of the service such charges (if any) as they may determine.

Under the provisions of the Chronically Sick and Disabled Persons Act, 1970, many of the permissive powers of Local Authorities have been withdrawn and statutory duties have been created. Some of this legislation is coming into force in 1970 and further implementation will take place later. In brief, Health and Welfare Authorities concerned are to be required to ensure that they are adequately informed of the numbers and needs of the substantially and permanently handicapped, and that those who might benefit by help should know what help is available. The Authorities are required to assess the needs and provide the necessary practical forms of help in the home as well as providing personal aids. Further statutory steps have been taken towards the removal of physical and architectural barriers to mobility, both in private dwellings and in public buildings.

Appendix M

DRESSING FOR SPECIFIC DISABILITIES

Cardiac cripples and bronchitis

With such patients, dressing and undressing is not so much a problem of mechanics as one of conservation of energy, and therefore no special adaptations to clothes are necessary. Whenever possible, the number of garments to be put on should be reduced, and heavy clothes should be avoided; for example, a light warm pullover should be worn rather than a jacket.

These patients are at their worst first thing in the morning and it is necessary to develop a streamlined routine which allows plenty of time and privacy: hurry and worry are exhausting. The major part of the routine of dressing can be carried out in the sitting position. Because of the likelihood of giddiness, patients should avoid struggling with head bent down, and therefore should place the foot up on a chair or stool to put on socks, shoes and trousers.

Hip lesions, arthritis, arthrodesis

Even when arms and hands are unaffected, patients with arthritis or arthrodesis of the hip experience difficulty in coping with all garments put on over the feet and pulled up to the waist, with socks, stockings or shoes and with calipers.

When one hip is fixed, it may be possible to put on stockings, socks or pants by lying on the bed on the unaffected side, flexing the knee on the affected side as far as possible and reaching back to pull the garment over the foot. When calipers are worn, the patient should not stand without them, and socks, shoes and calipers must therefore be put on while on the bed, or seated beside the bed. Most elderly disabled patients will need help to put on a full-length caliper; younger patients may learn to put it on themselves.

Putting trousers on over a caliper is difficult and it may be helpful to insert a zip in the inner leg seam from ankle to knee. This should open from the bottom up, so that it can be closed by pushing down the slide with a dressing-stick.

If a caliper is not worn, socks, stockings and shoes are put on from a sitting position on the side of the bed, with the help of a stocking aid and a shoehorn or long-handled reacher. Alternatively, if the patient's balance is good he may stand with his back to a chair, bend his knee and place his foot on the chair and reach back with one hand to pull on socks and shoes.

If lace-up shoes are worn, it is possible to do them up with a dressing-stick, or elastic laces may be used. In either case, one side of the top of the tongue of the shoe should be permanently stitched to the shoe's upper, and a long shoehorn used to position the shoe and steady it while the foot is pushed in.

Putting on pants and trousers may also require a long-handled reacher, but a skirt is best put on over the head and pulled down and adjusted when standing. If necessary, the placket opening can be lengthened.

Women may find 'petti-pants' helpful as they can be put on over the head or wide-legged pants can be adapted with a gusset opening.

Rheumatoid arthritis

Patients with severe rheumatoid arthritis have perhaps the greatest problems in dressing as it is impeded by stiff and painful joints, weak grip and deformity. The pain and stiffness is usually more severe in the morning when the major activity of toilet and dressing has to be tackled.

The characteristic limitations of movement in shoulders and elbows leads to difficulty in reaching beyond front mid-trunk range, that is, in putting on garments with inset sleeves, in pulling up over the shoulders, pulling up over the hips, tucking shirt into trousers or vest into pants, reaching neck fastenings, and reaching fastenings at back of neck and back of waist.

Since rheumatoid arthritis usually affects knees, ankles and hips and these joints may be stiff and painful, such patients often have difficulty in standing. They therefore have difficulties in putting on clothes for the lower half of their body as well as the upper half.

As a general rule, women will find clothes which can be put on over the head easier to cope with than those which open right down the front. Some patients prefer a vest and waist slip, while others find a 'princess-style' petticoat of heavier weight, or of brushed nylon, serves as vest and slip combined. All these clothes can be put on by the same method—the garment is gathered in both hands from the hem upwards and held open at the neck, the arms are raised as high as possible supporting the elbows on a table if necessary and the head bent forward and ducked into the garment; it is then wriggled and worked down, using a dressing-stick to adjust. Some patients with very limited shoulder movement become very adept at raising a garment over the head with a dressing-stick.

A Lycra brassiere with the back fastening sewn up is usually sufficient, or if a patient needs more support she can wear a front-fastening brassiere modified by a Velcro pull-through fastening.

If a light suspender belt is sufficient support, a maternity belt is the best buy, as its back suspenders are positioned well forward within easy reach. For those who need it, a front-fastening corset with Kempner pull buckles may be worn, or an all-in-one 'liberty bodice' type of corset which is soft and easy to pull on, and has elastic-shanked, button fastenings. It is impossible for anyone with weak and painful hands to pull up a roll-on type of girdle.

Patients with stiff and painful shoulders and limited elbow flexion find it difficult to get their arms into garments with inset sleeves. For this reason, a skirt which can be put on over the head and a loose-fitting jumper with raglan sleeves are the easiest outer clothes to wear. The sleeves of the jumper should be drawn well up on the arms before the garment is put over the head.

For those with very limited arm movements, the sleeve seams and side seams can be opened under the arm so that the bent elbow can more easily be pushed into the sleeve, and the opening fastened by pushing together dabs of Velcro. Lightweight quilted anoraks or woollen jersey coats with foam interlining and with raglan sleeves are particularly suitable. A spring-steel buttonhook will help with conventional fastenings, or Velcro may be substituted for buttons.

Men with severe rheumatoid arthritis have similar problems of dressing. They usually find that a loose-fitting terylene overshirt is easier to put on than a coat-style shirt, and also avoids the difficulty of tucking the shirt into trousers. Vests can be cut short to avoid tucking in, and underpants buttoned, or held with Velcro on to trousers, so that both garments can be put on as one. Trousers may be pulled on by the braces, but long-handled reachers may be needed to pull them over the feet. The main difficulty with socks is often found in pulling these over stiff ankles and a shortened gutter aid may help.

Hemiplegia

The functional disability of hemiplegia is not simply 'one-handedness' as other disabling features such as confusion, loss of sensation, loss of balance and loss of spatial sense may also affect the patient's ability to dress himself.

A prolonged period of training is often necessary, and the routine adopted should be simple and practised in a quiet, unhurried atmosphere. One process should be taught at a time, and it is suggested that managing clothes for toilet should be learned first.

A simple routine for a woman when going to the toilet is to take the back of the skirt and petticoat up together and tuck the hem into the waistband at the back, then lift and tuck into the waistband at the front. This leaves the hand free to cope with pants and with cleaning herself. The pants are pulled down over the iliac crests at both sides, and then down over the buttocks on the affected side first. If these manoeuvres are too difficult for older patients, adapted split knickers may be worn.

Men hemiplegics will find it helpful to wear braces both to pull the trousers up when dressing, and to loop over the affected forearm to prevent the trousers falling to the ground while going to the toilet. Underpants should be attached to the trousers by means of the braces, or by means of Velcro fastenings.

Button fly-fastenings are easier than zip fastenings to manage with one hand.

When a satisfactory toilet regimen has been achieved, the whole process of independent dressing may be tackled, starting on the bed with socks, stockings corsets and pants. The patients can then progress to sitting on the side of the bed with support available on the affected side, or sitting on a stable chair beside the bed.

Because of the likelihood of falling towards the paralysed side, everything which will be needed during dressing and undressing should be placed to the side of the unaffected hand. A table in front of the patient to take the weight of garments is often helpful.

Women will find the pull-front type of corsets the most easily managed, as the Kempner type of buckle can be loosely fastened first, and then tightened as the corset position is adjusted. The easiest method to put on the corset is by lying on the bed and rolling onto it. If the abdomen is drawn in when tightening the buckles, very little re-adjustment should be necessary when the patient stands.

Back suspenders should be repositioned, moving them well forward to the side of the corset. Suspenders can be fastened with one hand with practice and it is easier to fasten them sitting down when there is less stretch on the elastic. Alternatively, they may be fitted on to the stockings separately and then hooked on to the corset.

Front-fastening brassieres with adapted fastenings; Velcro pull-through systems, Kempner buckles or buttons on elastic shanks, can be more easily managed with one hand than the conventional garments.

For upper garments, the general routine to follow is: affected arm in first, out last. For over-the-head garments: affected arm in, head through, sound arm in. If some confusion is present, it may help to mark the sleeves for the affected arm with a coloured tag. Garments with some stretch in the material are easiest to manage, and all over-the-head clothes should in addition have wide neck openings.

Those patients with sensory disturbance can be helped by teaching the habit of looking to see that the sleeve is not twisted, and that the cuff is properly positioned. A tape loop sewn on the inside of the shirt cuff on the affected side can be looped over the thumb to hold the shirt down when putting on a pullover or jacket.

Skirts are best put on over the head and adjusted when standing. Fastening a waistband can be difficult, but drawing in the abdomen will make it easier to oppose the fastening with one hand. Velcro fastenings can be fastened loosely at first and then adjusted, or a horizontal-slide zip fastening may be used. In the presence of a vertical zip placket, the lower end of the zip may be held down against the body by the affected hand, or by leaning up against a piece of furniture, but zips in general are not easy to manage with one hand, especially when the placket flap or undergarments have to be tucked in. The final stages of arranging skirts or fastening trousers can usually be done standing, hooking the affected arm over a bar for support, or leaning on a solid piece of furniture.

For hemiplegic patients, as for patients with cardiac or bronchitic lesions, bending with the head down should be avoided, whether to put on socks or stockings or pull up pants and trousers over the feet. These garments can be put on by placing the foot of the affected side upon a stool, or across the opposite knee.

Trousers are pulled over the affected foot first, but should not be pulled above the knee, as it will then be difficult to put in the other leg. The trousers are pulled up most easily by braces which, as has been said earlier, can be looped over the affected arm before standing to prevent the trousers falling. If standing balance is very poor, the trousers may be pulled up over the seat by rolling from side to side in the chair.

A technique for pulling on heavy jackets or coats is as follows: Place the jacket on a table beside the seated patient, on his affected side. This will take the weight of the garment and prevent it slipping off again each time the grip is freed from the sleeve as it is pulled up. Pull the sleeve up the paralysed limb with the other hand, working it round the elbow joint and avoiding putting a hand up the sleeve in an attempt to pull the paralysed arm down. Persist in pushing the sleeve up, occasionally slipping the hand under the armhole of the jacket and pushing up into the armpit, and finally lifting it up on to the shoulder; once there, the danger of the jacket slipping off is less, but it can still do so, especially if there is a slippery lining and if the bulk of the garment has slipped off the supporting table.

Re-arrange the garment if necessary, so that the armhole will be accessible for the second arm and then, while holding the lapel on the affected side firmly down with the chin, turn away from the table and reach round to the back with the normal arm into the second armhole. 'Shrug' the jacket up on to the shoulders, and finally give an extra pull up over the point of the shoulder on the side of the paralysed arm.

Paraplegia

The main dressing problems of the paraplegic patients are due to spasm; danger of damage to skin; and incontinence.

It is safest to do most of the dressing of the lower half of the body on the bed, where spasm will not result in a fall and extremities are less likely to suffer skin abrasions. If there is no spasm, the dressing can be more easily carried out in the wheelchair.

Incontinence presents special difficulties. Underpants may have to be adjusted to wear over urinary appliances. Women may need special waterproof pants and disposable pads. When a urinary appliance is worn, it is helpful to have a zip inserted in the lower inside seam of the trouser leg (opening from the bottom upward), both for the ease of dressing and to empty the urine bag during the day.

Calipers, if used, should be put on while on the bed, and in this case men may need long zips in the inside trouser seams.

Smooth-fitting stretch-socks avoid abrasive wrinkles inside the shoes, but they should not be tight nor have elastic tops. The inside of shoes should also be inspected frequently for wear and abrasive snags.

A short coat, cloak or poncho, is more comfortable than a full-length coat in a wheelchair, as a long coat may ruckle under the seat and cause pressure on the skin of the buttocks. Leather reinforcements on the inner side of the jacket sleeves will protect them from hard wear from the propelling wheels of a chair.

Tetraplegia

The main dressing problems of a tetraplegic patient are due to inadequate sitting balance, loss of hand-grip, spasms, danger of skin abrasions, incontinence, and excessive sweating.

Dressing is usually a slow and exhaustive procedure and most tetraplegics will need help in dressing their lower half, and in putting on a spinal brace or corset if one is worn. If independent dressing is aimed at, it is advisable to avoid garments which need to be pulled on over the head, as sight is necessary to maintain balance for these patients.

When hand grip is impaired, strategically-placed tape-loops sewn into garments are invaluable; a finger or thumb may be hooked into the loop for pulling. Rubber thimbles on the index fingers can also help a patient to get a grip on garments. Sleeves can be pushed up or down by rubbing the forearm against the body. Dabs of Velcro can replace buttons, though a spring-steel buttonhook, if this can be handled, will make it possible to cope with buttons. Zips will need a key-ring attached to the runner tag.

The lower half may be most easily dressed with the patient sitting on the bed, supported by a backrest, thus leaving both hands free. Conversely, clothes above the waist are usually put on while sitting in the wheelchair in front of a table on which to support the elbows. If spasm in the legs is likely to throw the patient off balance while dressing, a quick-release restraining strap may be used across the knees.

To put on a jacket or cardigan, the patient lays it out on the table collar towards self and lining uppermost. Both hands are pushed into the sleeves, and the jacket thrown back over the head, at the same time ducking the head forward. The arms are then pushed through, and the garment is gradually pulled down and tidied.

Because of the danger of losing his balance, a patient should practice this repeatedly with someone in attendance, before it is attempted independently.

For a woman, a wrap-round kilt with half-length slip attached can be laid in the chair before transferring, if a self-operated hoist is used, but would of course be displaced if transfer is by sliding-board.

The question of whether or not it is better for a girl to wear slacks or a skirt must be considered in the context of her individual needs. A skirt is easier to put on, and easier for the toilet; slacks are warmer, can be grasped to lift the legs when transferring, and will prevent any embarrassment if a patient is frequently lifted from the wheelchair.

A tetraplegic patient will have great difficulty in securing the conventional stud-type suspender for stockings; the back one can in any case be dispensed with if she is always in a wheelchair. Stockings can be elastic-topped providing they are not tight.

A woman who has to go to the toilet on her own during the day, and has difficulty managing her pants, may dispense with wearing them and simply sit on a soft absorbent towel.

Ataxia—Inco-ordination

The patient with advanced multiple sclerosis has all the problems of the tetraplegic patient, including spasm which is often severe, plus an intention tremor and possibly impairment of sight. When this stage is reached, independent dressing becomes impracticable.

The patient with unwanted movement and inco-ordination such as the patient with athetoid cerebral palsy, on the other hand, can sometimes become completely independent in dressing even though the ataxia is severe, as this type of patient is not often easily fatigued, and persistent and repeated practice in a calm atmosphere will often give good results.

Whenever possible, fastenings should be avoided. Loose-fitting clothes of strong stretchy material which go over the head are better than those of jacket type. Raglan sleeves are easier to manage than inset sleeves. Buttons on strong elastic or tape shanks are most easily managed, as Velcro may be difficult to position correctly, and may prove to be not secure enough to stand up to the continual pull of athetoid movement. Zips are difficult to manage, and tend to get caught up in other clothes. Any vulnerable parts of garments, neck openings or pockets should be reinforced with tape or extra machine stitching. Outer jackets should be lined with slippery material.

Elastic-sided shoes, although easier to put on, may not be strong enough for this type of patient. Tying the laces of laced shoes is very difficult, but firm shoes may be necessary and they may have to be reinforced at the toes. The tongue of the shoe must be firmly sewn to the upper at one side to keep it in place while pushing the foot into the shoe. The loop-knot method of tying a bow may be achieved with practice, as an alternative to the one-hand method, when the long end of the lace is tucked into the shoe at the ankle. Patients with severe ataxia will most likely require assistance with tying their shoes.

Amputees

Single amputees whether upper or lower limb, have little difficulty in dressing, though practice will be required for the short above-knee and the 'through shoulder' amputee. Bilateral lower-limb amputees are usually able to dress and undress independently, though such patients are predominantly in the upper age range and may find the process slow and tiring. Double arm amputees will have considerable difficulties, and a bilateral above-elbow amputee will probably need some help.

Below-knee amputees will usually dress while seated on the side of the bed. Above-knee amputees will get dressed on the bed, lying back to position the socket at the ischial tuberosity.

Use of the right size of stump-sock and ensuring that no creases or folds are formed when putting it on are both important in the maintenance of a healthy condition of the stump. If left *in situ* when the prosthetic cup is in place, the sock should not be pulled too tightly over the stump end. Some amputees attach a piece of tape to the tip of the stump-sock, so that, when the sock is put on, the tape can be threaded out through the ventilation hole of the socket, enabling the wearer not only to pull the stump into the socket, but to pull the tip of the sock away from the end of the stump and by so doing to eliminate creases.

Many patients with one artificial leg find it easiest to dress the artificial limb with pants, trousers, and shoe before fitting it on the stump and before dressing the sound leg. Others, in order not to pass a dirty shoe through the clothes, put the shoe on last, that is after the leg has been passed through the clothing. Bilateral lower-limb amputees dress both artificial limbs completely before fitting them onto the stumps.

The sock on the artificial foot will wear out quickly if the shoe is a loose fit on the foot. Less damage is done if a thick undersock is used. When buying socks, it is advisable to buy more than one pair of exactly the same pattern, since the sock on the artificial foot wears out more quickly than the sock on the normal one. It is difficult to keep sock suspenders from slipping down on the artificial leg, but metal studs can be riveted or screwed onto the shin by the limb-makers, to hold the suspender in the proper place.

The sole of the shoe should be flexible in walking and should bend easily with the joint movement of the artificial foot. It will add to comfort if the shoe of the artificial leg is kept in good repair and not allowed to get worn down at the heel. Women with amputations above the knee should decide what height of shoe heel they intend to wear, and this should not be varied without reference to the Limb Fitting Centre, because the alignment and stability of the limb may be affected by such change. There is less risk for the below-knee prosthesis wearer in such circumstances, but any gross change of height of heel should be reported to the Limb Fitting Centre.

Stockings can be protected by stocking-guards. Women may also prefer to have a flock or matt finish to their limbs instead of a polished finish which tends to show through their stockings.

Trousers may need to be protected from damage either by a clothing pad of leather fixed to the back of the thigh-piece by the limbmaker, or by a lining inserted into the back of the trouser leg, to prevent wear by the artificial limb. Joints on artificial limbs should be provided with leather or plastic protective covers.

When a single artificial arm is used, the patient will quickly learn to put this on himself. The prosthesis is laid on a table and the stump is pushed well into it, the support harness being pulled up on the stump shoulder, and the axillary loop hanging down the back. The stump is then raised quickly. At the same time, the patient reaches back with the other hand through the axillary loop and the shoulders are shrugged as if putting on a jacket. It is easier for the artificial arm to be put into garments first when dressing, and taken out last when undressing. It is usually worn over a vest and under a shirt.

The usual procedure for putting on a pair of artificial arms is as follows. Lay the prostheses on a table or bed with the arms extended in front of the body, and with the back cross strap placed centrally. Thrust the dominant stump into the socket from the medial side, between the control strap and Y-strap. Place the harness across the shoulder on the dominant side, allowing the opposite prosthesis to dangle down the back. Turn the body so that the hanging prosthesis is supported on the table with the hook forwards. Reach with the non-dominant stump round the back, and push it into the socket. Shrug on to the shoulders.

This process can be readily learned by the below-elbow and above-elbow amputee with long stumps, but high above-elbow amputees, and through-shoulder amputees will need help in putting on their prostheses.

Clothes for these patients should be loose fitting, as they will have to withstand friction from the prostheses. Man-made fibres or wool-and-nylon mixtures are the best. Tucking clothes into trousers or skirts is almost impossible with artificial hands, so it is best to wear overshirts or overblouses.

It is particularly difficult for the above-elbow amputee to reach fastenings to the centre line of the body. Front trouser fastenings present a particularly difficult problem, but a zip fitted with a ring-tag can sometimes be managed with a short, curved dressing-stick.

Appendix N

SOLVING EATING AND DRINKING PROBLEMS

Activity	*Problem*	*Problem solving*
General		
Access to table in wheelchair	Close access to table in wheelchair	Desk arms on wheelchair. Dining-table of suitable height with sufficient clearance under for knees, and no obstructing cross-bars. Dining-table not too narrow, nor against wall, to accommodate footplates. Cantilever table. Tray table on wheelchair. Special tray on Monodrive etc.
Access for semi-ambulant	Stiff hips/knees	High dining-chair needed, correspondingly higher table. Tray on armchair
	Reach	Reach in horizontal plane is assisted by having table at such a height that the elbows and forearms can rest on the table.
Stability		Where any ataxia or inco-ordination, or spasm, important that furniture is heavy and stable.
	Access to table when sitting in bed	Suitable back rest, giving stability and leaving arms free. Overbed table. Bed tray.
	Lying	When necessary to eat lying flat, plate can be balanced on chest or on bed trays. A bed mirror is then useful to see plate.

Solving Eating and Drinking Problems—*continued*

Activity	*Problem*	*Problem solving*
Ease of cleaning	Spilling food	Formica-topped table. Plastic tablecloth. P.V.C. upholstery on chairs. Plenty of paper napkins available. If 'bib' is needed, it is unobtrusive if made of the same material as blouse/dress and backed with plastic foam and waterproof plastic material.
	Athetoid children	Plastic overall with sleeve or plastic bib and oversleeves with elastic cuffs.
Aids to arm/hand function		
Special table and accessories	Limited range of movement; table to mouth	Adjustable-height table, use elbow height for writing, raised for eating. Small box table, to required height stood on dining table, must be heavy based to give stability, or clip to table edge. Ditto with hole cut out for plate or bowl to drop in.
	Inability to scoop feed up from whole plate.	Turntable for plate.
	Weakness of elbow flexors	An elbow ring pad suitably placed on table will give pivot point for elbows without risk of pressure-sore.
Arm supports and splints	Partial paralysis of arms and fatigue	Mobile arm-supports—straight pivot or supinator. Accessories: T-bar; spork. Overhead slings; not often used over a chair now, but are used for some meals over a bed (mobile arm-supports are very difficult to position in bed)
	Weakness of wrist	Appropriate splint for wrist; usually wrist-extension support.
	Poor grasp	Appropriate hand splint. Opponens splints. Metacarpophalangeal flexion splint. Flexor-hinge splint.
Aids to control ataxia/tremor	Athetoid movements and tremor	Weighted cuffs 'damp down' unwanted movement in many cases. Stabilizing wrist in simple wrist extension splint may help.

Solving Eating and Drinking Problems—*continued*

Activity	*Problem*	*Problem solving*
		In few cases, and with much practice and supervision, friction arm-supports may help, but are not generally useful.
	Arm and hand tremor, plus tremor of head as in disseminated sclerosis	Use thick plastic spoon or plastic-coated spoon, to minimize cutting of lips and gums.
		Stabilize head with 'wing' head-rest and feed with spoon.
		Once head tremor becomes pronounced, much better to give up independent feeding. Risk of cutting face with spoon or fork must be assessed for each individual.
Plates and table-ware		
Stability	Plate moving on a table	Important that plate is held still. Non-slip mats. Rubber suction pads ('Octopus'). Damp Wettex cloth. Dicem.
	Inco-ordination and tremor	Heavy plate, on mats (as above), or plate fitting into cut-out in tray or table, or suction pads fitted to base of bowl.
Design	Inability to 'catch' food on plate	Ideally, plate with low rim at point of entry of spoon, and high rim on opposite side to push against, as Manoy Melaware.
		Clip-on plate buffer guard.
		Plate with deep rim, such as child's plate.
	Slowness in eating or swallowing	Specially-heated plate.
		Plate placed over soup plate of hot water.
Material	Arm and hand weakness	Lightweight plastic plates are easy to handle and can be stabilized on rubber mat.
	Inco-ordination and tremor	Heavy china plates give more stability, but plastic does not break easily when dropped.
	Egg cups	Suction-based egg-cups.
		Broad-based children's plastic egg-cups.
Cutlery	Inability to pick up and grasp cutlery	In severe cases, T-bar and spork.
		Long oppenens splint and cutlery clip.
		Various handles to aid grasp to suit

Solving Eating and Drinking Problems—*continued*

Activity	*Problem*	*Problem solving*
		individual, such as built-up handles, using rubber, felt or plastic.
		Extended handle with grip over back of hand.
		Careful selection of cutlery on the market.
		Much stainless steel too clumsy, heavy and slippery.
		Avoid cutlery which lies flat to table and difficult to pick up.
		A slight upward tilt at end of handle helps grasp.
		Select wooden handles well-shaped for grasp.
	Difficulty in bringing spoon to mouth at correct angle	Angled cutlery to suit individual. Some are available commercially or can be made with adjustable angle.
		Swivel spoon.
	Limited reach	Long-handled cutlery.
	Poor power in upper limb: spoon	A spork will catch food with less effort, but should not be used when there is any tremor—spoon only.
	fork	Sharp prongs require less effort to spear with; 4-prong usually easier than 'Danish'-type 3-prong.
	knives	Steak knife with saw or serrated edge.
	One hand	Cheese knife, rather than clumsy and expensive 'Nelson' knife.
		Fork with cutting edge, *e.g.* Eze eater by Nyecraft.
Drinking	Inability to lift: from table	Use straws, clipped on to cup.
		Tipping-cup on stand.
		Plastic mug, softer type, picked up in teeth.
	in wheelchair	Drop-in holder for tumbler fixed to chair at shoulder-level, with straw.
	in bed	Cycle-bottle carrier with long straw attached to bedside table.
	Difficulty in lifting without spilling	Children's 'training' beakers, with round, weighted bottom.
	Weakness in grasp and lifting	Only half-fill cup, it is the liquid that weighs most.

Solving Eating and Drinking Problems—*continued*

Activity	*Problem*	*Problem solving*
		Choice of mugs, etc. on the market: lightweight ridged, e.g. Bex tumblers and mugs. Select cups with large handles. Two-handled plastic container for tumbler.
	Slowness — need to keep drink warm	Insulated plastic picnic mugs.
	Lack of sensation and risk of burning, *e.g.* tetraplegics who tend to balance cup on wrist or forearm, or hold between palmer surface both wrists	Insulated plastic mugs. Plastic containers.
	Disabled person on own during day	Plastic stopper on thermos drilled, and plastic straw fitted. Drink will keep warm for several hours.

Appendix O

SOLVING TOILET PROBLEMS

Activity	*Problem*	*Problem solving*
Access to toilet	General safety	Level access. Non-slip floors. Floor in good condition, i.e. no ragged lino or carpet edge. Good lighting in approach and in room. Grab-rails.
	Outside toilet	Level, non-slip access or ramp. Car-port type weather protection.
	Housing: size of room	Reverse door to open outward. Fit sliding door. Review and when possible, remove all unessential furniture and fitting. If adjacent, remove part wall to make one room with bathroom.
	width of room	Use of narrow wheelchair for toilet purposes only.
	steps	Two shallow steps preferable to one deep one. Grab-rail. Ramp for wheelchair (seldom practical indoors).
	Toilet: type	High or low cistern; high gives more transfer space, low sometimes useful to lean against. Corbel type allows closer approach.
	placing	Pedestal should preferably be at least 12 in (30 cm) from rear wall and 12 in (30 cm) from the side-wall.
Ability to transfer on/off	Height of toilet-seat	Appropriate to individual (most disabled are better suited with a seat height at 19 in or 21 in (48–53 cm).

Solving Toilet Problems—*continued*

Activity	*Problem*	*Problem solving*
	Type of toilet-seat	Old-fashioned wooden bench-type preferable. Extension of bench, i.e. fixed sliding-board to individual height. 'Horseshoe' open front, easier for cleaning perineum, but may reduce stability. Back-rest may also be needed.
	Stiff hips	Seat higher at back than front.
	One stiff hip	Raised seat with cut-out for stiff hip. High box seat with arms at waist-level to push up when rising and to lean on for balance when seated.
	Type of wheelchair	Aim is to minimize distance between toilet-seat and wheelchair: swinging detachable footrest; detachable arms; positive brakes; hard-based cushion. Chairs with single cross brace allow very close approach forward to lavatory pan.
	Wheelchair cushions	Hard-based cushions aid transfer. Paraplegic cushion facilitates use of bottle or female urinal or small boat bedpan.
	Pulling up and balance: grab-rails	A horizontal grab-rail about 2 ft 8 in (81 cm) from the ground and a vertical rail at a comfortable distance in front of the pedestal are usually found to be suitable. When balance poor, e.g. tetraplegic, side rail to lean on when seated. A bar which will drop down in front so that the patient can lean forward is sometimes preferred. Grab-rail in approach passage way may be necessary for semi-ambulant and also for pulling commode chair into room.
	Very stiff patients or those with calipers tending to slide forward.	Foot-stop on floor.
	Crutches, stick	Foolproof method of hanging or clipping them within easy reach (if dropped, patients may not be able to rise from toilet-seat).

Solving Toilet Problems—*continued*

Activity	*Problem*	*Problem solving*
	Methods of transfer:	
	from wheelchair with good manoeuvrability	Individual's method of transfer adapted to space available. For wheelchair patients, an area of approximately 5 ft × 5 ft 9 in (160 × 180 cm) is often needed for toilet purposes. Others may manage in a space 2 ft 9 in × 5 ft 9 in (80 × 180 cm)
	from wheelchair in long narrow room	Approach facing pedestal and transfer forward, sitting facing wall. Low cistern is helpful to lean on. Approach toilet backward, transfer through zip-opening back of chair.
	Too narrow for wheelchair	Transfer to commode chair at doorway, or outside door. If privacy allows, arrange clothes before transfer to commode chair. Use wooden chair as bridge chair standing inside door, should have non-slip rubber stops on feet of chair. Grab-rails outside may be necessary, especially where transfer method is to stand, pivot and then sit down.
	Need to use wheelchair with front propelling wheels	Opening back canvas. Extended bench seat as bridge, approach at angle to front of pedestal. Sliding-board can be used but tends to slip on toilet-seat.
Manage clothes	Limited reach (*e.g.* rheumatoid arthritis, women:	
	pants down/up	Simple dressing-stick (need not be very long) to pull pants up/down. Wide-leg pants or split-pants; draw aside with dressing-stick to micturate. Tape loop sewn top of pants, loop over arm to prevent slipping down too far out of reach. No vest, wear thicker slip 'princess' style; for warmth use brushed nylon slip, or cotton interlock. Wear waist-length 'toplet'.

Solving Toilet Problems—*continued*

Activity	*Problem*	*Problem solving*
	skirt out of way	Raise skirt and slip together, draw towards front, roll and tuck into waist-band at front. Split back skirt and slip lining to skirt.
	suspenders	Back suspender moved to side of girdle so that one does not have to undo to sit on toilet-seat.
	Limited reach: men	
	trousers up/down	Wear braces, always loop over arm when lowering so that trousers do not fall to floor.
	pants up/down	Velcro into trousers, or tape loops onto braces.
	fly opening	Zip usually preferred; lengthen under crutch for wheelchair patients. Toilet stick, if necessary, ring in zip pull-tag.
	tuck in shirt	Shorten back of shirt and use dressing-stick. Wear overshirt.
	vest	Wear sleeveless pullover over shirt instead of vest.
	One hand: women	Wide-leg or split pants (as above). Vest (as above). Suspender (as above). Pull up skirt and slip at back first, tuck in back of waist-band, then front. Dress, pull right up and take hem in teeth.
	One hand: man	
	trousers/pants	As above.
	fly-opening	Buttons preferred.
	shirt-vest	As above.
	Paraplegic	Zip at lower inside seam of trousers for access to incontinence appliance. Cut-out at front of under-pants for access to incontinence appliance. If normal arms, no other problems.
	Wheelchair with upper-limb weakness: women	
	skirt	Split-back skirt and slip.
	pants	Split pants with overlap. If in chair all day, no pants, sit on nappy.
	Wheelchair with upper-limb weakness: men	
	trousers up/down	Zip opening at both side-seams, and continuous front waistband.

Solving Toilet Problems—*continued*

Activity	*Problem*	*Problem solving*
	Pants up/down	No pants.
	fly-opening	Zip from bottom upwards.
	shirt/vest	As above.
Cleaning perineum	Fittings:	
	toilet-paper	Paper placed within easy reach. Single sheets easier than roll for one hand.
	seat	'Horseshoe' seat, easier to clean self, especially for those with limited hip abduction.
	flush-handle	Flush-handle within reach. Pull-handle: lengthen chain, and crank-handle to hang forward.
	washing	Portable bidet-spray in lavatory pan, if in bathroom. Some disabled flush toilet while still seated on it. Closomat.
	Limited reach	Toilet stick—curved to suit individual, milled at end to hold paper. 'Tissue'-type paper folds over and clings best. Wipe from front backward. Turn stick and tap against pan to drop paper.
Menstruation	Painful periods, heavy loss, depression. Loss of sensation, unaware of onset.	Regulation or suppression of menstruation (*see* Chapter 4).
	Limited reach; weak hands; inability to cope with hygiene	Sanipants with tuck-in pads the easiest. For disabled women, it is much preferable to have lavatory in bathroom to facilitate washing perineum and hands, when necessary. Soak stained garments in cold water. Rinse with hibitane against odour.
Use of toilet at night	Outside toilet or toilet inaccessible	Commode beside bed. Right or left to suit individual.
	Urgency of micturition	Detachable arm on bed side. Paper available. Adequate lighting.
	Poor balance	
	Confusion	
	Cannot reach toilet without putting on calipers, etc.	Control of fluid intake—no drink after 8.00 p.m. Take bulk of fluids during morning.
	Emptying commode	Slide-out type easier than lift-out. Round steel easiest to keep clean.

Solving Toilet Problems—*continued*

Activity	*Problem*	*Problem solving*
		Use small trolley to carry, if necessary. If toilet is in bathroom, length of hose from hot tap to toilet is help in washing out. Leave a little hibitane in bottom of clean pan.
Incontinence	Micturition: men	Appropriate urinary appliance, *see* Chapter 4.
		Zip-opening on lower inside leg seam facilitates emptying bag. Tap enlarged when grip is impaired. Paraplegic cushion.
	Micturition: women	Urinary appliance seldom satisfactory. Paraplegic cushion with 'boat' bedpan, emptied frequently.
		Absorbent padding; protective pants. Indwelling catheter.

Appendix P

SOLVING BATHING PROBLEMS

Activity	*Problem*	*Problem solving*
Access to bath or shower	General safety	Level non-slip floor, etc., as for toilet. Non-slip bath-mat. Suitable grab-rails. Heated towel-rails must be low temperature
	Housing: small bathroom; approach passage too narrow, with awkward turn in.	Sliding-door as direct access from bedroom.
	Provision for overhead hoist	Check joists, or reinforce for overhead track. Consult electricity board for safety of electric hoist.
	Bath	Bath-side not blocked in, for approach of hoist or deep recess for wheelchair footplates.
	sufficient space to approach	Check manoeuvring space in bathroom for wheelchair.
	High rim to shower-pan	Transfer from chair placed outside shower-pan to seat inside.
		For ambulant patients, 2 or 3 shallow steps installed, up and over with ridged rubber surface and suitable grab-rail. When possible, install shower with gently-sloping tiled floor and a floor drain, but no rim. This can be installed downstairs, but seldom upstairs.
Transfer to bath or shower	Height of bath	*See* Chapter 6 on Transfers and Hoists. If transferring from wheelchair, the end of bath should be same height as chair or slightly lower.

Solving Bathing Problems—*continued*

Activity	*Problem*	*Problem solving*
		For semi-ambulant patients who step into bath, sink bath as low as practicable. For those dependent on hoist to transfer, and helper to wash, then raise bath to convenient height for helper—but consider other members of the family, *e.g.* children. A safety non-slip mat in the bath is helpful in all cases.
	Type of bath	Bath should preferably have a flat bottom, *e.g.* Module bath. Shorter baths are often safer as the patients cannot slip under water.
	Method: from wheel-chair to bath, side transfer	Close approach to bath—swinging detachable footrests. Positive brakes. Using overhead handle-grab, or rail on wall, place one or both legs over rim into bath, transfer to bath-rim, re-position legs, transfer down into bath.
	front approach to side of bath	Swinging detachable footrests. Positive brakes. Roll chair forward to side of bath, leave enough room to put one leg, then other over rim to bath. Release brakes; approach as close as possible, engage brake and using overhead hand-grip if necessary, transfer forward into bath. Using grab-rail on wall, if necessary, turn in bath.
	front approach to end of bath	When space allows, technique as for front approach to side of bath but using the end of the bath and also using overhead grab and/or grab-rail. Can be done with a wheel-chair with fixed footrests, using a bench as a bridge, with footplates under it. This approach avoids having to turn in the bath.
	getting up out of bath	Get out before letting water out to gain some help from the water buoyancy. Sit on seat in bath (various types are available, *e.g.* 'Washaw' or 'toilet-seat' type.

Solving Bathing Problems—*continued*

Activity	*Problem*	*Problem solving*
		Grab-rails slanted down towards centre of bath.
	Weak trunk, poor balance	May need helper for transfer, but once safe in bath may be able to wash self. Use a back rest in the bath, *e.g.* 'Rest-Easy' swivel back-rest. Wooden kitchen chair, or formed plastic garden chair, with legs cut down, stood in the bath. The chair must be stabilized by wood slats firmly over bath rim and crutch-tips on bottom of legs.
	Inco-ordination	Quick-release straps can be used to hold patient. 'Safer' plastic bath-seat which hooks on side of bath is particularly useful for athetoid children.
	Unable to transfer without lifting-equipment: hoists	Hoists on overhead rails can be fitted in small bathroom where a portable hoist is not practical. Simplest is track and trolley with bar handle-grip and can be used by one helper for the severely disabled such as tetraplegics. Hewitt Watson hoist with track and trolley. (*N.B.*—Special safety precautions are necessary when installing electric hoists in bathrooms. *See* Chapter 6.) Portable hoists, such as New Oxford, Hoyer, Zimmer can be used in moderate-sized bathrooms, but require clear space under the bath for the legs of the hoist; minimum clearance is 9 in for most hoists, but check is needed for newer models. Nylon net all-in-one bath slings are useful, and dry out easily. Back rest and/or head sling may be needed. Nylon strap-slings can be used and they scrub and dry easily.
	Transfers to bath: ambulant disabled	Seated side transfers from bathroom stool or extended bench. The best method when calipers are worn and balance poor without them.

Solving Bathing Problems—*continued*

Activity	*Problem*	*Problem solving*
	Shower in bath	Standing—shallow bath preferred. Vertical or ladder grab-rail. One or two steps up and over, with ridged rubber surface to steps. Bath seat or kitchen chair in bath. Use of hand shower. (*N.B.*—When vertical grab-bars are used they must have plastic or other non-slip winding. Wet hands slip very easily on smooth pole.)
	Transfer to shower: side transfers	A shower seat against wall and projecting beyond shower-curtain, acts as fixed slide-board and seat. A glideabout-type chair can be kept for taking showers, transferring from usual wheelchair by usual individual methods. A wooden kitchen chair, formed plastic chair or steel-framed canvas chair can be used. Special stools for amputees, or unilateral fixed hip can be made to individual need.
	grab-rails	Most suit individual need, but following will serve most disabled: Horizontal bar 3–4 in above wall side rim of bath, set out 3 in from wall; vertical bars, 2–3 ft in length at either end of horizontal; $1\frac{1}{2}$ in diameter; plastic winding or coating for non-slip grip.
Taps and fittings	Reaching taps: bath	Taps are more easily reached when fitted side centre rather than end of bath, but patients often tend to use them to pull up. Lever-type taps can be fitted, or long-handled tap-turner used. Soap, brushes, face-cloths, etc. readily available either on shelf across bath, or basket hung on side.
	shower	A thermostat is essential for shower used by disabled. Hand-operated shower hose, or same type in adjustable wallfitting preferred,

Solving Bathing Problems—*continued*

Activity	*Problem*	*Problem solving*
		not overhead rose. Tap within easy reach from shower-seat. Fitting for soap, brushes, etc. within easy reach.
Washing and drying	Washing Drying	Non-slip baby-soap. Bath-wrap towel on seat or wheel-chair to wrap right round. Smaller towel or mitten towel for rubbing down. Best to rinse all soap from hands and if possible dry them before holding grab-rail to pull out.
Local authority services.	Unable to take bath or shower with family help available	District nurse can visit regularly to give a patient a bed bath when necessary, or to help family to bath patient Bath service often available when skilled nursing not needed. Ensures regular inspection without being too obvious, thus making sure that no scratches or bruises or any abnormalities are left to get so bad that hospitalization is required.

Appendix Q

SOLVING WASHING AND GROOMING PROBLEMS

Activity	*Problem*	*Problem solving*
Access to handbasin	General (including safety)	Level access to handbasin or other source of hot water. Non-slip floors; flooring in good condition. Good lighting. Appropriate grabrails. Hot pipes lagged Low-heat towel rail. Warm room. Privacy. Stable bathroom stool.
	Housing: size of room	As for toilet. *See* Appendix O
	width of door	2 ft 3 in minimum
	steps	No step or threshold rim at entrance.
	handbasin	Height to suit individual (32 in chair); 36 in standing.
	type	Non-pedestal type, access for wheelchair. Support at side, if necessary, leaving clear knee-room. Waste-pipe insulated. Any sharp edges, *e.g.* nut on waste-trap covered to avoid abrasion of knees. Helpful to have shelf fitted up to side of handbasin to lean elbows on and to keep accessories to hand. Mirror above basin larger than average so that seated disabled and standing family can both use.
	handbasin:	For some patients, it is helpful to be able to wash while seated on toilet.

Solving Washing and Grooming Problems—*continued*

Activity	*Problem*	*Problem solving*
	placing	May be necessary to stand basin out from wall to accommodate wheelchair footplates, and stiff calipered legs if seated on stool to wash.
	Unable to use hand-basin or difficult access to bathroom	Plastic bowl on lapboard or low table or chair, though help may be needed to carry and fill bowl; disabled person can get on washing while helper does other chores.
		Plastic bowl is cut-out in shelf/table, cannot tip and is support for elbows.
Ability to reach	Stiff shoulders, elbows, trunk	Consider method before aids, *e.g.* support on shelf.
		May be easier to wash perineum while seated on toilet.
		Long-handled sponge, comb, safety razor, etc. made to individual need, *e.g.* enlarged handle, handle curved to grip back of hand, friction grip surface.
		All accessories, soap, face-cloth, shaving tackle, etc. kept within close range and reach.
	Drying	Dry Terry towelling is probably the best; if possible it should be warmed before use, and then it will dry without rubbing. It may help to have one end of towel firmly fixed to towel rail. Most disabled have difficulty handling a large towel, two small ones are better. 'Mitten'-end towels made from roller-type Terry towelling, (like oven cloth), helpful for weak grip.
	Stiff hips, knees	Some disabled can wash and dry feet at long range, using aids, *e.g.* long-handled bath-brush. May need help, but this can be minimal if bowl with hot soapy water put for feet to soak, lift out onto hot Terry towel.
		Need help caring for toenails regularly (chiropody service).

Solving Washing and Grooming Problems—*continued*

Activity	*Problem*	*Problem solving*
Ability to grip	Weak, painful hands: washing	Terry towelling mitten may be easier than face-cloth. Wide tape sewn over back of sponge—slip hand through. Pimple rubber, curved handles on aids to suit individual. Nailbrush suction to handbasin.
	teeth	Soak dentures. Toothbrush with adapted handle, if necessary. Suitable plastic mug (2-handled; non-tip). For inco-ordination or tremor, or weak arms, rest both elbows on shelf, hold brush in right hand, grip right wrist with left hand then move head rather than hand to brush round mouth.
	shaving	Electric razor with clip-on double handle grip. Electric-razor stand with stiffish ball-and-socket joint, move face over razor.
Care of nails	Hands	Filing is much safer than cutting or clipping, especially when any inco-ordination or loss of sensation is present. File suitably fixed, or with enlarged handle. Nails best kept short, to avoid snagging and breaking during transfers and to avoid abrasions to the skin. If difficulty is experienced in cleaning the nails, soak well in hot, soapy water and rub against piece of Terry towelling in bottom of bowl.
	Feet	If patient cannot safely reach feet and cut nails, it is better not to attempt to use aids; will probably need regular help in washing and it is best to have regular help with toenails. There is usually Welfare Department provision for chiropody if bunions, corns or ingrowing nails need attention.
Care of hair	Women:	Short hair style preferable, easier to wash, can be brushed often. A 'perm' is not necessarily helpful, for unless the hair is well set after

Solving Washing and Grooming Problems—*continued*

Activity	*Problems*	*Problem solving*
		washing, it can 'friz' and look worse than a straight simple style.
	Washing hair	Wash in bath with hair-sprayer on taps. Care of scalp and prevention of dandruff by washing frequently with special shampoo after application of scalp lotion. Wash brush and comb whenever hair washed.
Care of skin	Dry skin	Many disabled tend to have dry scaly skin, especially on legs and feet. Hibitane baths are useful. Soak feet in warm soapy water. Dry well but carefully, as skin is often thin and brittle from prolonged inactivity and poor circulation.
		Massage with oil (arachis oil more readily available and cheaper than olive oil) or use calamine cream as an alternative.
	Pressure areas	Especially buttocks when chairbound. Sit and sleep on sheepskin. Regular inspection of skin; patient can check self by using hand mirror.
		Wash every day, dry very well, either with rolling movement on bed or chair doing one side at a time sitting on towel. Dust lightly with talcum powder. Folds of buttocks and in groins are better with oily ointment such as zinc cream or a barrier cream rubbed in sparingly.

Appendix R

SOLVING COMMUNICATION PROBLEMS

Activity	*Problem*	*Problem solving*
Spoken word	Sensory dysfunction: hard of hearing; deafness	Visual: lip-reading, written word; pictures and signs. *See* Royal Institute for the Deaf publications.
	Motor dysfunction: respiratory complications; lack of volume, etc. (*e.g.* Parkinsonism)	Alphabet and sign-board writing. Speech amplifier.
	contact beyond immediate environment	Adapted telephone (*see* G.P.O. pamphlet). Remote-control system (*e.g.* Possum). Intercom call systems. Remote-control door answer and opener. Call-bell and call-lights.
	Cerebral dysfunction: aphasias	Speech therapy. Follow-up practice.
Written word	Sensory dysfunction: partially sighted	Magnifiers. Large-print books.
	blindness	Tactile: braille, tape recorders, talking books. *See* Royal National Institute for the Blind publications.
Reading	Motor dysfunction: inability to handle books and papers	Simple aids: rubber thimble, paper clips, etc. Reading stands and newspaper racks. Mechanical page-turners.
	Cerebral dysfunction: Dyslexia	Speech therapy. Follow-up practice.
Writing	General:	Suitable tables: surface, height, tilting, wheelchair table.

Solving Communication Problems—*continued*

Activity	*Problem*	*Problem solving*
	inability to hold pencil and paper	Simple aids: penholder, clip-board, magnet board. Splints, *e.g.* flexor-hinge splints.
	loss of arm function	Mobile arm-supports. Slings.
	amputee	Prostheses: conventional; powered. Use of feet and mouth.
	Cerebral dysfunction: agraphia	Speech therapy. Follow-up practice.
Typing	Slight loss of function in arm and hand	Suitable table. Arm sling.
	Inco-ordination	Keyguard. Simple aids: weighted cuff; non-slip mat.
	Severe loss of function in arms and hands	Mobile arm-supports. Electric typewriter. Continuous-fold paper. Aids for feeding-in paper.
	Total loss of function in arms and hands	Mouthstick; headstick

Appendix S

ASSESSMENT FOR WORK: CLERICAL AND OFFICE WORK

Preliminary tests

Writing: copying from typed material and from dictation.
Graded spelling tests.
Reading: three grades, followed by questions to test comprehension.
Simple arithmetic.
Expression: reading aloud;
discussion after reading;
write letter about subject discussed.
Ability to use reference books: *e.g.* telephone directory, trade catalogue, etc.

Office work—necessary processes involved

Telephone: manner and voice;
handle telephone and write message;
ability to take messages correctly.
Filing: Correct filing of cards;
recall of information (understanding of system);
ability to handle small draw file, ledger file, using punch and stapler, foolscap drawer file, lateral filing.
Entering data on file cards.
Figures: neatness of filling-in figures;
correctness of filling-in figures;
adding columns correctly.

Adding machines
Typing
Shorthand

Appendix T

ASSESSMENT FOR WORK: COOKERY

Cooking is a skilled job and as such needs to be analysed and assessed for each patient according to his/her own individual circumstances, that is whether catering for a family or living alone.

The first necessity is to assess heights and placing of kitchen equipment in relation to the physical disability and the home conditions and then to try out basic cooking procedures in order to select those most suitable. For example: frying as a procedure carries an inherent risk but for a patient with ataxia or tremor it can be positively dangerous and such a patient should be encouraged to use grilling as an alternative method of cooking similar foods.

In the form below, eleven basic cooking techniques are checked against functional and economic factors. To assess the safest and most suitable cooking methods for the individual patient, a selected set of recipes are tried for each appropriate technique. The therapist can then advise as to the most suitable methods for cooking at home, taking into consideration any special diet and the patient's economic circumstances.

Classification of Cooking Techniques according to the Factors Needing Assessment for Individual Patients. Based on the Hazards and Physical Demands of the Activity.

	Accident Risk			Lifting			Preparation								Supervision		
							Amount			Effort			Timing				
	Low	Medium	High	Light	Medium	Heavy	Minimal	Medium	Maximal	Intermittent	Medium	Sustained	In advance	Immediate	Minimal	Medium	Constant
Hot beverages			√		√		√			√				√			√
Uncooked	√			√				√			√		√		√		
Grill	√			√			√			√			√				√
Boil, serve cold	√				√			√		√			√		√		
Boil, serve hot		√			√			√		√			√		√		
Casserole		√				√		√		√			√		√		
Bake	√				√				√			√	√		√		
Steam			√		√			√			√		√			√	
Roast			√			√	√			√			√			√	
Fry			√	√				√			√			√			√
Pressure cook			√			√		√		√			√				√

Appendix U

CARE OF MEDICAL SHEEPSKINS

Frequent washing is recommended and sheepskins should be changed as follows: for general use every 7 days; for patients who sweat heavily, every 5 days; for patients with open wounds, every 2–3 days.

Hand washing and domestic washing-machines

(1) Soiled skins should first be sponged thoroughly in cold water.

(2) Hand wash gently in warm, not hot water, using detergent recognized as being satisfactory for washing wool, or soap; or: agitate as slowly as possible for about 10 minutes (washing-machine).

(3) Rinse well in fresh warm water until all soap is removed.

(4) Do not wring; put through squeeze-roller or spin-dryer to remove surplus water.

(5) Hang out to dry, preferably in the open air.

WARNING.—Do not attempt to dry skins over hot-water radiators or too close to heaters. High temperature will cause the pelt to harden and spoil the skin.

(6) Where necessary, the wool pile may be restored by combing and brushing with wire-brush.

Hospital laundries

(1) A pre-rinse in cold water to remove any soiling.

(2) 10–15-minute wash in warm water.

(3) A non-ionic detergent should be used such as Renex or Lissapol.

(4) Rinse in warm water, and follow with 5-minute cold rinse to which a quarternary ammonium compound such as cirrasol or cetrimide has been added.

(5) Hydro-extract and tumble dry in a moderate temperature.

Appendix V

CHECKING A FLEXOR-HINGE HAND-SPLINT

Fitting

(1) Is the head of the ulna free from pressure?

(2) Is desired available passive range of movement permitted at wrist, metacarpophalangeal and interphalangeal joints?

(3) Does the palmar piece conform to the palmar arch?

(4) Does the forearm piece conform to the forearm?

(5) With a wrist-driven splint, does the forearm piece stay in position during wrist extension?

(6) Do the splint joints approximate anatomical joints?

(7) Are the supportive bars correctly positioned and conforming to the anatomy?

(8) Does the thumb post hold the thumb in approximately 45-degree abduction or as close to that position as the passive range of movement will allow?

Comfort

(1) Is the splint comfortable? If not, can it be made more comfortable by (*a*) less correction; (*b*) re-adjustment of the spring tension; (*c*) improving fit.

(2) Can the patient wear the splint long enough without discomfort for useful function.

Function

(1) When relaxed, is hand as near the functional position as the passive range of movement will permit? (10-degree wrist extension).

(2) Is patient able to position forearm in full pronation in order to pinch-grip effectively and pick up objects from a flat surface?

(3) Do the index- and middle-finger pads have maximum contact with the thumb pad?

(4) In pinching, are thumb and finger pads clear from metal of the finger cages?

(5) Does the splint permit maximum functional grasp?

(6) Is release of grasp adequate for function?

(7) Are the ulnar fingers positioned so that they do not interfere with pinch or grip?

(8) Can the patient apply and remove the splint?

(9) Do corrective parts obtain maximum correction within the patient's tolerance?

(10) Does the amount of pinch-force represent an effective proportion of the available wrist-extensor power?

(11) Is release of pinch adequate for function?

Information helpful in evaluating functional benefit of splint

(1) Source of muscle-power driving splint. Strength of muscle driving splint.

(2) Prehension force without splint.

(3) Prehension force in splint.

(4) Finger opening in splint (inches).

(5) Passive range of movement:

	Recorded optimum
Forearm	Full pronation
Wrist	40-degree flexion
	40-degree extension
Thumb	40-degree abduction
	Full metacarpophalangeal and intercarpophalangeal extension
Fingers	0–90-degree metacarpophalangeal flexion extension
	20–90-degree intercarpophalangeal flexion extension.

Appendix W

FUNCTIONAL CLASSIFICATION OF DISABILITY

Wheelchair patients

(1) With normal arms.

(2) With impaired use of arms: (*a*) Impaired reach; (*b*) Weakness of grip; (*c*) Ataxia (unsteadiness and inco-ordination of movement).

Ambulant patients

(1) Both legs affected, but not arms.

(2) Both arms affected.

(3) Both legs and both arms affected.

(4) One leg and one arm affected.

(5) One leg affected.

(6) One arm affected.

(7) Stiff back and hips (cannot sit or stoop).

(8) Problems of small size; children, dwarfs.

(9) Limited exercise tolerance; early fatigue, that is, certain heart, chest and nervous disorders.

(10) Muscular weakness, and limited physical endurance.

Patients where extra caution is required

(1) The elderly.

(2) Generalized inco-ordination of movement.

(3) The blind and partially-sighted.

(4) The deaf and hard of hearing.

(5) Epileptics.

Bibliography and References

General

The Disabled in Society (1967). Peter Townsend. London; Royal College of Surgeons

Proceedings of a Symposium on the Motivation of the Physically Disabled (1968). Ed. by P. J. R. Nichols. London; National Fund for Research into Crippling Diseases

Aspects of Rehabilitation (1967). London; National Fund for Research into Crippling Diseases

The Rehabilitation, Training and Resettlement of a Disabled Person (1956), (Piercy Report) Cmd. 9883. London; H.M.S.O

Principles of Rehabilitation (1963). W. Russell Grant. Edinburgh; Livingstone

Help for the Handicapped (1958). London; National Council of Social Services

Services for the Disabled (1961), (2nd edn). Ministry of Labour. London; H.M.S.O.

Rehabilitation and Care of the Disabled in Britain (1965). British Information Service. London; Central Office of Information

Help Yourselves (1966). P. E. Jay, E. Walker and E. Ellison, S.R.O.T., M.A.O.T. Sponsored by the British Council for Rehabilitation of the Disabled. London; Butterworths

Stigma. The Experience of Disability (1966). Ed by P. Hunt. London; Geoffrey Chapman

Consumer's Guide to the British Social Services (1967). Phyllis Willmott. Pelican Book A871. Middlesex; Penguin

Equipment for the Disabled (1966), (2nd edn). Ed by M. Agerholm. London; National Fund for Research into Crippling Diseases

Clinical Problems

Still's Disease

B. M. Ansell (1965). 'Still's Disease.' In *Progress in Clinical Rheumatology*. Ed by A. St. J. Dixon, page 95. London; Churchill

B. M. Ansell. 'Rheumatism in Childhood" In *Modern Trends in Rheumatology*. Ed by A. G. S. Hill, page 18. London; Butterworths

Poliomyelitis

J. Trueta, A. B. Kinnier Wilson, and M. Agerholm (1956). *Handbook on Poliomyelitis*. Oxford; Blackwell

Cerebral palsy

G. A. Pollock (1962). 'Surgical Treatment of Cerebral Palsy.' *J. Bone Jt Surg*. **44B,** 68

K. S. Holt (1967). *Assessment of Cerebral Palsy*. London; Lloyd Luke

Neurological conditions

D. Williams (1966). 'Management of the Chronic Neurological Patient.' *Br. med. J*. **2,** 1554

P. Sandifer (1967). *Neurology in Orthopaedics*. London; Butterworths

Paraplegia

V. Benes (1968). *Spinal Cord Injury*. London; Cassell

J. J. Walsh (1965). *Understanding Paraplegia*. London; Tavistock Publications

Paraplegia. The official journal of the International Medical Society of Paraplegia is published quarterly by Livingstone (Edinburgh) and contains articles of all aspects of paraplegia and tetraplegia

Hemiplegia

W. S. Fields and W. A. Spencer (Eds), (1967). *Stroke Rehabilitation* Missouri; Warren H. Green Inc.

R. Harris, M. Bruck, and E. P. Copp (1964). 'Rehabilitation and Resettlement in Hemiplegia' *Ann. phys. Med*. **7,** 209

J. B. Millard (1966). 'Rehabilitation and the Hemiplegic Patient.' *Ann. phys. Med*. **8,** 244

P. R. Lee, S. Groch, J. Untereker, K. Monahan, and H. A. Rusk (1958). *Rehabilitation. Monograph XV*. New York; Inst. of Phys. Med. and Rehab.

G. F. Adams and L. J. Harwitz (1963). 'Mental Barriers to Recovery from Strokes.' *Lancet* **2,** 533

Spina bifida

Proceedings of a Symposium on Spina Bifida (1966). London; National Fund for Research into Crippling Diseases

W. J. W. Sharrard (1964). 'Posterior Iliopsoas Transplantation in the Treatment of Paralytic Dislocations of the Hip.' *J. Bone Jt Surg*. **46B,** 426

W. J. W. Sharrard (1967). 'Paralytic Deformity in the Lower Limb.' *J. Bone Jt Surg*. **49B,** 731

E. P. Quibell (1967). 'Principles and Problems of Rehabilitation in Spina Bifida.' *Proc. R. Soc. Med*. **60,** 769

Rheumatoid arthritis

J. H. Kellgran, M. R. Jeffrey, and J. Ball (1963). *The Epidemiology of Chronic Rheumatism*. Oxford; Blackwell

Reports on Rheumatic Disease (1959–1968). Issues Nos. 1–34. London; Arthritis and Rheumatism Council for Research in Great Britain and the Commonwealth

General Care

Pressure sores

D. Norton, R. McLaren, and A. N. Exton-Smith (1962). *An Investigation of Geriatric Nursing Problems in Hospital*. London; The National Corporation for the Care of Old People

Control of menstruation

E. A. Hamilton and P. J. R. Nichols (1968). 'The Problem of Period Control in Disabled Women.' *Ann. phys. Med.* **9,** 289

C. E. Flowers, N. Vorys, V. Stevens, A. T. Miller, L. Jensen (1966). 'The Effects of Suppression of Menstruation with Ethynodiol Acetate upon the Pituitary, Ovary and Endometrium.' *Am. J. Obstet. Gynec.* **96,** 784

Late onset of respiratory insufficiency

E. A. Hamilton and P. J. R. Nichols (1970). 'Late Onset of Respiratory Insufficiency.' *Ann. Phys. Med.* **10,** 223

Sheepskins

M. R. Ewing, C. Garrow, and N. McHugh (1961). 'Sheepskin as a Nursing Aid.' *Lancet* **2,** 1147

Aids and Appliances (general)

Aids for the Disabled (1968). London; B.M.A. Planning Unit Report No. 3

S. Licht (Ed), (1966). *Orthotics etcetera*. Connecticut; E. Licht

E. M. Smith and R. C. Juvinall (1963). 'Theory of Feeder Mechanics.' *Am. J. phys. Med.* **42,** 113

S. G. Chyatte, C. Long, and P. J. Vignos (1965). 'The Balanced Forearm Orthosis in Muscular Dystrophy.' *Archs phys. Med.* **46,** 633

Wheelchairs

H. H. Kamenetz (1969). *The Wheelchair Book*. Springfield; Thomas

Owner's Manual (1965). Everest and Jennings (Zimmer Orthopaedic Limited)

D. W. Jolly (1964). 'Symposium on the Wheelchair.' *Paraplegia* **2,** 20

Upper-limb functional splints

M. Anderson (1968). *Functional Bracing of Upper Extremities*. Springfield; Thomas

R. L. Bennett and A. R. Stephens (1955). 'Assistive and Adaptive Apparatus for Upper Extremities.' *Phys. Ther. Rev.* **35,** 626

C. B. Wyn Parry (1966). *Rehabilitation of the Hand* (2nd edn). London; Butterworths

Architecture

S. Goldsmith (1968). *Designing for the Disabled* (2nd edn). London; Royal Institute for British Architecture

F. Walter (1968). *An Introduction to Domestic Design for the Disabled.* London; Disabled Living Activities Group: Central Council for the Disabled

Access for the Disabled to Buildings (1967). British Standard Code of Practice: 96, Part I. London; British Standards Institution

Furniture

S. Bramwell Jones (1968). 'The needs of the Disabled; a Guide to the Selection of Household Furniture and Equipment.' *Br. Hosp. J Soc. Serv. Rev.* **78,** 155

S. Bramwell Jones (1969). 'The Household Needs of the Disabled; a Guide to the Selection of Furniture and Equipment.' *Br. Hosp. J. Soc. Serv. Rev.* **79**, 679

Education

W. W. Taylor and I. W. Taylor (1967). *Services for Handicapped Youth in England and Wales.* New York; International Society for Rehabilitation of the Disabled

The Handicapped School Leaver (1964). Report of a Working Party. London; British Council for Rehabilitation of the Disabled

P. Hendersen (1968). 'The Educational Problems of Meningomyelocoele.' *Hosp. Med.* **2,** 909

Training and work

J. K. Arthur (1967). *Employment for the Handicapped.* Berks.; Abingdon Press

Central Office of Information (1965). *Rehabilitation and Care of the Disabled in Britain.* London; H.M.S.O.

R. W. Conley (1965). *The Economics of Vocational Rehabilitation.* Baltimore; Johns Hopkins Press

A. C. Gogstad (1968). *Evaluation of Factors Determining the Results of Vocational Rehabilitation.* Norwegian Monographs on Medical Science; Universitets-forlaget

J. F. Montgomerie (1958). *The Handicapped Person.* Edinburgh; Scottish Council of Social Service

J. F. Montgomerie (1960). *Jobs for the Handicapped.* Edinburgh; Scottish Council of Social Service

Working Party Reports and Conference Proceedings

British Council for Rehabilitation of the Disabled. *The Handicapped School Leaver* (1965). Dr. Elfed Thomas, B.Sc., Director of Education for the City of Leicester. Professor Thomas Ferguson, M.D., B.Sc., University of Glasgow

Ministry of Labour and National Service. *Rehabilitation and Resettlement of Disabled Persons* (1943). Mr G. Tomlinson, M.P. Cmd. 6415. London; H.M.S.O.
Ministry of Labour and National Service. *The Rehabilitation, Training and Resettlement of Disabled Persons* (1956). The Rt. Hon. Lord Piercy, C.B.E. Cmd. 9883. London; H.M.S.O.
National Youth Employment Council. *The Future Development of the Youth Employment Service* (1966). London; H.M.S.O.
Ministry of Labour and National Service. *Services for the Disabled* (1961). London; H.M.S.O.

Index

W